Truth Decay

Printed in the United States of America

ISBN 0-9742077-1-3

First Printing 2002

Printed on Recycled Paper

Books from Tuberose Publishing

The Care & Feeding of a Human Being:
Vol. #1 ***The Care***
Vol. #2 ***The Feeding***

The Vital Vegetarian Cookbook

Critical Condition

Advanced Medical Awareness

Herbal Alchemy

Children's Health

Truth Decay

Tuberose Publishing
Box 1706
Brooksville, Florida 34605
www.tuberose.com

The information in this book has been compiled from the best of the available literature from the most astute and eloquent researchers, educators, and practitioners that have been looking in the same direction for the truth in health-related issues. This is an amalgamation of many of those who have gone before, as natural healers, and to the many patients that brought a healing lesson to share with us.

"The Constitution of this Republic should make special provisions for Medical Freedom as well as Religious Freedom. To restrict the art of healing to one class of men and deny equal privileges to others will constitute the Bastille of medical science. All such laws are unAmerican and despotic."

–Benjamin Rush, M.D.
A signer of the Declaration of Independence
and this nation's first Surgeon General.

"When you are constantly moving forward, searching for the cutting edge, everyone behind you always believes you have gone too far. The further back from the cutting edge they are, the more extreme and, indeed, insane, you appear, to be. In this way, one person's "madness" can be another's common sense."

- David Icke -

Special thanks to Susan Stockton for her excellent editting skills.

Warning: *The statements made in this book have NOT been evaluated by the F.D.A. or the A.D.A.*

We must legally warn you that if you are ill, have any disease, are pregnant or nursing, you should consult your medical doctor before attempting any natural or herbal program.

Contents

Introduction

This book is not intended as an authoritative text, but as an introduction to and overview of the hazards associated with the practice of conventional dentistry and the evolved field of *holistic* or *biological* dentistry. This information has been compiled from the teachings of many researchers, practitioners, and patients. There is an abundance of scientific research and peer-reviewed articles that can be studied by the serious inquirer. Included is a list of books and information sources available for study.

The renouned German physician Dr. Reinhard Voll estimated that nearly **80% of all illness is related entirely or partially to problems in the mouth.** The reason the teeth are such a threat to health is that, in addition to their connection to every organ and gland in the body, they can harbor infections without symptoms. There's no pain or discomfort. Yet, there may be chronic infection eroding the body's immune response–wearing out the immune system. This infection is very difficult to detect. Few people today have escaped the problems of dental cavities and gum infection. **About 98% of Americans have some areas of diseased gum tissue in their mouths**, over half of these are also experiencing a progressive "bone loss." Fortunately, cavities and *pyorrhea* (gum disease and bone loss) are both 100% **preventable** and **reversible**.

The mouth is a hostile environment. It's warm, moist, and full of nutrient-laden saliva, decaying teeth, and soggy gums, which makes it a haven for bacteria. Teeth are subject to sudden *changes of temperature* created by extremes such as coffee and ice cream. *Mechanical stresses* challenge the mouth in the form of chewing ice and a combination of hard and soft foods. It is attacked chemically by foods that are highly *acidic* and highly *alkaline* with overtones of *salinity* and *sugar*. All these conditions provide corrosive influences, necessitating artificial replacements supplied by the dentist. Mercury amalgam fillings are the **major source of mercury exposure** for the general public, at rates **six-times higher** than from fish and seafood.

Oral toxicity has been the cause of much anxiety, depression, hyperactivity and suicidal behavior as well as other psychological conditions. The sufferers then are referred to psychiatric physicians who place them on powerful psychoactive drugs and treat them with electro-shock therapy.

These procedures cause the same symptoms that are being addressed, as well as **permanent brain damage**. Symptoms start in childhood with the treatment of tooth decay, caused by a poor diet and consumption of acid-forming sugar, phosphoric acid in sodas, etc. Kids are given "chrome caps" on their baby teeth, thus starting the sequence of toxic, damaging mayhem. Because the metals affect the nervous system, they are labeled as *ADHD, hyperactive, learning disabled,* etc. and so starts their demise.

The root canal procedure is a fatally flawed procedure. The very nature of the procedure itself prevents it from achieving its supposed primary goal: a non-infected, sterile tooth. There is a high risk of keeping in the mouth a dead tooth that can harbor anaerobic bacteria, viruses and fungi, where neither the body's immune system nor antibiotics can fight them off. Sooner or later the root canaled tooth's bacteria and their toxins can invade the body, weakening the immune system, the nervous system, the heart, etc. yet often without the medical doctor even thinking to suspect the role that is being played by an infected, toxic tooth.

If the detrimental effects of root canals on the public health are major, then the effects of jawbone cavitations (osteonecrosis) are even more colossal, given the apparent widespread incidence of jawbone osteonecrosis. The routine manner in which dentists extract teeth, including wisdom teeth, will routinely result in the formations of cavitations. Not a single patient (out of thousands examined) who has had all four wisdom teeth removed was found to be free of cavitations. In fact, most had four, and nearly all the rest had three. extensive cavitations will be found in the jawbones of most of our older citizens who are wearing full dentures. Younger adults should also be checked: cavitations are also routinely triggered by the presence of root-canaled teeth, toxic crowns and other dental toxins, periodontal and other infections, and by accidents and other trauma to the jawbone. Relying on x-rays for the diagnosis of cavitations is inadequate. Injection of *Sanum* remedies will not remove what is, effectively, gangrene in the jawbone.

Organized dentistry is filled with statements that vastly underestimate the amount of mercury released from dental amalgams. Organized dentistry usually claims that amalgam surfaces give off 0.067 to 0.057 micrograms/day/sq cm of surface, but this claim has failed numerous scientific examinations

Professor Boyd Haley, Chair of the Chemistry Department at the University of Kentucky (www.toxicteeth.net), has measured the release of mercury vapor and found the release to be 7.54 micrograms/day/sq cm of surface when undisturbed and 45.49 micrograms/day/sq cm of surface when brushed using a medium bristle toothbrush (758 times higher than the ADA's estimate of mercury emission). The major contributor to mercury body burden of American citizens is from dental amalgam. Dentists are required to handle dental amalgam as a hazardous material before it goes into teeth, and scrap amalgam must be handled as toxic, hazardous waste when it comes out of teeth

Dental clinics serve as the largest single source of mercury pollution. The mercury from dental fillings can be converted by bacteria in the oral and intestinal cavities into methyl mercury, making it far more toxic to humans and other living things. Another troublesome chemical reaction occurs when methyl-thiol, which is a toxin produced in periodontal disease, reacts with ionized mercury to form extremely dnagerous mercury-thiol compounds that behave similarly to methyl mercury and can pass the intestinal and blood-brain barriers.

Mercury harms brain tubulin, the most important protein in the brain, and is severely toxic to neurons. Boyd Haley warns that our brains have no protective mechansim against the damage done by the mercury vapor given off from dental amalgams. Even low levels of mercury exposure can damage human nerve cells, Haley warns, and cause all of the signs of Alzheimer's disease, a leading cause of disability and death. Far more than any other toxin, mercury produces all the hallmarks of Alzheimer's disease: greatly decreased glutathione levels, neurofibrillary tangles, abnormally aggregated tubulin, increased hyper-phosphorylation of protein-Tau, and increased production of beta-amyloid protein, which makes up amyloid plaques.

Mercury has been linked to Alzheimer's more than any other toxin, including Aluminum, Haley warns, and the rate of Alzheimer's disease is growing and is projected to increase much more in coming decades. Haley, a world's expert on human toxicity issues, urges that dental amalgams, which are half mercury, be banned. Doctors have missed the mercury diagnosis for a long time because they only did a straight blood test and not a chelation challenge test.

Fritz Loscheider, Ph.D., is Professor Emeritus in the School of Medicine, University of Calgary and is former head of the Department of Medical Physiology there. Dr. Lorscheider was part of a research team at Calgary that linked low level mercury to rapid neuron death. He presented a stunning video showing a nerve cell dying within a few hours after being exposed to a drop of low-levels mercury solution. The research was published in 2001 in Neuroreports, a peer-reviewed journal. The paper and the video can be viewed on the website www.neuroreports.com/30mar01. That study was just the latest of a series of studies that link mercury in low concentration to impairment and death of nerve cells and that link mercury to all the markers of Alzheimer's disease, a leading cause of disability and death.

Younsters who die of unexplained heart attacks, such as the young athletes that die in high school on exertion during athletic events, have 22,000 times more mercury in their hearts than normal. Autistic babies appear to be a subset of the population that is unable to excrete mercury from nerve cells. Based on the many factors that influence the toxicity of mercury--genetic, hormonal, chemical, and environmental--it is not known what the tolerable level of mercury is for each individual, as it can vary dramatically from person to person. Dental mercury is, by far, the greatest source of mercury entering sewage waste treatment systems, accounting for 40% of the load. One in eight women of reproductive age in the U.S. has blood mercury levels that pose a risk to the developing fetus.

Diabetes, from mercury toxicity, has hundreds of symptoms; it masquerades under many different medical aliases, and its symptoms are treated by many different medical specialists. In 1995 diabetes, then being treated by numerous competing medical specialists, accounted for **over 40% of the deaths from all causes** according to data reported in *American Demographics*. In the 1930s and 1940s, many of the medical specialties that we know today emerged from what had been up to then the general practice of medicine. This reorganization was greatly influenced by the emergence of *diabetes*, now known as *hyperinsulinemia*. From an incidence of 0.0028% per capita in the late 1800s, diabetes soared **over a thousand times** to become a serious epidemic by 1950. Thus the "heart specialist," the "endocrinologist," the "hepatic and biliary specialist" as well as many other medical specialists began to compete for market share in the treatment of diabetes.

It became fashionable, for example, to declare that diabetes increased cardiovascular risk, where formerly it was well understood that heart failure was a direct consequence of *un*treated or *poorly* treated **diabetes**. Since then, each of the medical specialties have their own proprietary *name* for their own proprietary *symptom set* which they recognized as their own proprietary *disease* and treated with their own ineffective proprietary *protocol*.

Our modern medical Babylon includes in their list such symptoms of this disease as *atherosclerosis, elevated cholesterol, hypertension, elevated glucose, elevated insulin, stroke, cardiomyopathy, kidney and liver failure, neuropathy, retinopathy, male impotence, blindness glaucoma, gangrene*, and many other debilitating symptoms. Several forms of *cancer* are a result of a failure to effectively treat diabetes in its early stages. None of the treatments by any specialist is directed toward *curing* the disease. They are all aimed at *suppressing* the proprietary *symptom set,* that the attending physician feels responsible for treating. Many of the treatments often leave the patient **worse** off than *before*.

Insulin has three sufur-containing cross-linkages and the insulin receptor is a *tyrosine kinase* containing sufur bonds, which are a preferred targets for binding by both mercury and lead. The metals inactivate insulin's ability to trigger the naturally occurring hormonal effects which would lower blood sugar. Mercury is causing *chronic hyperinsulinemia*. As a consequence, blood glucose levels become so elevated that the glucose "spills over" into the urine, and is converted into *triglycerides* (fat), which contribute to cardiovascular illness.

Despite these high blood glucose levels, cells "starve" since insulin-stimulated glucose entry into cells is impaired. This leads to *ketosis*, which is an acid condition. Since ketone bodies are acids, their high concentration puts a strain on the buffering capacity of the blood and exess hydrogen ions in the urine. Alkaline minerals, including sodium, potassium, calcium, and magnesium, as well as water, are depleted, leading to dysregulation of the **thyroid** and **adrenals,** and **dehydration,** with loss of blood volume, as well as the conditions already metioned. **The mercury burden in the body comes primarily from dental amalgam, or in infants and children, from *thimerosol*** (ethyl mercury), used as a preservative **in vaccinations.** Mercury fillings are placed in teeth made unhealthy by the **refining of foods**, particularly flour and sugar.

When you have a root canal, or even a big filling, or crown or anything that is not compatible with the body, it **sets up an interference field, blocking or altering the energy pathway passing through it**. It will affect different parts along that meridian, different organ systems in the body, and usually will cause it to have a problem as well. If the tooth is removed, the energy does tend to pass through it; however, without the tooth in the bone, it is still altered. Without stimulation from a tooth, blood circulation and lymphatic drainage will be impaired, and the bone and tissue surrounding the extraction site can become diseased (cavitations) and die. Infections in the teeth and toxins have no place to go but down; down into the jawbone and into the rest of the body, creating systemic pathologies.

Teeth

The oral cavity is the special province of the dentist. It contains more than teeth and gingivae. Examination of the lips, the tongue, the floor of the mouth, the buccal mucosa, the palate, the temporomandibular joint, the fauces and even the tonsils and the throat should be a routine part of the dental examination. Recognition of early pathologic changes in the oral cavity of systemic as well as local origin is the responsibility of the dentist and a part of the dental health service.

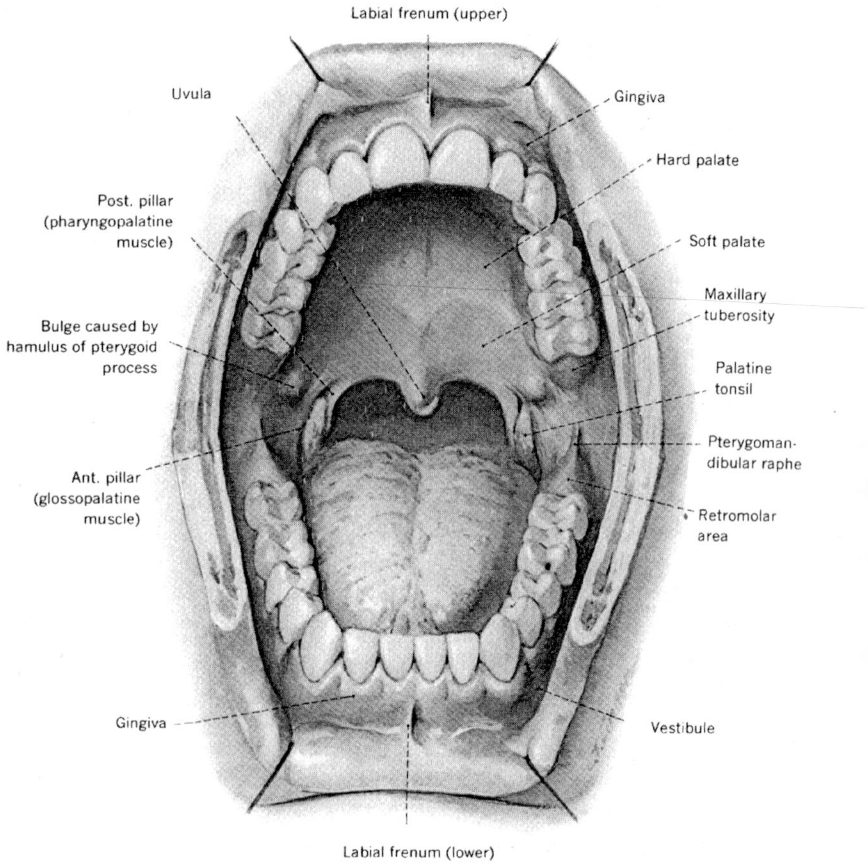

The Oral Cavity

A systematic examination of the oral cavity should include the structures lying on the floor of the mouth. This area is readily visible when the tongue is raised. The inferior (ventral) surface of the tongue is smooth and glistening and free of papillae. It is covered with a thin mucous membrane through which some of the underlying structures can be seen. The sublingual region is extremely vascular. The small vessels are superficial and covered by only a thin layer of mucosa. Soluble drugs (nitrates and sulfa and other drugs) placed under the tongue are absorbed into the general circulation rapidly in a manner analogous to absorption from intraperitoneal injections. The floor of this space is the mylohyoid muscle.

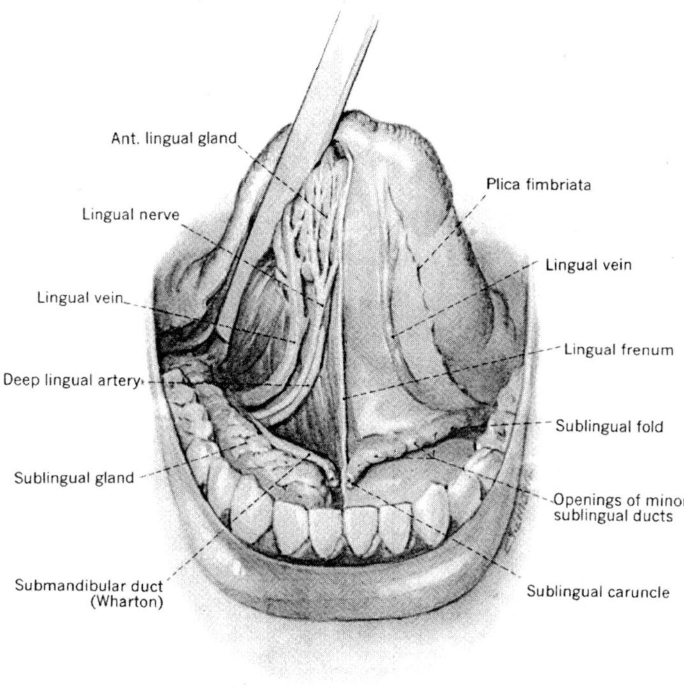

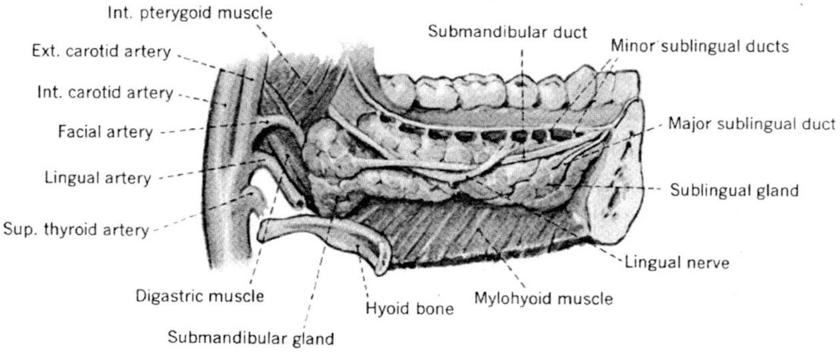

The Floor of the Mouth

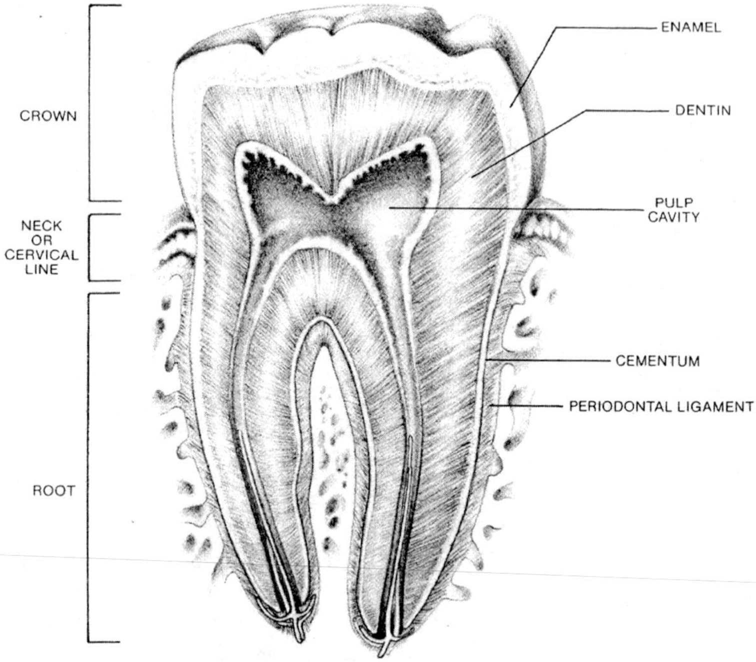

1st molar-buccolingual view

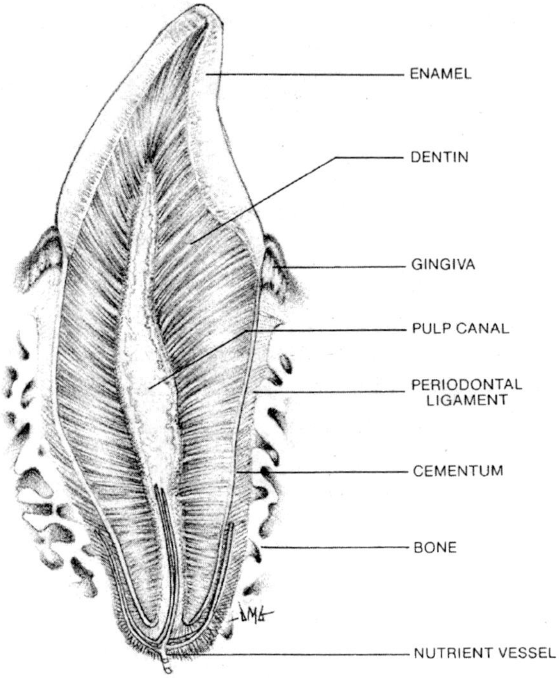

Incisor-sagittal view

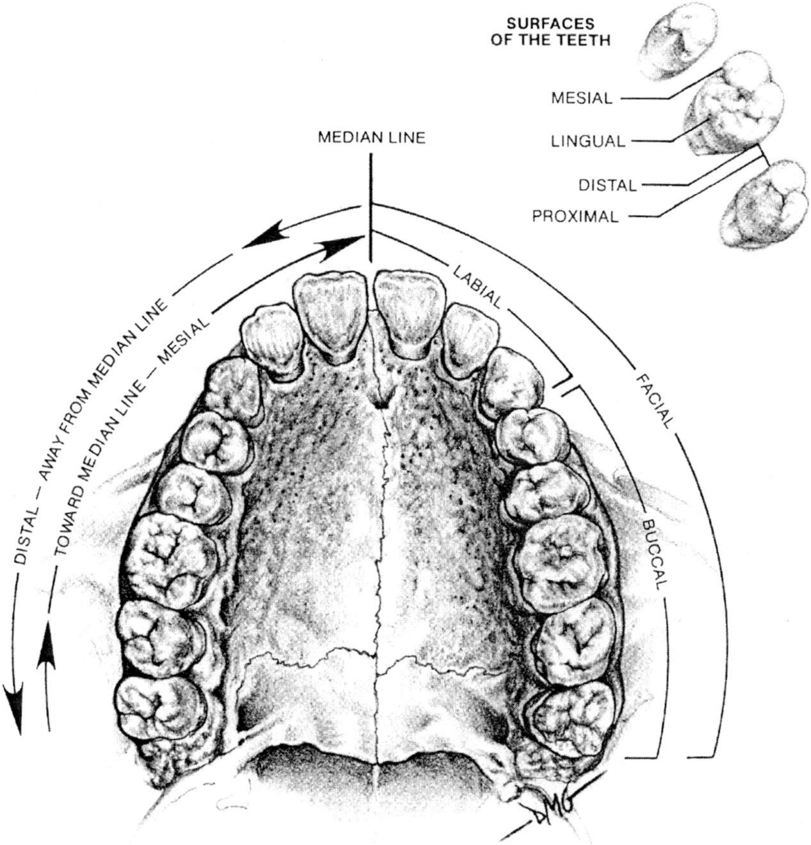

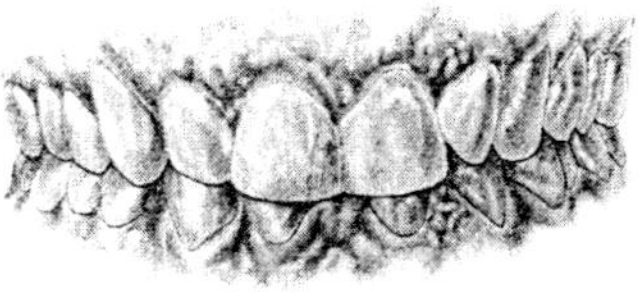

Closed Bite

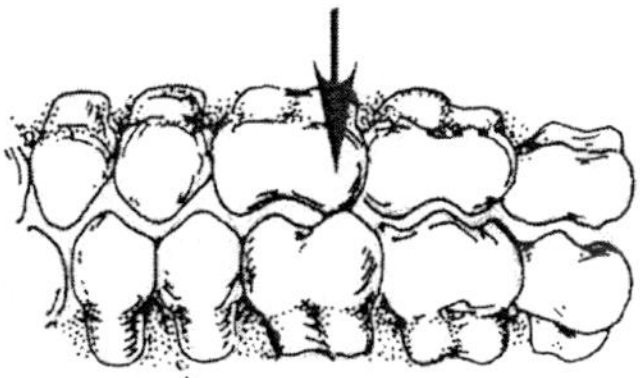

Prematurity

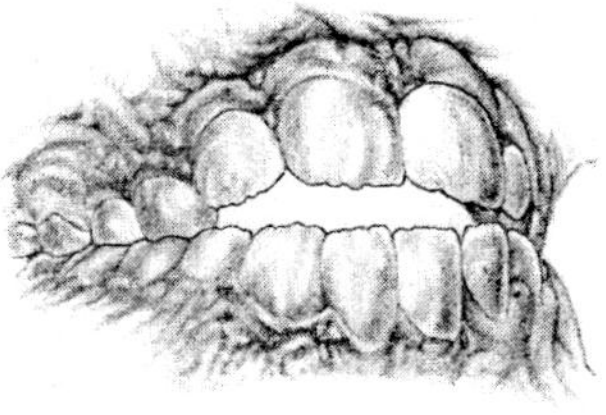

Open Bite

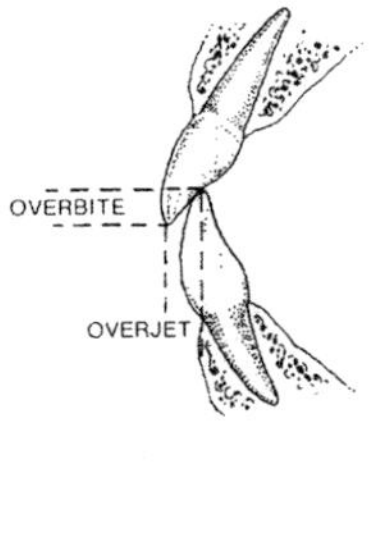

The integrity of the permanent arch depends on the care given to the deciduous teeth. Prevention of dental disease and protective dental treatment should start with the deciduous dentition.

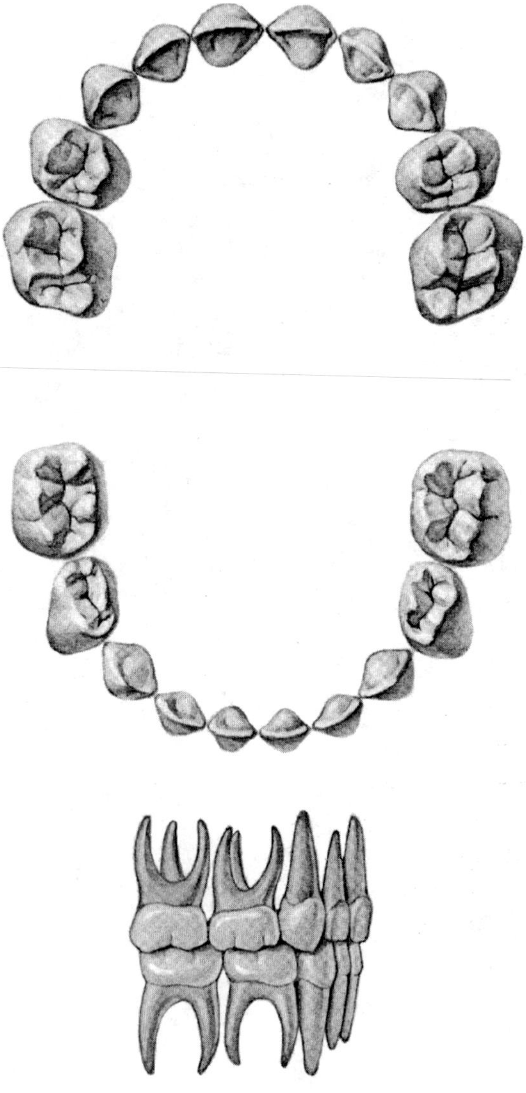

The Deciduous Arch

The integrity of each arch depends on the normal curvilinear arrangement of the teeth, with each tooth in contact with its adjacent neighbors. A break or irregularity in the contact line, which is caused by the loss or displacement of a single tooth, or a part of a tooth, results in the imbalance of the entire arch (malocclusion). The teeth of opposing arches interdigitate in such a manner that the upper arch overlaps and confines the lower, and each tooth is opposed by two teeth of the other arch (except the upper third molars and lower central incisors).

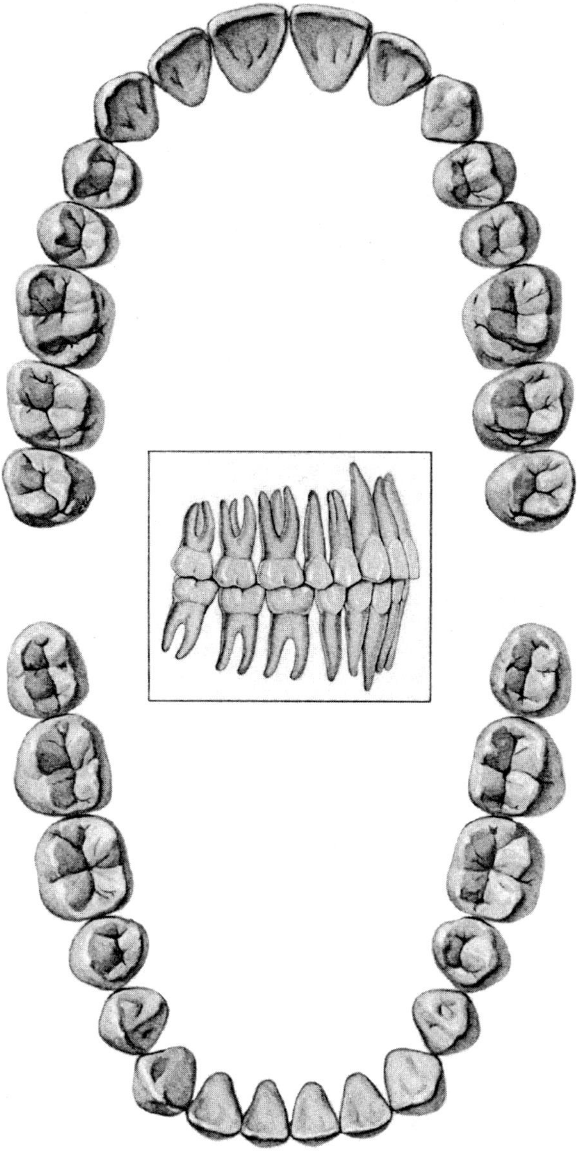

The Permanent Arch

The teeth are drawn as if they were transparent in order to show the three-dimensional relationships of the enamel, dentin and pulp.

Enamel. The enamel is a hard structure covering the crown of the tooth. It is the hardest tissue in the body and is composed almost entirely of inorganic salts (97%). The function of the enamel is to resist abrasive wear.

Dentin. The dentin is a calcified tissue forming the main bulk of the tooth. It consists of about 67% inorganic salts and is penetrated by tubules containing protoplasmic processes coming from cells (odontoblasts) in the pulp. It is these protoplasmic processes within the dentinal tubules that may transmit a sensation of pain to the nerves in the pulp when they are irritated by the action of bacteria, chemical or thermal changes, or by the dental bur.

Pulp. The central cavity of the tooth is filled with a soft tissue, the pulp, which is the remains of the formative organ of the dentin. Two regions may be recognized: (a) The pulp chamber in the crown. (b) The pulp canals in the root.

Cementum. The cementum, which is relatively very thin, covers the surface of the roots. It is shown as a thin line. Its function is to embed the periodontal fibers and thus hold the tooth within its bony socket.

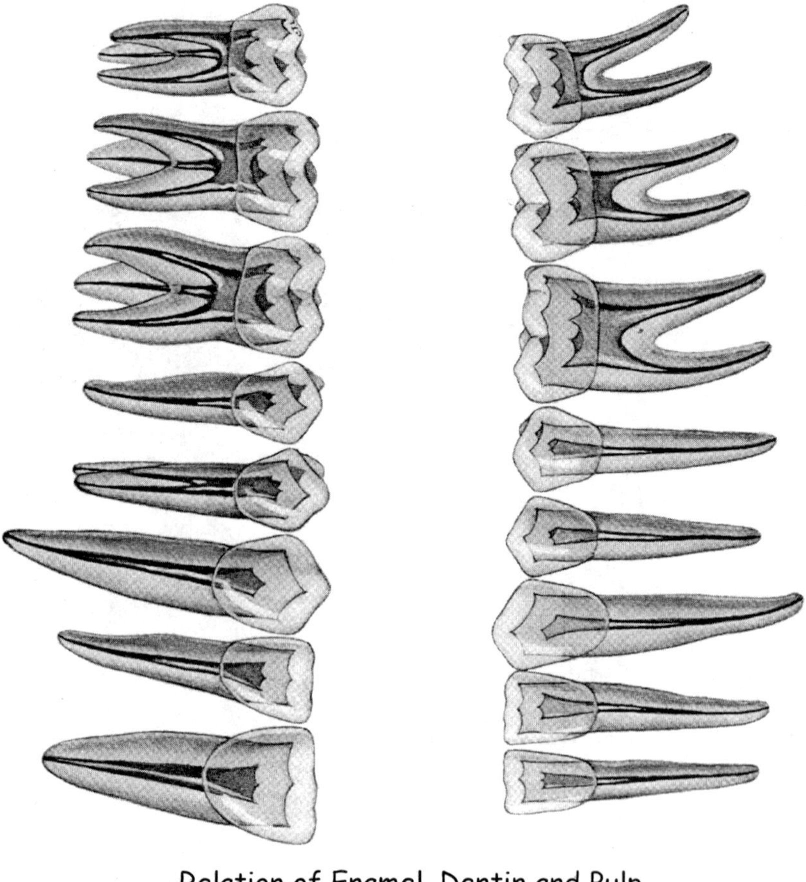

Relation of Enamel, Dentin and Pulp

Each tooth undergoes the following successive periods of development during its life cycle: ***I. Growth:*** (A) *Initiation*: Beginning formation of the tooth bud from the oral epithelium. (B) *Proliferation*: Multiplication of cells and elaboration of the enamel organ. (C) *Histodifferentiation*: Specialization of cells. The cells of the inner epithelium of the enamel organ become ameloblasts; the peripheral cells of the dentin organ (pulp) become odontoblasts. (D) *Morphodifferentiation*: Arrangement of formative cells along the future dentino-enamel (and dentino-cemental) junction to outline the future crown (and root). ***II. Calcification:*** Hardening of the matrix by deposition of calcium salts. ***III:Eruption:*** Migration of the tooth into the oral cavity. ***IV: Attrition:*** Wearing of occlusal and interproximal contact surfaces during function.

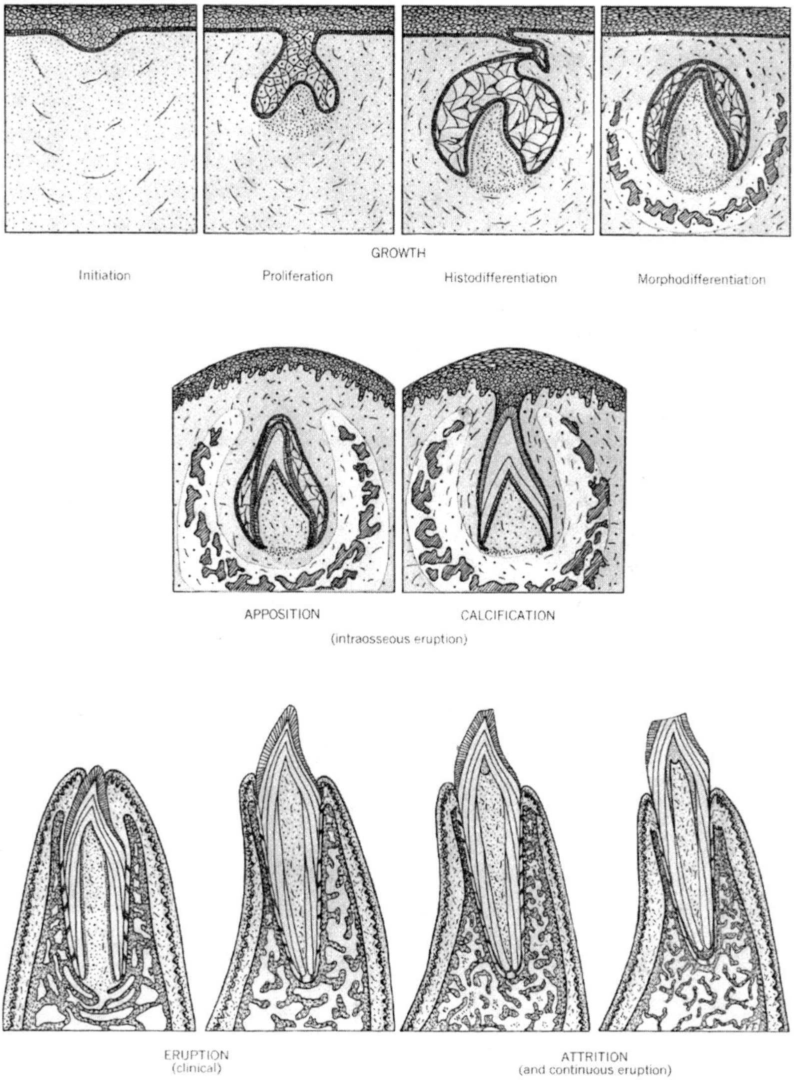

Life Cycle of the Tooth

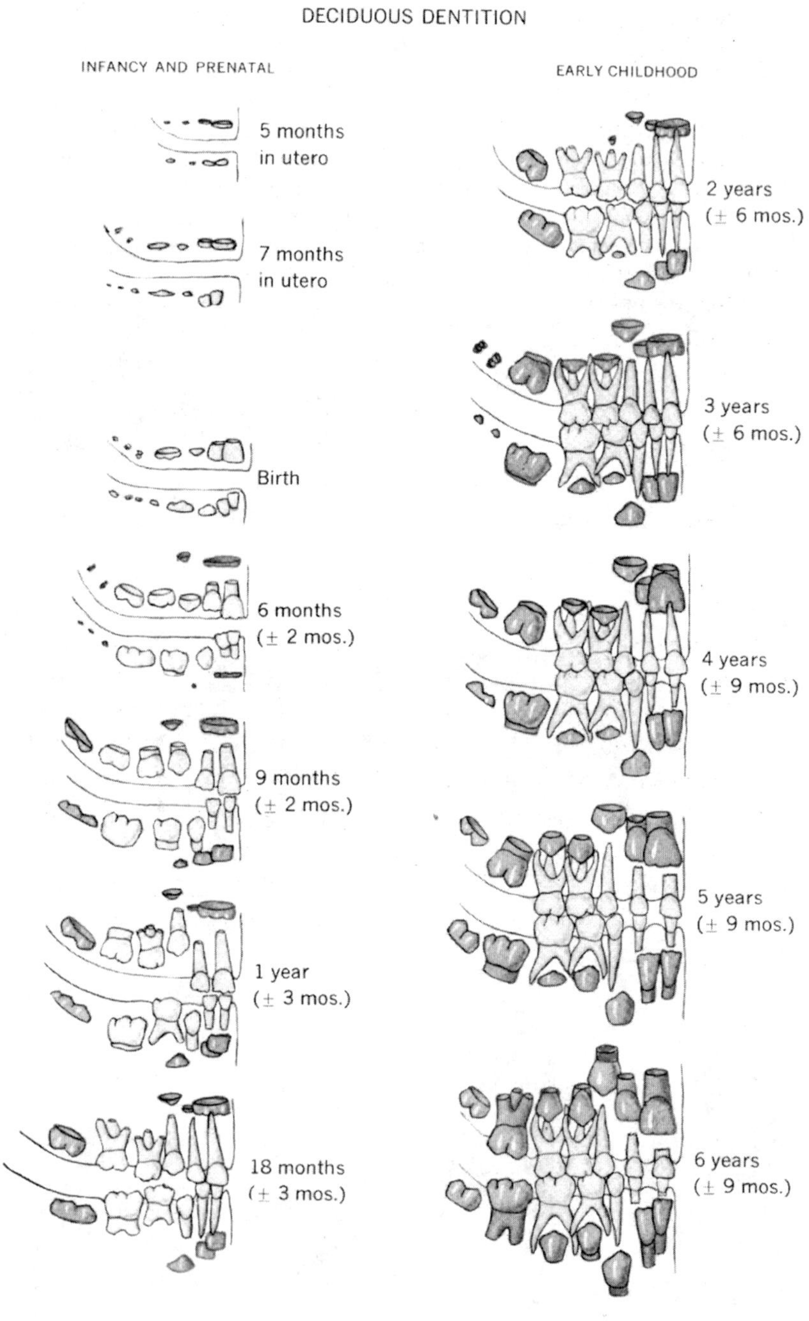

Development of Human Dentitions

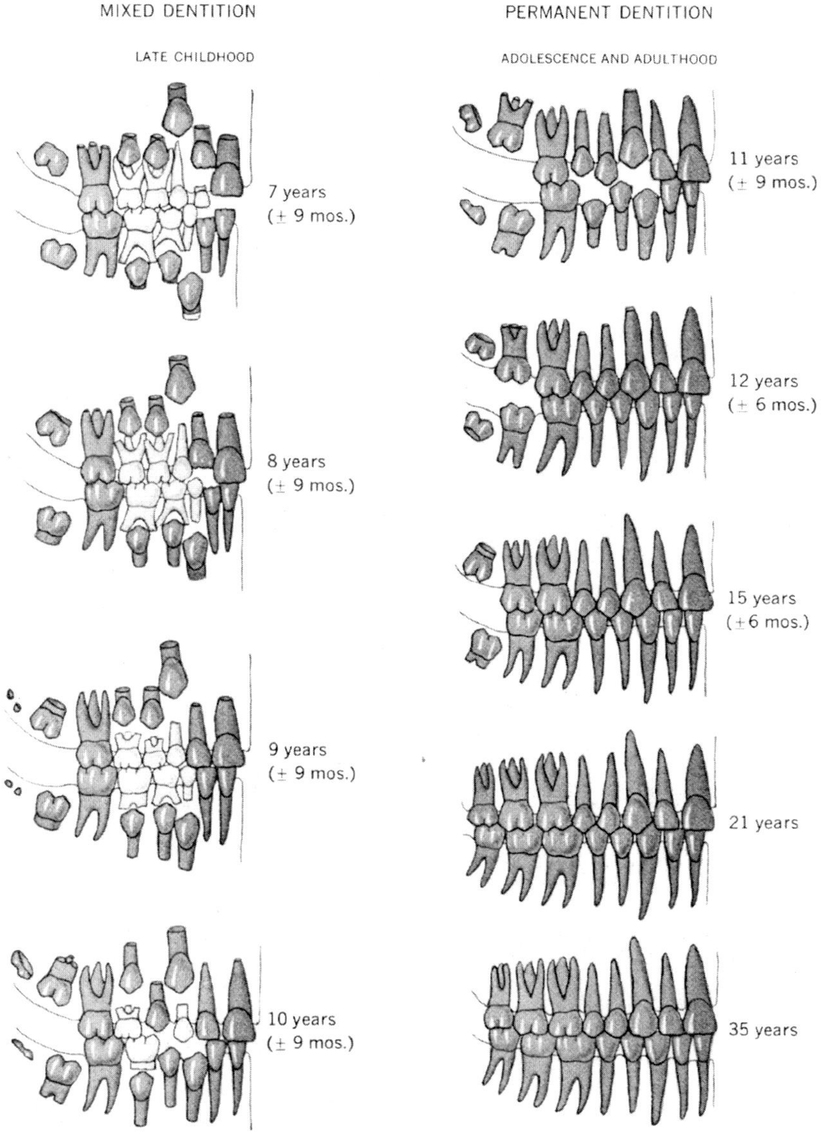

Development of Human Dentitions

The teeth are shown on a chronologic grid to assist in the clinical analysis of the chronology of developmental defects of the teeth, particularly hypoplasia. The levels of the developmental rings and periods are indicated on the right.

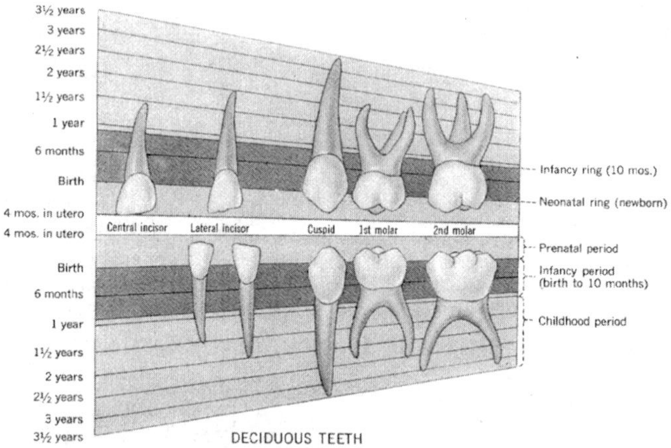

DECIDUOUS TEETH

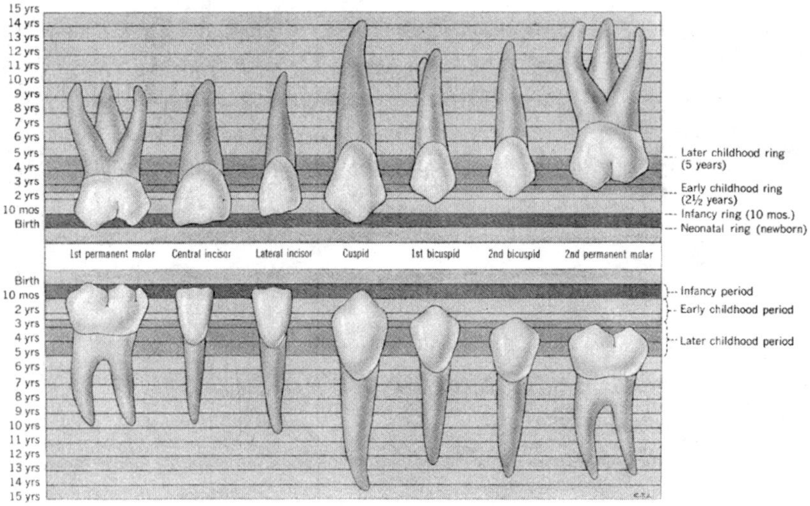

PERMANENT TEETH

Chronology of Crown and Root Development

Tooth eruption is the process whereby the tooth migrates from its position within the bony crypt inside the jaw, to its final position in occlusion within the oral cavity. This movement begins as soon as the crown is completed and the root begins to form but does not depend upon growth of the root since teeth can migrate without root formation and usually travel a distance much longer than the length of the root. In spite of many theories as to its mechanism, the source of the force which causes the tooth to migrate is still unknown. Eruption is a developmental process which is peculiar to teeth. It is continuous through life and is still active even after the teeth are in occlusion. It compensates for the occlusal wearing of the teeth and results in supra-eruption when an antagonist is lost. Eruption is the most easily disturbed of all the developmental processes since it is markedly influenced by local factors.

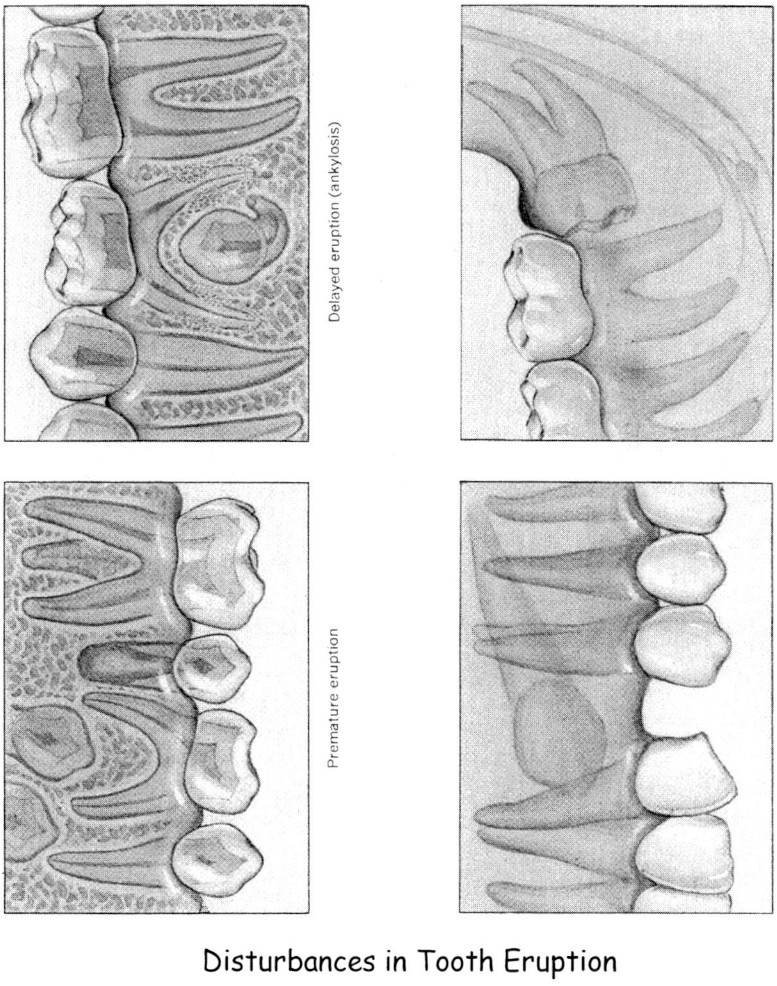

Disturbances in Tooth Eruption

Dental caries is a progressive lesion of the calcified dental tissues (enamel, dentin or cementum) characterized by loss of tooth structure resulting from a solution of the inorganic and digestion of the organic tooth substances. The exciting cause appears to be a mixed bacterial infection beginning at the surface and progressing toward the pulp.

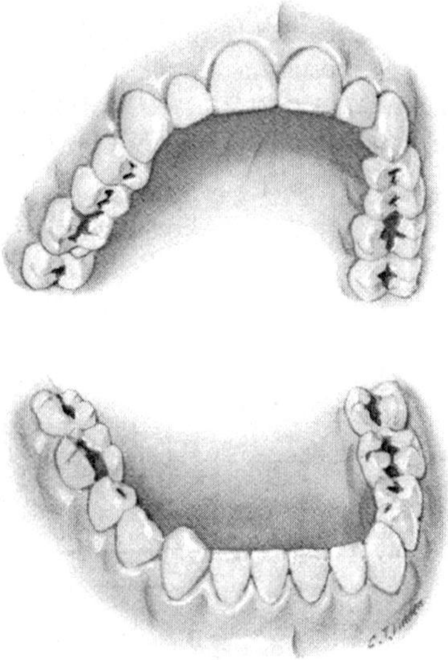

Simple caries

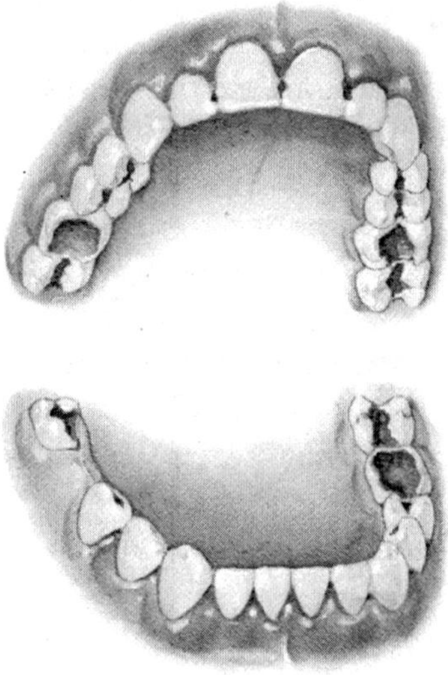

Neglected caries

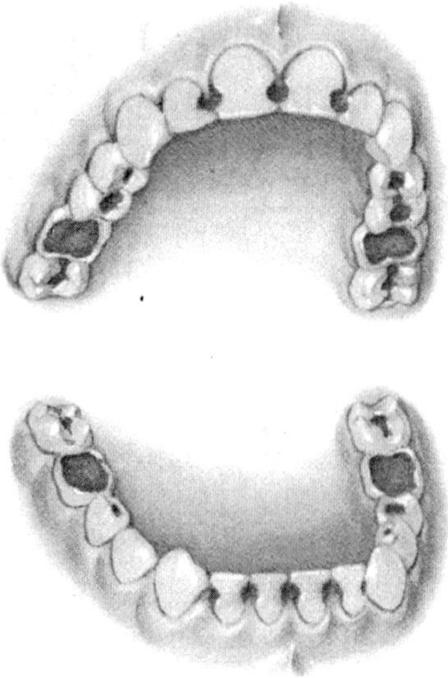

Teen-age caries

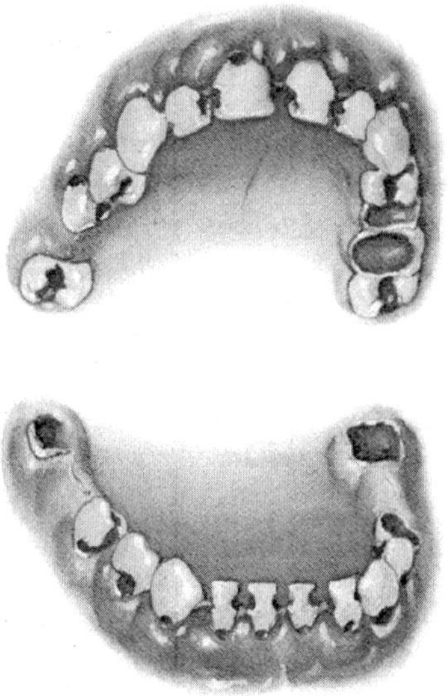

Rampant caries

Dental Caries

1. Bacterial colony in groove or on surface of tooth.
2. Decalcification of enamel by products of acidogenic organisms.
3. Cavitation of enamel.
4. Beginning dentin invasion
    (a) Decalcification
    (b) Proteolysis of organic matrix
5. Continued dentin invasion.
6. Invasion deep into the dentin and approaching the pulp.
7. Pulpitis.
8. Death of pulp.
9. Localized periapical granuloma, cyst or abcess.
10. Spreading periapical infection.

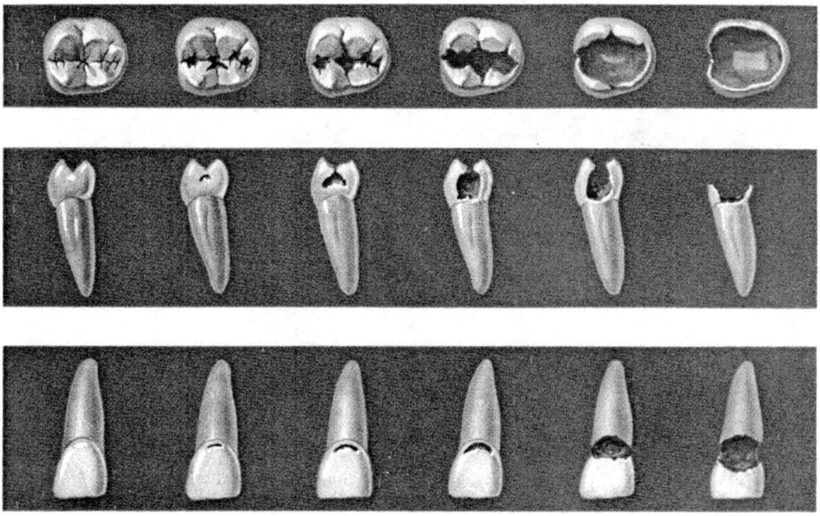

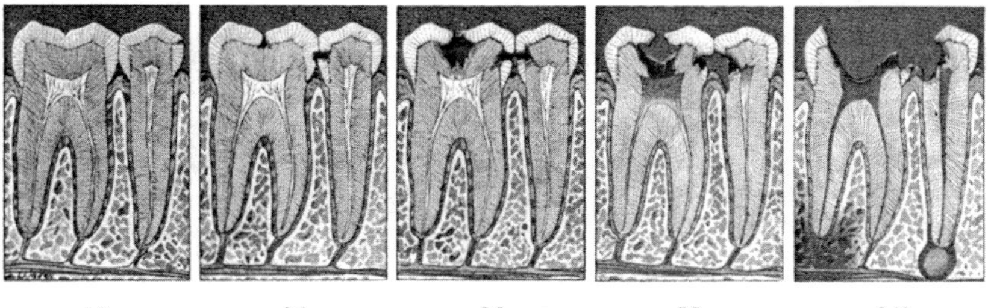

Ten Stages in the Progress of Dental Caries

Erosion is a progressive smooth wearing of the tooth structure generally at the gingivolabial or buccal level. This lesion, which may be wedgeor cup-shaped, is characterized by a smooth, hard, highly polished surface, increased sensitvity and no evidence of bacterial action. It begins in the young adult and rises during middle age. Erosion generally begins in the cuspid-bicuspid region and spreads anteriorly and posteriorly. It commonly begins in the cementum at the cemento-enamel junction and produces a wedge-shaped defect. The exact etiologic factors are unknown. The following conditions have been held responsible: (1) Chemical erosion by acid secretions from the labial or buccal mucosal glands. Generally found in nervous, sensitive individuals who are chronic worriers. (2) Mechanical wear resulting from incorrect toothbrushing (cross-brushing) with an abrasive dentifirice. Increased gingival festooning is present. (3) Combinations of 1 and 2. Dental erosion usually proceeds at a more rapid rate than can be explained by incorrect toothbrushing alone and follows a pattern which differs from that produced by toothbrushing. (4) Excessive use of citrus fruits.

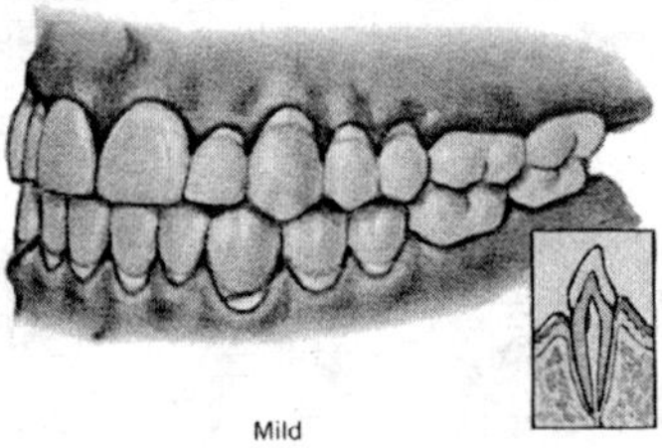

Mild

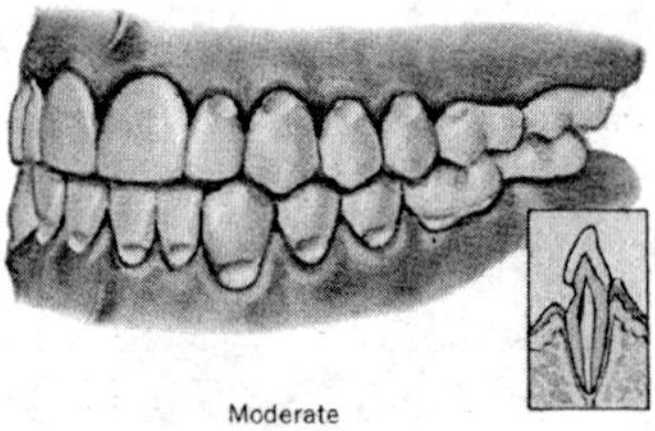

Moderate

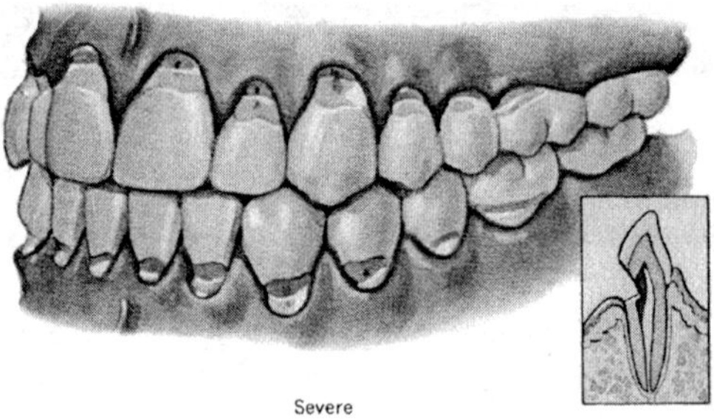

Severe

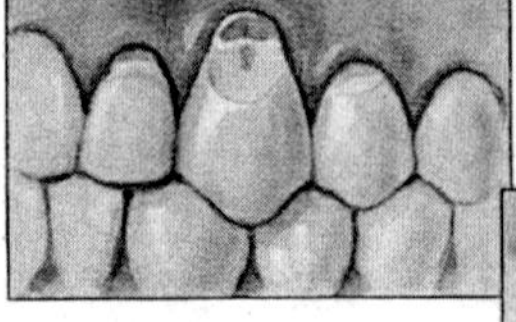

Notched

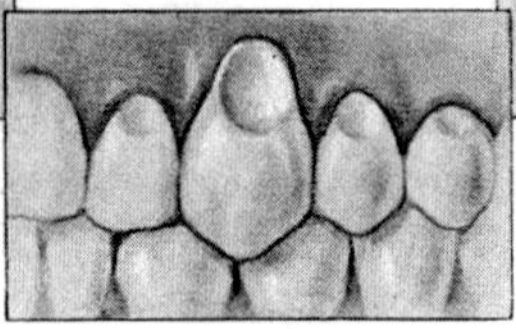

Dished

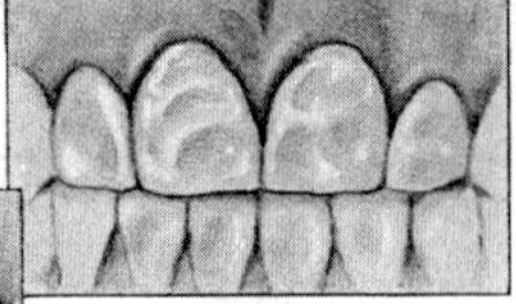

Figured

Dental Erosion

Disturbances of the periodontal tissues (gingivae, periodontal membrane, cementum and alveolar bone) supporting and investing the teeth occur in from 75 to 80% of the adult population. The incidence rises with age. More teeth are lost as a result of periodontal disturbances than from caries. Periodontal disease can be caused by: (1) Local conditions such as calculus, filth and irritation (Simple gingivitis); (2) Systemic conditions that lower tissue resistance (Systemic gingivitis); (3) Combinations of local and systemic conditions (Complex gingivitis).

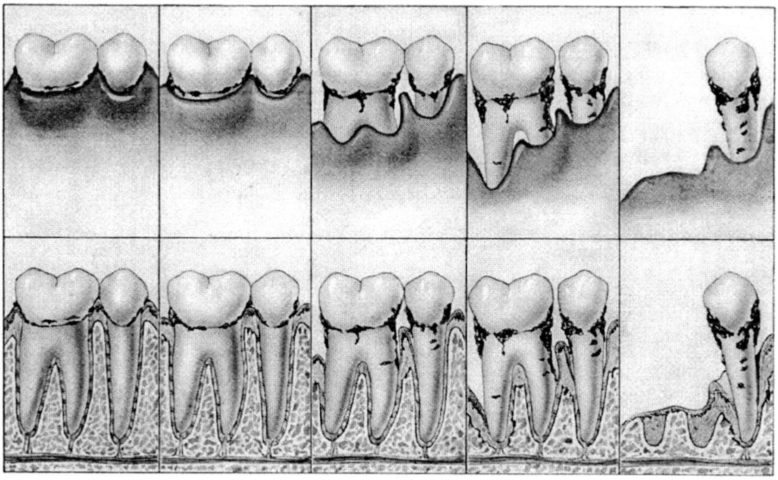

Filth gingivitis

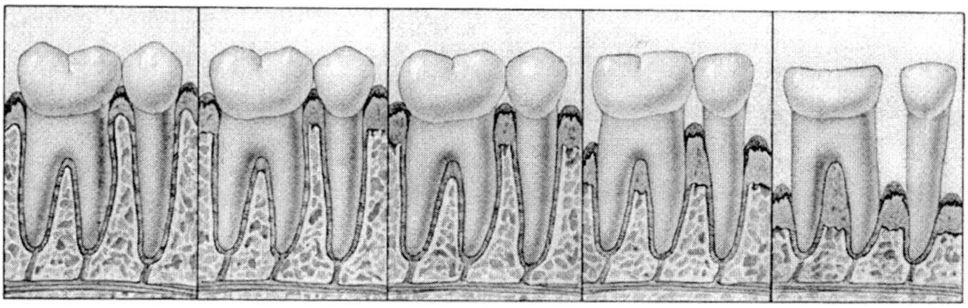

Alveolar crest atrophy

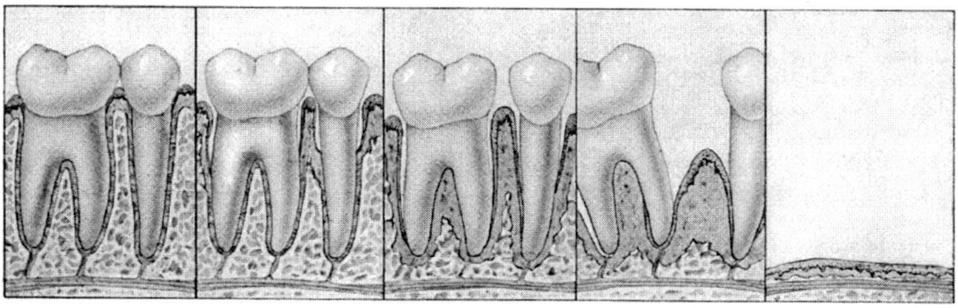

Diffuse alveolar atrophy

Progress of Periodontal Disease

The dental arch is not a static structure, but rather one that is in a state of dynamic balance among the various forces acting upon it. The removal of a single element in the arch upsets this equilibrium and may result in the breakdown of the entire dental apparatus. The resulting malocclusion leads to improper mastication of the food. Cleansing with the toothbrush is difficult and the normal cleansing action of the food does not occur. The irregularities in the alignement and occlusion of the teeth, therefore, are important predisposing factors in the progress of dental caries and periodontal disease.

The first permanent molar is the keystone of the dental arch. The extraction of a lower first molar without immediate replacement, especially after eruption of the second permanent molar, may result in shifting of the teeth, malocclusion, periodontal injury and caries.

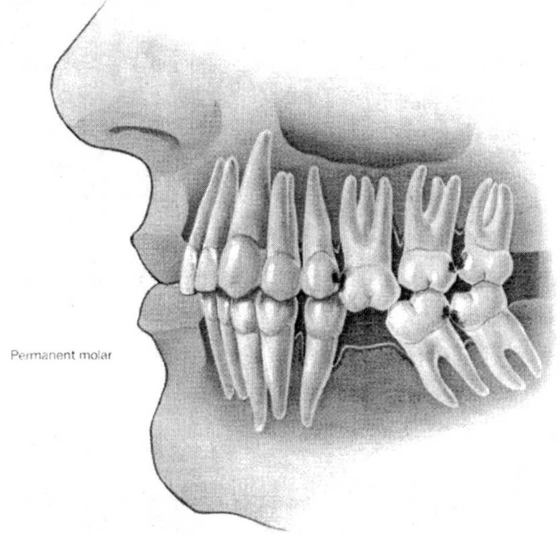

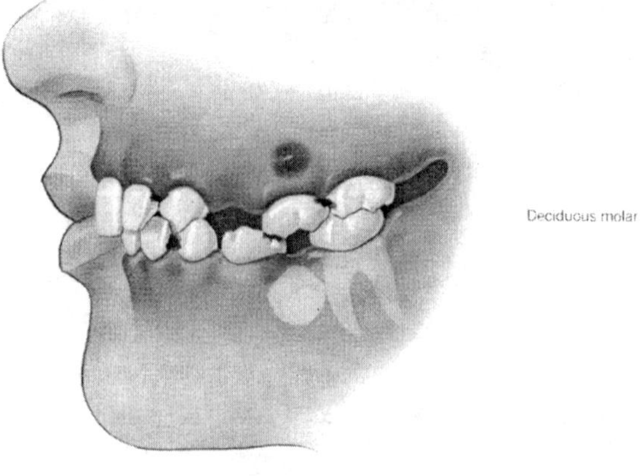

The Effects of the Loss of a Tooth

Crossbite is the result of a reversal in the normal *labio-lingual* or *bucco-lingual* relationship between the upper and lower teeth. In normal occlusion, the upper teeth overlap the lower. In crossbite the reverse occurs. Crossbite of single teeth usually results when a retained deciduous tooth (or tooth root) deflects the erupting permanent tooth from its normal path, as illustrated. This occurs most often in the upper incisor region. Crossbite may also occur in the cuspid, bicuspid and molar areas. However, the etiology of crossbite in first permanent molars is often obscure since these teeth do not have deciduous predecessors. It may be related to tongue habits since it is often accompanied by a partial submergence of the lower molar.

ANTERIOR CROSSBITE

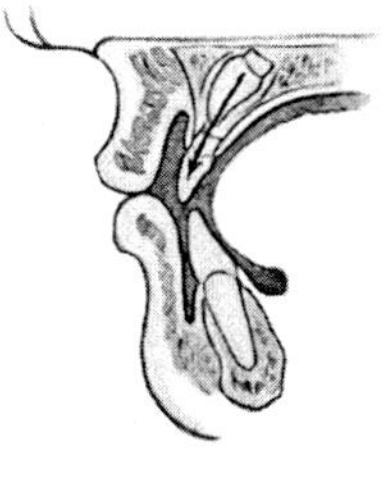

Normal eruption

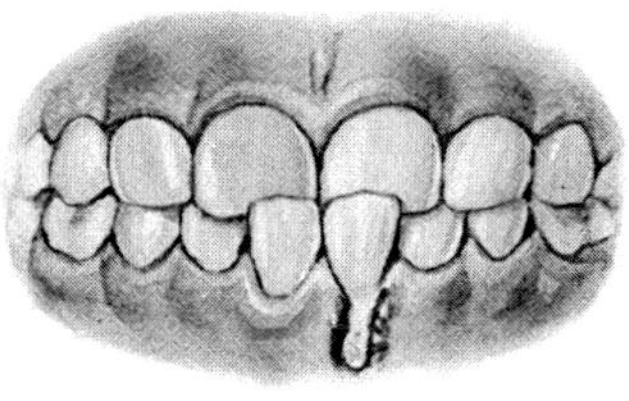

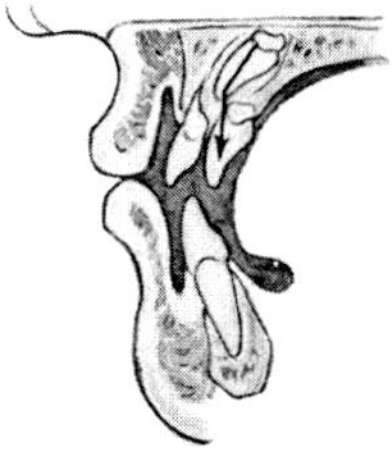

Deflected eruption

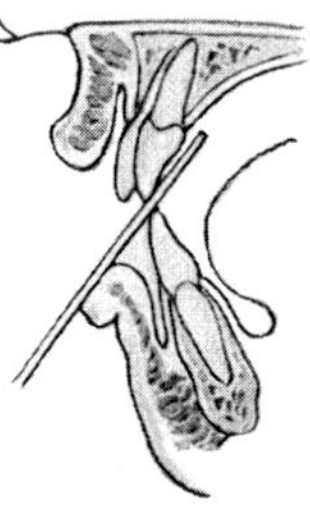

Tongue blade correction

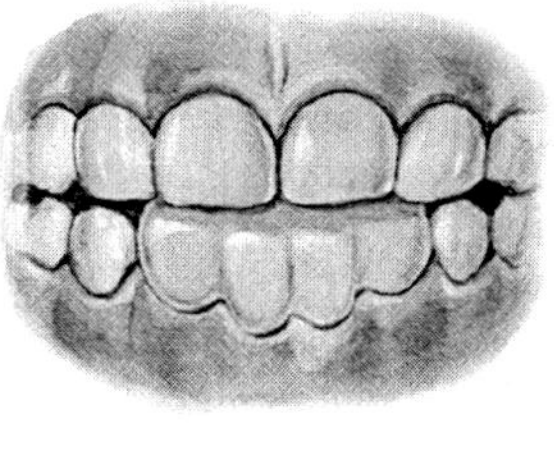

Bite-plane

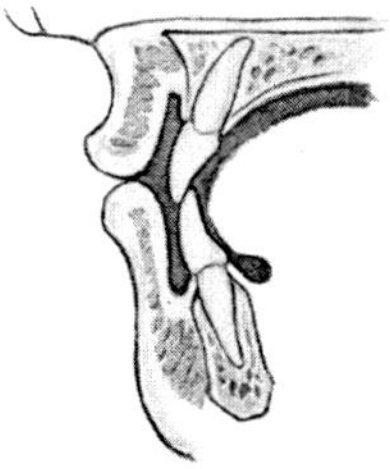

Corrected

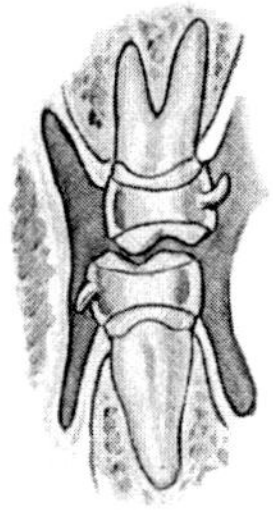

Molar crossbite

POSTERIOR CROSSBITE

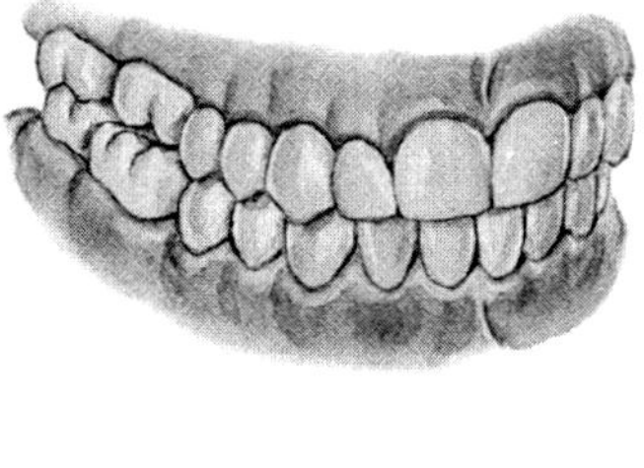

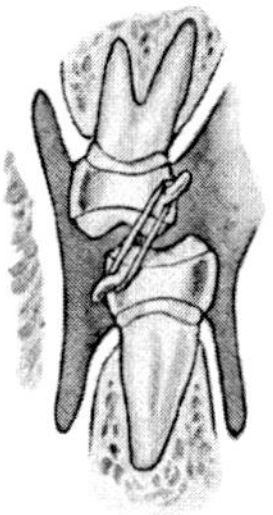

Corrected

Crossbite

The Twelve Cranial Nerves

Nerve		*Function*
1. Olfactory	Sensory–from olfactory cells in nasal mucosa. Smell.	
2. Optic	Sensory–from ganglion cells in retina. Vision.	
3. Oculomotor	Motor–	to all ocular muscles except lateral rectus and superior oblique. also contains parasympathetic fibers to sphincter of pupil, ciliary muscle.
4. Trochlear	Motor–	to superior oblique muscle which rotates eyeball outward and downward.
5. Trigeminal	Motor–	to muscles of mastication, tensor tympani, tensor veli palatini, mylohyoid and anterior belly of di gastric.
	Sensory–	*Ophthalmic branch* to cornea, ciliary body, iris, lacrimal gland, conjunctiva, nasalmucosa, eyelid, eyebrow, forehead and nose. *Maxillary branch* to skin of cheek, lower lid, side of nose, upper jaw, teeth and mucosa and maxillary sinus. *Mandibular branch* to lower jaw, teeth ad mucosa.
6. Abducens	Motor–	to the lateral rectus muscle. Rotates the eyeball outwards.
7. Facial	Motor–	to facial muscles, muscles of scalp and ear, stapedius, stylohyoid and posterior belly of digastric. Also contains parasympathetic fibers to submandibular and sublingual salivary glands and lacrimal, nasal and palatine glands.
	Sensory–	(N. Intermedius)–from taste buds in anterior two-thirds of tongue. General sensation from lateral of soft palate and adjacent pharynx and external auditory meatus.
8. Acoustic	Sensory–	from spiral ganglion of chohlea (auditory division). Hearing.
9. Glossopharyngeal	Sensory–	from taste buds in posterior third of tongue. Sensation from fauces, tonsils, pharynx and soft palate.
	Motor–	to pharyngeal musculature and parasympathetic to parotid gland.
10. Vagus	Motor–	to all muscles of the larynx. parasympathetic to heart, lungs, bronchi, G.I. tract.
	Sensory–	from heart, lungs, bronchi, trachea, larynx, pharynx, G.I. tract, external ear.
11. Spinal accessory	Motor–	cranial portion to pharynx, uvula and levator veli palatini. spinal portion to sternomastoid and trapezius muscles.
12. Hypoglossal	Motor–	to tongue.

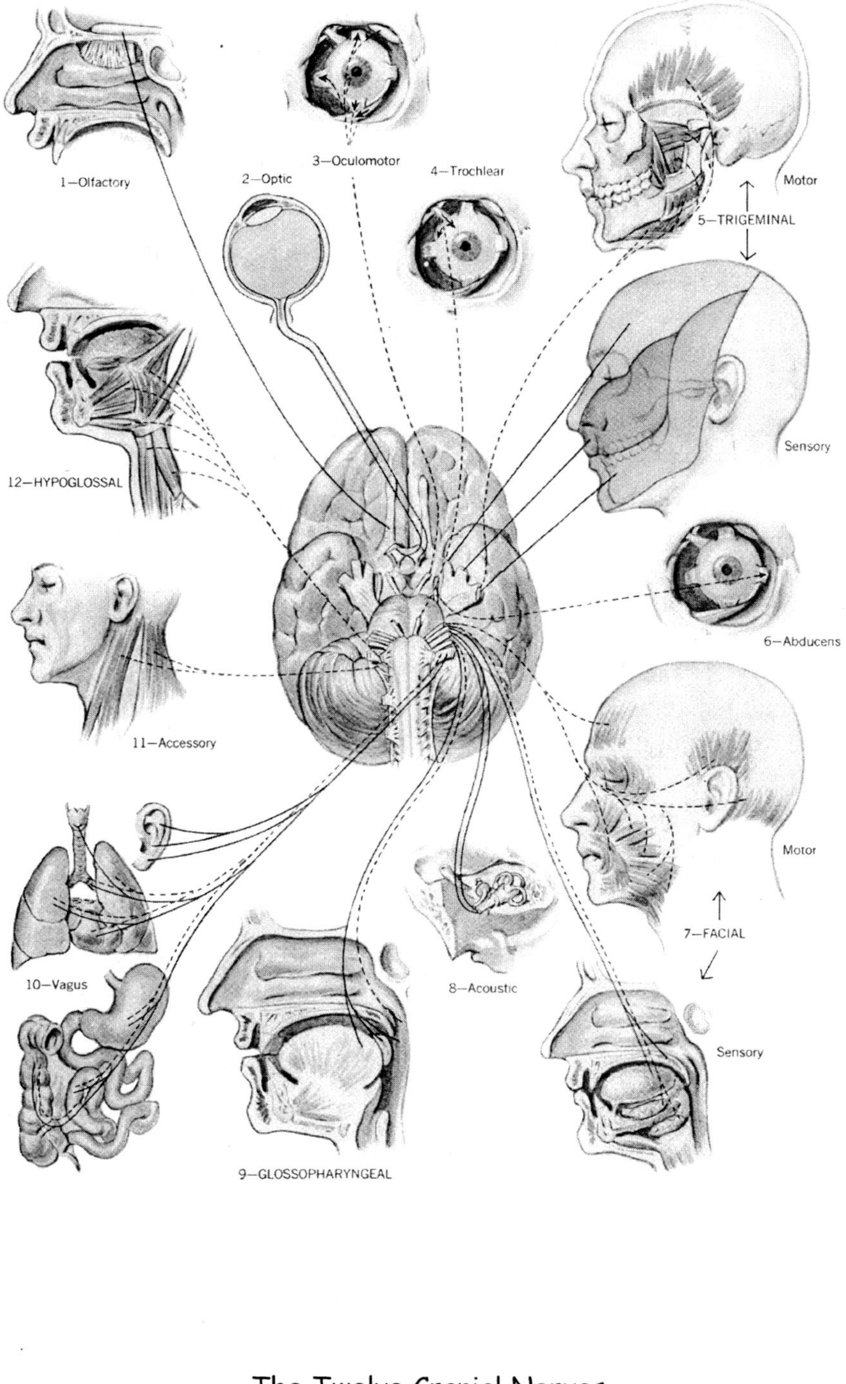

The Twelve Cranial Nerves

Different Types of Dental Restorations

1. **Sealants**–white filling materials in a "flowable" form. Used ot fill the decay-susceptible groves of the back teeth (usually children 6-18) as a preventive procedure.

2. **Fillings**–composite (white) filling materials. Placed directly into the tooth. Used where the existing fillings or areas of decay are small enough that the remaining tooth structure has not been overly weakened.

3. **Inlays**–used in similar situations as fillings except a pre-made piece of ceramic material is bonded into the tooth. This results in superior physical properties, possibly providing a lifespan of 2 to 3 times longer than a composite filling. Inlays are a top-quality alternative to the composite filling. Traditionally gold alloys have been used for inlays, but now ceramics are excellent.

4. **Onlays**–used in situations where the tooth is fractured or has been severely weakened, the onlay is similar to the inlay described above except that the ceramic covers the entire or most of the biting surface. Unlike a crown, it does not cover the entire visible tooth structure, so there is no need to grind away all sides of the tooth unless there is a specific reason (like decay).

5. **Crowns (Caps)**–the largest tooth restoration, a crown sometimes cannot be avoided. It covers all sides of the tooth as well as the end. It is used when there is limited tooth structure left, when an existing crown must be replaced, or when tooth is an "anchor" tooth for a fixed bridge. In cases where it is impossible to get proper moisture control (below the gum line or near the back of the mouth), a cemented crown may substitute for a bonded one.

6. **Veneers**–thin porcelain facings that cover the front side of teeth. Used cosmetically to change the length, color and shape of teeth.

7. **Bridges**–used to replace missing teeth when sufficient "anchor" teeth are available on each side of the gap. Numerous systems are available, including fiber-reinforced ceramics, zirconium-based ceramics and porcelain fused to metal bridges.

8. **Implants**–titanium posts surgically placed into the jawbone. Implants are used to support a dental p[rosthesis (from a single crown to full denture) once the bone grows around the post (usually three months after placement).

9. **Removable Partial Dentures**–used to replace missing teeth when insufficient teeth remain to support fixed bridges or a patient does not test well for bridge materials. Partial dentures can be metal or acrylic-based. Acrylic-based partials are bulkier and do not stay in place as well as metal partials.

10. **Removable Full Denture**–used when no teeth remain. Caution: most, but not all, acrylic bases contain cadmium, a toxic substance, as a color stabilizer.

Teeth

A tooth consists of the *crown* and the *root* portions, divided by the cervical line. A cross section of a tooth reveals its four tissues–*enamel, cementum, dentin*, and *pulp*. The pulp is soft tissue furnishing blood and nerve supply to the tooth, while the other three are hard tissues. The crown has a cutting edge, which, in the case of the incisors, is an *incisal ridge*; for the rest of the teeth there are *cusps*. A cusp may be singular, as in the canine teeth, or there may be two or more cusps as in the pre-molars and molars. *Intercuspation* occurs when the cusps of the teeth of the upper (maxilla) and lower (mandible) jaws come together.

Surfaces of Teeth

The crowns of the incisors and canines have a ridge which is the cutting surface, plus four other surfaces. The pre-molars (bicuspids) and molars have the *occlusal* surface as their cutting surface, along with four other surfaces. All surfaces which face the tongue are *lingual* surfaces. The outer surface of the pre-molars and molars is called the *buccal* surface, and the outer surface of the incisors and canines is called the *labial* surface. The outer surface of the entire arch is referred to as the *facial* surface. The surfaces of the crowns which face adjoining teeth in the dental arch are called *proximal* surfaces. They are further distinguished as *mesial* or *distal*, which refers to direction in the dental arch. The proximal surfaces facing the middle of the arch are called mesial surfaces, while those facing the extremes are called distal surfaces.

General Terms

When the teeth of the mandibular and maxillary arches come into *intercuspation* in a functional arrangement, it is called *centric* or *central occlusion* (CO). When this intercuspation is abnormal, the result is *malocclusion*. The term *centric relation* (CR) refers to the *condyles* of the mandible in their functional position in the *mandibular fossae*. There is considerable discrepancy in the literature regarding the definition of centric relation. *Prematurity* refers to a first tooth contact which deviates the mandible from centric relation prior to complete intercuspation, producing a "slide," which is part of malocclusion. Most authorities state that *centric relation* must be in harmony with *centric occlusion*.

A *crossbite occlusion* is where the opposing upper and lower teeth are reversed from the usual occlusion. This places the lower posterior or incisor teeth outside the upper dental arch. There may be an *anterior* (forward) or a *posterior* (backward) crossbite. When posterior, it may be *uni-* or *bi-lateral*. *Overbite* and *overjet* refer to the relation of the central incisors when the teeth are in centric occlusion. Normally, the incisal edges of the *mandibular incisors* occlude against the lingual surface of the *maxillary incisors* in such a way that approximately one-third of the mandibular incisor crown is overlapped by the upper incisor. This vertical overlap is called *overbite*. The projection of the upper incisors beyond their antagonists in a horizontal direction is called *overjet*, sometimes referred to as *horizontal overlap*.

*Closed bit*e refers to excessive overbite where little or none of the lower incisors are visible during centric occlusion. *Open bite* refers to failure of some teeth to contact when in centric occlusion. The term *freeway space* or *interocclusal distance* refers to the distance between the occluding surfaces of the maxillary and mandibular teeth when the mandible is in its *physiologic rest position*. The physiologic rest position is the position of the mandible when the muscles of mastication are inactive. They have no electrical activity as observed on electromyography.

Periodontal Ligament

The periodontal ligament has great importance in the overall consideration of the *stomatognathic* system (all structures from the shoulder girdle up). Understanding this structure's role in the system requires a thorough understanding of its *histology* (microscopic study of the structure of tissues) and its role in the relation of tooth to bone. The periodontal ligament is composed of fibers, blood vessels, lymphatics, nerves, and cellular elements. It anchors the tooth from its *cementum* to bone, *alveolar* tissue (tooth sockets), and other teeth. When there is no stress placed on the tooth, the fibers of the periodontal ligament are relaxed and somewhat wavy. When force is applied to the tooth, the tension applied to these relaxed fibers provides a shock absorber mechanism to the attachment of the tooth. There are three types of fibers:

Gingival fibers–connect the cementum to the gingiva.

Transspetal fibers–connect to adjacent teeth.

Alveolar fibers–connect the tooth to the bone.

1. **Alveolar crest fibers** connect the cervical cementum to the lamina dura.

2. **Horizontal fibers** run at right angles to the long axis of the tooth from cementum to bone.

3. **Oblique fibers** run from the cementum in an oblique fashion so that they angle from bone to the apex of the tooth. These are the most important and numerous of the periodontal fibers. The oblique arrangement gives additional strength ot the tooth. As force is exerted on the tooth toward the apex, the oblique fibers tighten, thus pulling the alveolar socket closer to the tooth. The periodontal ligaments and associated structures are called the *periodontal transmission mechanism*, which adapts to the forces applied to the tooth. When function and adaptation of the periodontal transmission mechanism are lost, there will be loss of the tooth.

4. **Apical fibers** run from the apical region of the root to the bone.

5. **Inter-radicular fibers** run from the crest of the inter-radicular septum to the bifurcation of the roots.

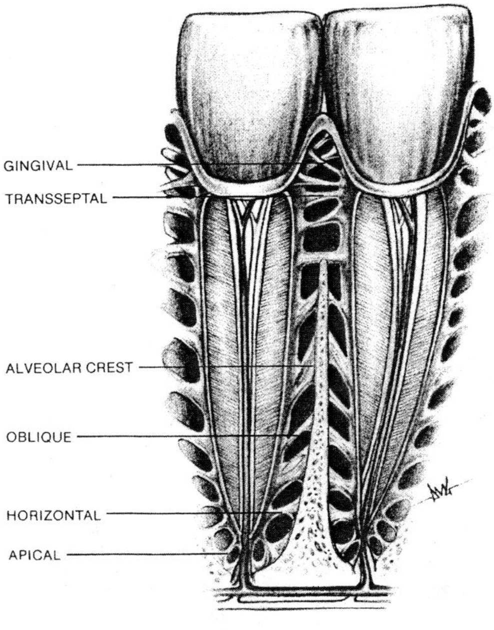

Periodontal Ligament

Function

The periodontal ligament has four basic functions: (1) supportive, (2) nutritional, (3) formative, and (4) sensory. The supportive function is the mechanical stabilizing effect of the fibers' attachment from the cementum to the tooth's supporting structures. The suspensory arrangement of the ligament cushions and acts as a shock absorber for forces applied to the tooth. The alveolar socket is tightened around the tooth when force is applied axially on the tooth. As the tooth is forced into the alveolar socket and the oblique fibers tighten the bone against the tooth, the periodontal space narrows, thus squeezing the blood and lymph vessels and forcing fluids out of the space. As pressure on the tooth is reduced, the space re-opens, drawing new fluid into the area; thus a hydraulic piston arrangement supplies nutrition to the area and removes waste products.

The formative function is to repair tissue in the normal renewal process or for pathological reasons. The periodontal ligament is the source of *osteoblasts*, *cementoblasts*, *fibroblasts*, *osteoclasts*, and *phage cells*. The neurological function, though, deserves the greatest consideration in this discussion. The far-ranging effects on the nervous system from disturbance in the dentition are unknown. There is evidence that remote problems can be caused directly through the nervous system to areas such as the arm. The work of Westrum, et al. suggests a cause and effect relationship in alteration of the dentition and changes in the nervous system. These studies may relate only to the pathological conditions of the dentition, or they may expand to functional conditions.

The nerve receptors of the periodontal ligament are *nociceptors* and *proprioceptors*. Activity within the stomatognathic system initiated by the procrioceptors in the periodontal ligament is much the same as with proprioceptive function and dysfunction in other areas of the body. A proprioceptor signals the status of position, stress, etc., through the *afferent* system. If necessary, a reaction to the changing conditions is sent over the *efferent* system. The nociceptors of the periodontal legament send information about the area's environment over the afferent system. Stimulation to these receptors may lead to conscious and/or reflex reaction. The proprioceptors are sensitive enough to determine the thinnest piece of paper placed between the teeth. It is through this mechanism that malocclusion is sensed, which may cause the entire stomatognathic system to change.

The least amount of malocclusion–which may only be a very slight contact by a single tooth in advance of the others–is perceived and integrated into muscular activity. This is to change the muscular pattern and avoid premature contact, saving wear and tear on that tooth; this this is an ideal situation. Sometimes the muscles cannot find a mandibular position free of prematurities. Another mechanism protective of the teeth is reflex from the nociceptor. An example of this action is when one is eatng cherries and bites o a stone. There is immediate reflex opening of the jaw to avoid injury to the teeth.

The opening reflex is also present in normal chewing. There is a difference in the muscular activity between those with natural dentition and those with dentures. The jaw-closing muscles are completely depressed during mouth opening in the presence of natural dentition. These reciprocal relationships are not as evident in denture wearers. This fine regulation of mastication is from the feedback control of the afferent system to regulate the efferent activity causing mandibular motion. Stimulation to these receptors may lead to conscious and/or reflex reaction. Proprioceptors from the teeth, muscles, and temporomandibular joint contribute afferent supply to the motor nucleus of the trigeminal nerve and also to higher centers to moderate volitional control.

The normal jaw-opening reflex is initiated by stimulation of the receptors in the periodontal ligament. This reflex is an inhibition of the mandibular elevators after tooth contact, sufficient to stimulate the receptors in the periodontal ligament. Measurement of the maximum bite force of individual teeth reveals a difference from tooth to tooth. This appears to be due to the limitation of bite force controlled by muscle inhibition as a result of stimulation to the periodontal ligament proprioceptors.

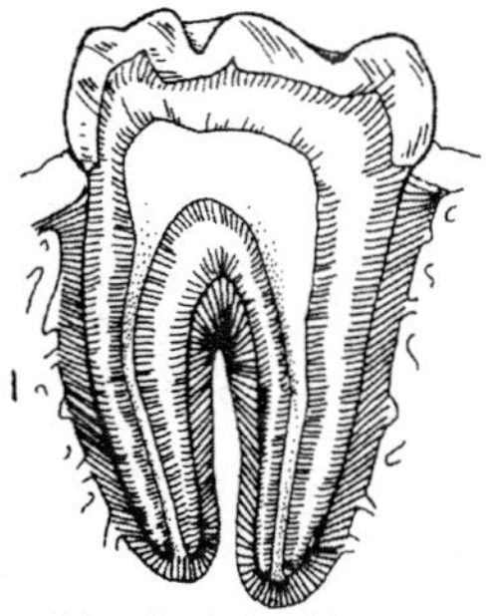

Relaxed periodontal ligament.

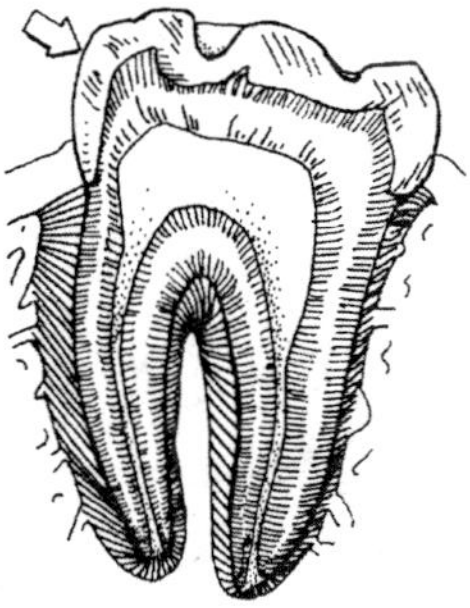

Force applied which is somewhat absorbed by the periodontal ligaments.

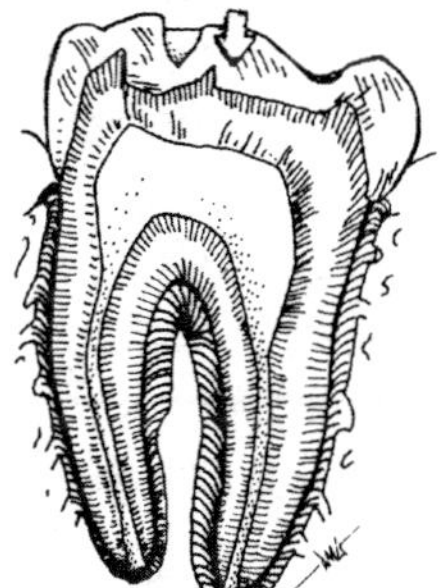

Axial force tightens the bone around the roots because of the angle of the oblique fibers.

Plaque

Normally our mouths are covered with millions of microscopic bacteria. These microscopic monsters live in a sticky film of protein and mucus called *plaque*, where they feed on leftover food particles. These bacteria produce acid as a result of their feasting and it is this acid which cuts into tooth enamel, creating cavities. Bacteria also pour out volatile sulfur compounds that cause embarrassing bad breath. Plaque can only be removed by mechanical scrubbing to break it up so it can be rinsed away. Only by physically cleaning off the adhesive plaque can it be removed. Unfortunately, there is no magic mouthwash that will break up or dissolve plaque.

Normal brushing removes these bacteria from our teeth, but many bacteria escape by hiding in the spaces between teeth where the toothbrush cannot reach. Brushing does not reach between the teeth to clean out the poisonous plaque and the toxic rotting food matter that seeps between your teeth. That putrefying waste stays there for days or weeks until you mechanically clean it out.

The plaque containing the bacteria eventually hardens into a substance known as tartar. Unlike plaque, tartar cannot be removed by brushing, but must be removed by your dentist or hygienist. Over time, levels of more dangerous types of bacteria build up within tartar. These bacteria produce toxins that irritate and inflame the gums. If left untreated, gingivitis progresses to gum disease called *periodontal disease, pyorrhea, periodontitis or gingivitis*—a condition where bacteria and their toxins invade not only the gums but also the bones and the structures supporting the teeth. This causes bone loss, loose teeth, and teeth that fall out.

Eighty percent of Americans have gum disease to some degree. Periodontal disease damages the small blood vessels running through the gums. Through these damaged blood vessels, bacteria and their toxins gain access to the blood stream. Once here, recent evidence indicates that the bacteria and toxins may contribute to major medical problems including premature delivery of infants, strokes, and heart attacks. When we floss, we rid our mouth of the bacteria that lead to gingivitis and periodontal disease, thereby saving our teeth and protecting our health.

Flossing

Flossing may not be easy. It takes 2-3 weeks of consistent daily flossing to get used to flossing. In the beginning it bleeds, it hurts, the floss snaps and gets stuck, and it is difficult only in the beginning because your gums are diseased and infected. But the bleeding, discomfort and difficulty go away as your gums heal and get healthy. Just like learning to ride a bike, it is difficult, you get bumped and bruised, but if you keep at it, you can do it. It takes perseverance, but once you make it over the 2-3 week hump, flossing becomes easier. You can do it if you try.

The best floss to use is *Glide*. It glides between the teeth easier than regular floss and makes flossing easier. Or, as an alternative, get some round toothpicks and break several in the middle until you get a thin sliver that will fit between the teeth. Stick it in each space between the teeth and work it in between each of the teeth. Or use on e of the plastic picks available at the drugstore.

Tongue Scraping

The top surface of your tongue is coated with a furry layer. The germs, bacteria or bugs and old food live in this furry layer and multiply. When you scrape your tongue, you milk these live and dead germs out of that furry layer. Your breath will be fresher in the morning will taste better.

Brushing

Brush your teeth slowly and reach way back in your mouth to clean the molars. Be patient, slow and methodical in brushing the teeth. Brush along the gumline because that is where harmful dental plaque grows. Feel the bristles getting under the gums. Clean both the insides and the outsides of your teeth all the way around. Follow an even pattern. Brush all the way around the outsides of the uppers, from one side to the other. Then do the insides of the uppers all the way around from one side to the other.

Then do the bottom teeth the same way, outsides then the insides all the way around. Take your time. Be patient, not in a hurry. Use a clock and do it for 2-3 minutes. Try to reach every area. Get to the hard-to-reach areas in the back. Repeat cleaning the uppers and lowers again. Use a toothpaste of your choice. **Avoid tartar-control toothpastes**, they make the teeth sensitive. **Avoid fluoride-containing toothpaste**, as this is a toxic poison.

Also, **avoid sodium laurel sulfate**, as this is also toxic to the body, creating nitrates and dioxins in the body. Research has proven that **brushing and flossing with just water is 95% as effective as using toothpaste**.

Use soft toothbrushes only. Hard toothbrushes feel like they are doing a better job, but the bristles are too big to fit under the gums and hard bristle brushes damage the teeth and gums. **Replace your toothbrush every three months.**

Flushing

After the flossing and brushing breaks up the plaque, it must be flushed away and the poisons and toxic rotting waste products rinsed out of the deep spaces under you gums (pockets). Buy an under the gum water-jet irrigator. This shoots out a water jet under pressure from the tip of the tiny hose that will flush between the teeth and under the gums. The gums surround the teeth like a rubber band and prevent liquids from reaching into the pockets. Simply rinsing your mouth will not get under the gums and into the pockets. Swishing mouthwash around will not get the mouthwash under the gums.

Fill the water tank with hot filtered water. Add one dropper full of "under the gum irrigant" to the water and stir well. Or use two tablespoons of baking soda mixed very well in the hot water. A few drops of *Aodine* detoxified iodine can likewise be mixed with the water as can a colloidal silver solution to disinfect the area under the gums.

Start at low pressure. Put the hose tip in your mouth and turn it on. Point it towards the gums of the upper teeth and into the space between the gums and the teeth. Slowly move the tip around the gum line on the outer sides of the teeth flushing under the gums and between the teeth. Then do it all the way around the insides of the uppers. Then do the lower teeth. Every few days turn up the pressure a little more until you eventually get u to high pressure. Do these things once a day, after your last meal but before bed, so the food and plaque don't cause damage overnight. In the beginning, it is going to take you a little longer to do this routine, but once you get it down and get good at it, it will go fairly quickly.

Damage to Teeth

A tooth is made of three parts, first is the outer layer of enamel which is inert and is what you see when you look into the mouth.

Secondly the inside of the tooth and most of the root is made of dentine which is a living tissue with its own nerve and blood supply. Dentine is perforated by millions of tiny holes called tubules, there are 3 miles of tubules in a lower front tooth and it is fluid flowing through these tubules which can cause hot and cold sensitivity of teeth and creates a vast market for sensitivity toothpastes.

Thirdly there is the pulp in the middle of a tooth in a space called the root canal. As well as containing nerve endings it contains blood vessels, lymph and connective tissue. There is a constant bathing of the dentine component of the tooth from the pulp with nutrients and fluid flowing out along the tubules into the surrounding periodontal tissues. This is essential to maintain healthy teeth. **When fluid flow reverses, decay starts in teeth.**

Any injury, *chemical, bacterial* or *thermal* can cause these tissues to swell, but as there is little room for swelling in the center of a tooth, **an increase in pressure due to this swelling often cuts off the blood supply to the tooth and all the vital tissue in the tooth dies.** You may often experience a throbbing pain as the body tries to pump blood into the tooth to help this inflammatory process.

The pulp and the tissue in the tubules become necrotic and it is now when problems start. With multi rooted teeth it is possible for the pulp in one root to die but other roots stay vital as they have separate blood supplies. This causes problems for dentists trying to diagnose whether a tooth is alive or dead. Eventually the necrotic tissue in the one root will slowly kill off the vital tissue in the other roots and the tooth is then described as dead or *non-vital*. This may or may not be painful and the degree of pain felt may vary from a slight twinge, to tenderness to bite on, to a full blown toothache which you cannot believe is happening to you.

The pain is dependent on your response to the irritation and whether there is bacterial infection of the pulpal material. Bacteria cause putrefaction of this pulpal material producing gas, which increases the pressure inside a tooth and pain. White blood cells stream into the pulpal area of the tooth attacking the bacteria and producing pus. more swelling and more pain.

The inflammation then spreads out of the tooth via the small foramina through which the blood and lymph pass into the tooth and affects the bone holding the tooth. Swelling here causes pressure in the bone which again is painful, and will continue until it perforates into the surrounding soft tissue or the dentist intervenes.

The dentist then has the choice to take the tooth out or to do a root treatment. Today in this technological age the dentist will offer to treat the abscess, deal with the pain and save the tooth. This is where opinions split as to what is best to do. Do we look to save individual teeth or do we look to treat the whole patient.

The standard way to root-treat a tooth is to drill a small hole into the tooth to gain access to the root canal. If the tooth is not fully dead or there is a great deal of inflammation then this procedure can be uncomfortable though often the tooth and the pulp are dead so no pain is felt. Through varying techniques of instrumenting the root canal and flushing irritant fluids down the canal the dentist hopes to remove as much of the necrotic tissue and bacteria as he can. Then a sterilizing liquid is sealed into the root for a few days in an attempt to further treat the infection and necrotic tissue. Antibiotics are often given to treat the infection outside the tooth.

If the pain goes, a further visit is arranged where the dentist opens up the tooth again to finish the root treatment. They should first take an X-ray with an instrument down the tooth to establish whether they are fully down the canal and have not left any area untreated. If this is satisfactory they fill up the space where the pulp was with and inert material so no future infection can take place.

Millions of this type of treatment are done every year with an apparent success rate of over 90% (i.e. no pain and healing on x-ray so the dentist and the patient are happy). This unfortunately masks a problem which can still be occurring. It is now recognized by more and more dentists that **it is impossible to clean out all of the necrotic tissue or to completely sterilized a tooth.** As mentioned before there are 3 miles of tubules in the smallest tooth of your mouth and no dentist claims to clean or sterilize all of these. **This then leaves areas of dead tissue in the tooth to continue decomposing and being infected.** White blood cells don't travel into tubules nor do antibiotics filter into these areas so the tubules become a safe haven for bacteria and possibly fungi.

They survive and feed off the necrotic tissue and whatever filters into the dentine tubules. The bacteria which colonize these tubules started as normal aerobic bacteria often from the mouth, but when they are sealed into the tooth their environment changes and they pleomorphize to become anaerobic and potentially much more harmful. Their metabolism changes and their waste products become much more toxic.

Until recently there was no scientific way of measuring the toxicity of these teeth but now using photoaffinity labelling, researchers are able to test the toxins from teeth against metabolically important enzymes such as pyruvate kinase, creatinine kinase and the results are disturbing. Of 40 root treated teeth tested 25% showed no toxins. 50% showed toxicity as great as hydrogen sulfide and most worryingly 25% were more toxic than hydrogen sulfide. Research is now looking at what these compounds could be and how we can test for them in the mouth rather than once a tooth has been extracted.

The root canal procedure is a fatally flawed procedure. The very nature of the procedure itself prevents it from achieving its supposed primary goal: a non-infected, sterile tooth. There is a high risk of keeping in the mouth a dead tooth that can harbor anaerobic bacteria, viruses and fungi, where neither the body's immune system nor antibiotics can fight them off. Sooner or later the root canaled tooth's bacteria and their toxins can invade the body, weakening the immune system, the nervous system, the heart, etc. yet often without the medical doctor even thinking to suspect the role that is being played by an infected, toxic tooth.

Of equal interest is the relationship of root filled teeth to traditional Chinese medicine and body energies. All teeth are linked to the body via acupuncture meridians and having a root filled tooth, a large amalgam filling, a crown, or anything that is not compatible with the body, on a meridian may set up an interference field, blocking or altering the energy flow (the chi ') passing through this meridian and cause a disease in an organ or body function remote from the tooth. For example a front upper incisor is on the Kidney/ Bladder meridians and having a root treated tooth here may cause gynecological problems, kidney problems, impotence, and sterility if you follow a Chinese medicine theme. These teeth also relate to spinal segments and joints, the front incisor relates to the coccyx and posterior knee and to L2, 3, S 3, and 6.

If the tooth is removed, the energy does tend to pass through it; however, without the tooth in the bone, it is still altered. Without stimulation from a tooth, blood circulation and lymphatic drainage will be impaired, and the bone and tissue surrounding the extraction site can become diseased (cavitations) and die. Infections in the teeth and toxins have no place to go but down; down into the jawbone and into the rest of the body, creating systemic pathologies. Some dentists are trained to look for these areas on X-rays and Cavitat procedures and when these areas are treated they can also bring considerable improvements in patients health. This energetic relationship between teeth and the rest of the body is opening whole new avenues of dental care and the chance for dentists to work with other complementary health workers.

Kinesiology is one technique where you can localize a problem tooth to see whether it affects overall body strength. If you then hold a remedy for necrotic pulp and the strength returns then there is a good chance that this tooth is affecting health. The use of an Electro-acupuncture or electro dermal screening device can, on an energetic level, determine if individual teeth are stressing that particular person and which tissue or area is being affected.

History

History

The first metal fillings, which had some longevity, were called *fusible metals*. D'Arcet's "mineral cement" was first used in dentistry, composed of 8 parts bismuth, 5 parts lead, 3 parts tin and $^{1}/_{10}{}^{th}$ part of mercury to expedite the fusing process. This was used in France and first appeared in the U.S. around 1820. A problem with this material was that **it had to be melted and then poured into the cavity**. Around 1826, Taveau of Paris introduced the use of a "silver paste" for permanent fillings. The silver paste he proposed was a simple combination of silver and mercury. Silver coins were subsequently used instead of purified silver. The coins were filed down and sufficient mercury added to the filings to make a paste or *plastic mass*. The residual mercury was then pressed out, and the residue was placed in the cavity where it soon hardened.

With the refinement of silver paste, using silver coin filings that contained other metals (like copper) used in the manufacture of the coins, silver amalgam was born and presented to the world. However, this new silver paste exhibited some very undesirable properties when hardening. The mixture would expand after setting, and **it was not unusual for the patient to return with a fractured tooth** or the filling protruding above the cavity, interfering with the closing of the jaw. As a result, most dentists went back to using gold foil or other substances, which, although not having the plastic quality of amalgam, were preferable to coping with the problems presented by silver paste. The maleability of amalgam was its greatest asset and, eventually, scientific experimentation would have produced a formula without the side effects of the original formulations. But, activity in New York prevented this from happening for 60 years and started what is referred to as the *First Amalgam War*.

In 1833, two brothers named Crawcour appeared in New York City and began a dental practice. They were two adventurers, with no training, experience or skill in dentistry. They exploited the use of amalgam by an unprecedented advertising campaign. The advertising promoted a new material that was much more affordable than gold and did not require the same amount of painful preparation as did gold. Although they had no professional credentials, the fierce and ruthless Crawcours soon built a thriving dental practice. They were so successful, their office became filled with the best patients of the area's foremost dentists. As a result, the dental profession started a relentless crusade against them.

Amalgam was denounced not only as a poor filling material but also as the cause of mercurial poisoning, diseases of the gums and numerous other disastrous ills. The campaign was so effective that the Crawcours were finally defeated. The amalgam war continued within the dental profession for another 25 years. **Organized dentistry denounced the use of amalgam.** In the initial period of the war, the American Society of Dental Surgeons was founded by Dr. C. A. Harris in 1840, at the same time he opened the first dental college in the U.S., the Baltimore College of Dental Surgery. One of the first resolutions passed by the American Society of Dental Surgeons was that "the use of *lithodeen* mineral paste, and all other substances of which mercury is an ingredient, were **hurtful both to the teeth and all parts of the mouth** and that **there was no tooth in which caries could be arrested and the organ rendered serviceable by being filled**, in which gold could not be used."

Members signed pledges promising not to use amalgam upon threat of expulsion from the Society. **Some members were actually expelled because they used amalgam.** Regardless, there was a sizeable minority, particularly those dentists working for the poorer people, who ignored the resolution. Their patients could not afford gold foil fillings, and although amalgam was an unsatisfactory filling material, it was better than anything else they could find for the fees they were able to collect. Additionally, there was a basic resentment by many of the prominent dentists that a dental society had the power to make them sign pledges or suspend them for failing to sign.

In 1855, in order to put an end to these internal conflicts, most of the resolutions prohibiting use of amalgam were withdrawn. The controversy over amalgam finally broke up the American Society of Dental Surgeons. Around the same time, Dr. Elisha Townsend of Philadelphia proposed an amalgam consisting of 4 parts silver and 5 parts tin, which were melted together. This was then reduced to filings and mixed with mercury to make a plastic mass for use in filling cavities. Others also experimented and developed new formulas for amalgam that hopefully would overcome the expansion problem.

Under the leadership of Dr. J. Foster Flagg, the first organized movement supporting amalgam was begun in the late 1870s. The movement known for its claims that amalgam was a valuable filling material and reports of it being injurious to the health of the patient were unfounded and untrue.

Most experiments done to prove this were inconclusive, and the profession remained doubtful as to advising the use of amalgam for fillings. This was all changed by the efforts of one Dr. G. V. Black. As a teacher, lecturer and scientific researcher, Black probably contributed more to the progress of dentistry than any other single individual. This notable achievement was the "perfecting" of dental amalgam in the early 1900s.

The 2nd Amalgam War started shortly after and is attributed mostly to the efforts of Professor Alfred Stock of Germany. Dr. Stock taught chemistry at the Kaiser-Wilheim Institute of Chemistry, and in 1926 he published his personal experiences with mercury, which had destroyed a major part of his life. His exposure to mercury was in the laboratory in the course of teaching and experimentation over 25 years. Dr. Stock's 1926 article identified silver amalgam fillings in the mouth as a source of mercury vapor. He outlined the experiments that confirmed his findings.

Dr. Stock concluded his article by saying, **"Dentistry should completely avoid amalgam for fillings or at least not use it whenever this is possible.** There is no doubt that many symptoms–**tiredness, depression, irritability, vertigo, weak memory, mouth inflammations, diarrhea, loss of appetite** and **chronic catarrhs**–often are **caused by mercury,** to which the body is exposed from amalgam fillings, in small amounts, but **continuously**. Doctors should give this fact their serious consideration. It will likely be found that the thoughtless introduction of amalgam as a filling material for teeth was a **severe sin against humanity**."

He identified amalgam as **an unstable alloy** that **continuously gives off mercury in the form of gas ions** (*methylation*) and **abraded particles**. Stock's articles created scandal among the metallurgists, doctors, dentists and chemists and were reported in great detail in the press. Stock's research findings related to amalgam and mercury have been confirmed. **The American Dental Association,** which came into being at about the same time the American Society of Dental Surgeons was being dissolved, **supported the use of silver amalgam then as the filling material of choice and still does today.**

Hal Huggins

Hal A. Huggins DDS, MS, the world's most controversial dentist because of his stand on trying to convince dentistry to stop the use of mercury in fillings, has been in practice 42 years in Colorado Springs.

He is a leading pioneer in identifying toxic dental materials and balancing body chemistry. Over the past four decades, he developed a multidisciplined health care model that has been influential in improving autoimmune diseases such as MS, Lupus, Parkinson's, and Alzheimer's. Other symptoms such as chronic fatigue, depression, and memory and digestive problems have also responded.

Dr. Huggins earned a post-doctoral Master's with emphasis on immunology and toxicology from the University of Colorado. Controversial in his stand against deception in dental regulations and practices, Dr. Huggins has been on the cutting edge of dentistry since the beginning of his practice. Once the darling of the American Dental Association and a speaker at many of the major dental conventions, his vigorous stand against silver (mercury) amalgams finally resulted in his losing his dental license in 1996 for "refusing to place or recommend placing silver amalgams and refusing to recommend or place root canals".

During the past 42 years, Dr. Huggins has lectured over 1400 days in 46 states and 13 foreign countries to professional and lay groups and has given over 1000 radio, TV and print media interviews. He has published over 50 articles concerning nutrition, child growth and development, mercury toxicity, root canals and cavitations, and has authored several books.

In his spare time, Dr. Huggins has discovered astounding research that has rocked the dental profession in the USA and in other countries. His studies led to the breakthrough that many people suffer immune suppression due to the presence of their dental fillings. This challenged the 160 year old assumption that silver-mercury fillings as well as other toxic metals were safe simply because they had been used previously.

Through his research in the toxicity of mercury and other dental materials, he found out that chronic fatigue and a wide array of auto-immune diseases may be linked to these materials. He developed a system that improves the quality of the immune system and allows many of these diseases to disappear, but it requires a series of blood studies and several hours of preparation before fillings are replaced. Dr. Huggins developed a blood test to determine which dental materials are "compatible" with an individual's immune system (different in each person, just like drug reactions) which disclosed that many dental materials cause immune reactivity in over 90% of the people tested.

To accommodate the numerous requests for referral dentists that his office receives daily, Dr. Huggins formed the *Multi-Discipline Alliance* of professionals who are trained to follow the Huggins Protocol. He is also a consultant in three countries at centers practicing the *Huggins Protocol.*

I.A.O.M.T.

In the fall of 1985, thirteen dedicated and concerned dentists met quietly in Banff, Alberta, Canada to assess what might be done to advance the science and clarify the technical issues of toxic substances used in dental materials. One of their primary concerns was in the area of mercury used in the common silver filling. From that quiet beginning has come an international, professional Academy with a mother chapter in North America and several others located throughout the world. The IAOMT (IAOMT.org) is a Canadian non-profit organization dedicated to funding solid peer-reviewed scientific research in the area of toxic substances used in dentistry, as well as providing continuing education and carefully reviewed procedures, protocols and methodologies to reduce risk for patients and professionals.

The fundamental mission of the International Academy of Oral Medicine and Toxicology is to promote the health of the public at large. Essentially, the Academy continually examines and compiles scientific research relating to the biocompatibility of oral/dental materials. Scientific research, published in esteemed medical jounals, has cast serious doubt on the postulated safety of dental mercury amalgam! (The I.A.O.M.T. has significantly financed this research). The I.A.O.M.T. has substantially assisted cataloguing the scientific research on dental mercury amalgam, which contradicts the ANECDOTAL position that 150+ years of use proved its safety!

Germany has now banned the use of conventional amalgam and has advised against the use of mercury amalgam in pregnant women, in children under 6 years of age, in anterior teeth, and in endodontic therapy. Their most recent proposed change (October 1994) will preclude the placement of mercury amalgam in all women of child bearing age! (The I.A.O.M.T. provided the scientific documentation for this proposal). The Swedish government is moving towards a total ban of mercury amalgam, which is in direct opposition to the single-minded effort of established organized detistry! (The I.A.O.M.T., through its membership, has been instrumental in the imitation process of this government's direction).

In May 1992, the I.A.O.M.T. members personally presented scientific information on dental mercury amalgam to the 400 members of the U.S. Congress! (Congress is now investigating the controversy about dental mercury amalgam). The I.A.O.M.T. has presented the documented scientific studies demonstrating adverse effects from dental mercury amalgam to government officials; to state boards of dentistry; to deans of dental schools and to officers of organized dentistry! The I.A.O.M.T members have made scientific presentations on the bio-incompatibility of dental mercury amalgam to government officials and health professionals in numerous countries!

Active I.A.O.M.T. chapters now exist in Canada, the United States, the United Kingdom, Germany, Australia and Brazil! The I.A.O.M.T. provides accurate scientific information to its members through newsletters and two scientific meetings each year! The I.A.O.M.T. has established a "Standards of Care" program for clinical practitioners. Straying afield from the "Standards of Care" program may be a threat to your licensure and personal livelihood! By providing scientific credibility to those questioning the use of dental mercury amalgam in dentistry, the I.A.O.M.T. has contributed significantly towards establishing the individual **right of choice** for both the practitioners and patients!

D.A.M.S.

The acronym DAMS stands for *Dental Amalgam Mercury Syndrome*. Sounding the warning about mercury in dentistry has been a major part of their work. DAMS, Intl. is the main non-profit group that educates the public on the hazards of conventional dental materials and practices. DAMS Intl. also sugggests solutions: how to safely remove the toxic hazards from the mouth and recover one's health.

In addition to their informative information packet, they provide books and videotapes on a variety of dental related topics, as well as a list of progressive dentists and other health care practitioners in your area. It is a difficult task to identify competent dentists and other health care practitioners who can be part of your dental-health care solution. They do the best they can and are always adding, editing and sometimes removing names from their lists. They don't claim that the lists are perfect guides, but they believe they are helpful as a starting point. They acknowledge that there may be other knowledgeable practitioners in your area that they do not yet know about.

DAMS welcomes feedback about the practitioners that others contact, and about knowledgeable practitioners who could be added to their lists.

For more information contact Leo Cashman (president) at:

Dental Amalgam Mercury Syndrome
P.O. Box 7249
Minneapolis, MN 55407-0249

800-311-6265 or
612-721-1144

Price/ Pottenger Nutrition Studies

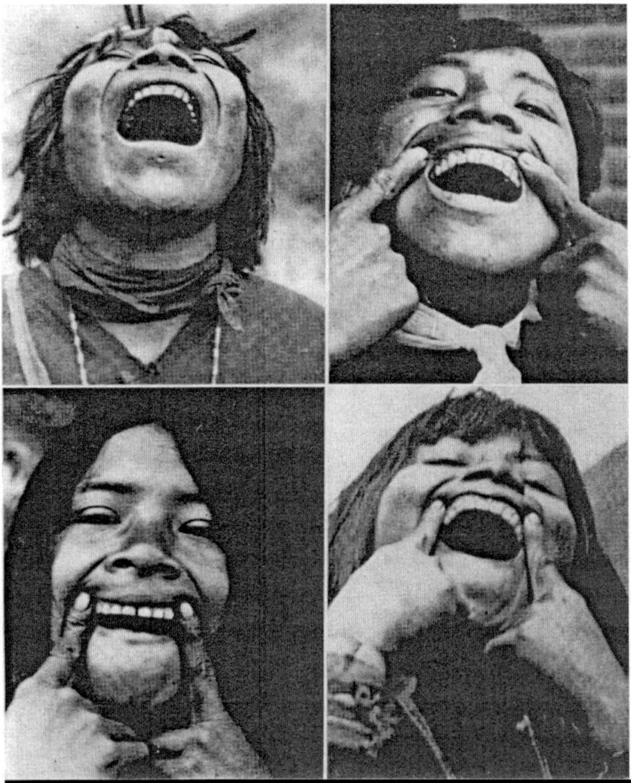

Indian Children on Traditional Diet

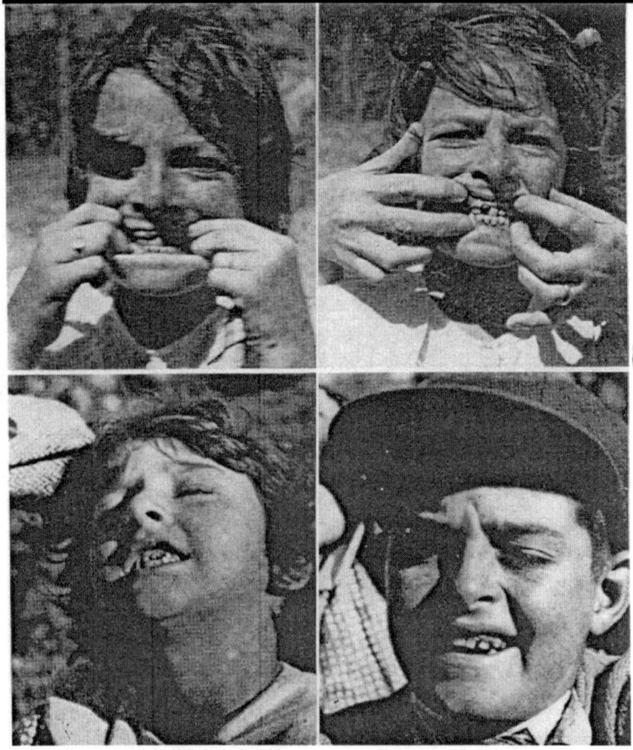

Children on Refined Flour and Sugar Diet

Price/Pottenger Nutrition Studies

Weston Price

Price noticed that his patients were suffering more and more chronic and degenerative diseases. He also noticed that his younger patients had increasingly deformed dental arches, crooked teeth, and cavities. This definitely concerned him: he had not seen such things just ten or fifteen years ago. Why was it happening now? Price also noticed a strong correlation between dental health and physical health: a mouth full of cavities went hand in hand with a body either full of disease or generalized weakness and susceptibility to disease. In Price's time, the *White Scourge,* tuberculosis was the major infectious illness. He noticed that children were increasingly affected, the ones with the **lousy teeth**. Dr. Price had heard rumors of native cultures where so-called primitive people lived happy lives, free of disease. He hit on an idea: why not go find these people and find out (1) if they really are healthy, and (2) if so, find out what they're doing to keep themselves healthy. Being rather well off financially, he and his wife started traveling around the world to remote locations. They were specifically looking for healthy peoples who had not yet been touched by civilization—at that time, such groups were still around.

Price's work is often criticized for being biased. Critics claim that he ignored native peoples that were not healthy; therefore, his data and conclusions about primitive diets are unfounded. These critics are missing the point and motivation for Dr. Price's work. Dr. Price was not interested in examining sick people, as he'd seen enough of them in America. Price was looking for *healthy* people, to find out what made them so, and see if there were any patterns among these people. During his nine years of journeys, Price did, indeed, come across groups of primitives who were having problems for various reasons. He made note of these groups, what appeared to be their difficulty, and then passed them over. Again, he was not interested in sick people. Price often found that the health problems were caused by food shortages (especially a lack of animal products), droughts–things people living off the land must face from time to time. Contact with white European civilization was also a significant factor in their illness.

Dr. Price and his wife went just about everywhere in their journeys. They traveled to isolated villages in the Swiss Alps, to cold and blustery islands off the coast of Scotland, to the Andes mountains in Peru, to several loca tions in Africa, to the Polynesian islands, to Australia and New Zealand, to the forests of northern Canada, and even to the Arctic Circle. In all, Price visited fourteen groups of native peoples. After gaining the trust of the village elders in the various places, Price did what came naturally–he counted cavities and physically examined them. Imagine his surprise to find, on average, less than 1% of tooth decay in all the peoples he visited! He also found that these people's teeth were perfectly straight and white; they had high dental arches and well-formed facial features. And there was something more astonishing: none of the peoples Price examined practiced any sort of dental hygiene; not one of his subjects had ever used a toothbrush! For example, when Price made his first trip to isolated Swiss mountain villagers, he noticed right away that the children's teeth were covered with a thin film of green slime, yet they had no tooth decay. What a difference from the children in his native Ohio!

Dr. Price also noticed that, in addition to their healthy teeth and gums, all the people he visited were hardy and strong, despite the sometimes difficult living conditions they had to endure. Eskimo women, for example, gave birth to one healthy baby after another with little difficulty. Despite the Swiss children going barefoot in frigid streams, there had not been a single case of tuberculosis in any of them, despite exposure to TB. In general, Price found no incidence of the very diseases that plague us *moderns* with our trash compactors and cellular phones: cancer, heart disease, diabetes, hemorrhoids, multiple sclerosis, Parkinson's, Alzheimer's, osteoporosis, chronic fatigue syndrome (it was called neurasthenia in Price's day), etc. Dr. Price also noticed another quality about the healthy primitives he found: they were happy. While depression was not a major problem then, it certainly is today: ask any psychiatrist.

While certain natives sometimes fought with neighboring tribes, within their own groups, they were cheerful and optimistic and bounced back quickly from emotional setbacks. These people had no need for antidepressants. Lest you think Dr. Price made all of this up, he was sure to take along with him one modern invention that would forever chronicle his research and startling conclusions: a camera. Dr. Price and his wife took pictures — 18,000 of them. Many of the pictures are contained in Price's masterpiece *Nutrition and Physical Degeneration* (available from the Price Pottenger Nutrition Foundation). The pictures show native peoples from all over the world smiling as wide as the Mississippi river, their perfect teeth shining bright.

What The People Ate

In addition to examining the natives, Dr. Price also gathered considerable data about their distinctive cultures and customs, and these descriptions fill many of the pages of his book. Price took great care to observe what these people were eating, for he suspected the key to good health and good teeth was in good food. He was surprised to find that, depending on the people in question and where they lived, each group ate very differently from the other. For example, the Swiss mountain villagers subsisted primarily on unpasteurized and cultured dairy products, especially butter and cheese. Rye also formed an integral part of their diet. Occasionally, they ate meat (beef) as cows in their herds got older. Small amounts of bone broths, vegetables and berries rounded out the diet. Due to the high altitude, not much vegetation grew. The villagers would eat what they could in the short summer months, and pickle what was left over for the winter. The main foods, however, were full fat cheese, butter, and rye bread.

Gaelic fisher people of the Outer Hebrides ate no dairy products, but instead had their fill of cod and other sea foods, especially shellfish (when in season). Due to the poor soil, the only grain that could grow was oat, and it formed a major part of the diet. A traditional dish, one considered very important for growing children and expectant mothers, was cod's head stuffed with oats and mashed fish liver. Again, due to the extremely inhospitable climate, fruits and vegetables grew sparsely. Price noted that a young Gaelic girl reeled in puzzlement when offered an apple: she had never seen one! Eskimo, or Innu, ate a diet of almost 100% animal products with hefty amounts of fish. Walrus and seal, and other marine mammals also formed an integral part of the diet. Blubber (fat) was consumed with relish.

Innu would gather nuts, berries, and some grasses during the short summer months, but their diet was basically all meat and fat. Price noted that the Innu would usually ferment their meat before eating it. That is, they would bury it and allow it to slightly putrefy before consuming it. Innu would also eat the partially digested grasses of caribou by cutting open their stomachs and intestines. The Maori of New Zealand, along with other South sea islanders, consumed seafood of every sort — fish, shark, octopus, sea worms, shellfish — along with fatty pork and a wide variety of plant foods including coconut and fruit.

African cattle-keeping tribes like the Masai consumed virtually no plant foods at all, just beef, raw milk, organ meats, and blood (in times of drought). The Dinkas of the Sudan, whom Price claimed were the healthiest of all the African tribes he studied, ate a combination of fermented whole grains with fish, along with smaller amounts of red meat, vegetables, and fruit. The Bantu, on the other hand, the least hardy of the African tribes studied, were primarily agriculturists. Their diet consisted mostly of beans, squash, corn, millet, vegetables, and fruits, with small amounts of milk and meat. Price never found a totally vegetarian culture. Modern anthropological data support this: all cultures and peoples show a preference for animal foods and animal fat.

Hunter-gatherer peoples in Northern Canada, the Florida Everglades, the Amazon, and Australia consumed game animals of all types, especially the organ meats, and a variety of grains, legumes, tubers, vegetables, and fruits when available. Price noted that all peoples, except the Innu, consumed insects and their larvae. Obviously in more tropical areas, insects formed a more integral part of the diet. Price noted that *the natives of Africa know that certain insects are very rich in special food elements at certain seasons, also that their eggs are valuable foods. A fly that hatches in enormous quantities in Lake Victoria is gathered and used fresh and dried for storage. They also use ant eggs and ants.* Bees, wasps, dragonflies, beetles, crickets, cicadas, moths, and termites were consumed with zest also, particularly in Africa.

Price also noted that all cultures consumed fermented foods each day. Foods such as cheese, cultured butter, yogurt, or fermented grain drinks like kaffir beer (made from millet) in Africa, or fermented fish, as with the Innu, were an important part of native diets. Curiously, all native peoples studied made great efforts to obtain seafood, especially fish roe, which was consumed *"so that we will have healthy children."* Even mountain dwelling peoples would make semi-annual trips to the sea to bring back seaweeds, fish eggs, and dried fish. Shrimp, rich in both cholesterol and vitamin D, was a standard food in many places, from Africa to the Orient. The last major feature of native diets that Price found was that they were rich in fat, especially animal fat. Whether from insects, eggs, fish, game animals, or domesticated herds, primitive peoples knew that they would get sick if they did not consume enough fat. Explorers besides Dr. Price have also found this to be true.

For example, anthropologist Vilhjalmur Stefansson, who lived for years among the Innu and Northern Canadian Indians, specifically noted how the Indians would go out of their way to hunt down older male caribou, for they carried a 50 pound slab of back fat. When such animals were unavailable and Indians were forced to subsist on rabbits, a very lean animal, diarrhea and hunger would set in after about a week. **The human body needs saturated fat to assimilate and utilize proteins, and saturated animal fats contain high amounts of the fat-soluble vitamins, as well as beneficial fatty acids with antimicrobial properties.** Of course, the foods that Price's subjects ate were natural and unprocessed. Their foods did not contain preservatives, additives, or colorings. They did not contain added sugar (though, when available, natural sweets like honey and maple syrup were eaten in moderation). Their diets did not include white flour or canned foods. Their milk products were not pasteurized, homogenized, or low-fat. The animal and plant foods consumed were raised and grown on pesticide-free soil. Their animals were not given growth hormones or antibiotics. These people always ate organic.

What The Samples Showed

Dr. Price was eager to chemically analyze the various foods these primitives ate. He was careful to obtain preserved samples of all types for analysis. Basically, the diets of these healthy peoples contained ten times the amount of fat-soluble vitamins, and at least four times the amount of calcium, other minerals, and water soluble vitamins than Western diets at that time. No wonder these people were so healthy! Because of the consumption of fermented and raw foods (including raw animal products), Price noted that native diets were rich in enzymes. Enzymes assist in the digestion of cooked foods.

Price noted that all peoples had a predilection and dietary pull towards foods rich in the fat-soluble vitamins. He considered butter from pasture-fed cows, rich in these vitamins as well as minerals, to be the premiere health food. Fat-soluble vitamins (A, D, E, K) are found in fats of animal origin, like butter, cream, lard, and tallow, as well as in organ meats. And to dispel a common myth about native peoples, they did live long lives. Price took numerous photos of healthy primitives with heads full of gray hair. While we don't know how old they were since they didn't have calendars, they were, by appearances, well past 60. The Australian Aborigines had a special society of the elderly. If there were no old people among them, they would have had no need for such a group.

Stefansson also reported great longevity among the Innu. It is true that death rates at younger ages were higher among some groups, but these mortalities were from the dangerous lifestyle these people lived, not from their diet. When you live in the Arctic Circle, for example, constantly fighting the elements, polar bears, ice flows, and leopard seals, you run the risk of an early death.

Another common misconception that modern nutrition holds about native peoples and their high meat and fat diets is that they suffered from all sorts of degenerative diseases, especially osteoporosis and heart disease. The facts, however, do not support these contentions. Although some studies done in the past few decades have tried to show the high rates of osteoporosis among the Innu as due to their high protein diet, other studies have shown no such thing. The work of Drs. Herta Spencer and Lois Kramer conclusively proved the protein/calcium loss theory to be nonsense. As it turns out, the negative studies on the Eskimo were done, not on Innu following their traditional diet, but among modernized Innu who had adopted modern eating habits and alcohol. Alcoholism is a major factor in bone loss. Certainly, Dr. Price would have noted that bone loss was a problem if it had been, especially since he was examining teeth, which are made of calcium, but he did not. While in Switzerland, Price got permission to dig up skeletal remains of some villagers: The bones were sturdy and strong. There are pictures in Price's book of these bones (and skulls showing mouths of perfect teeth free of decay). Price found no incidence of any major diseases, including heart disease.

This is not to say that native peoples did not have any problems, for such is certainly not the case. Price learned of native remedies for a host of minor ills such as headaches, colds, wounds, and burns. But as far as degenerative diseases go, he found nothing, as these diseases were unknown. This brings up the other major finding of Dr. Price's research: the effects of a modern diet on native peoples. Let us now turn to this.

The Roots Of Disease

When Dr. Price visited the various primitive groups, he noted that white European civilization had begun making inroads into the areas where they lived. Some of the native peoples opted to leave and move into areas where it was more *modern.* Dr. Price also had the opportunity to compare white colonialists who were living alongside, or close to, the native peoples he was studying.

What he found with his study was what he thought he would find: disease and dental decay. When people read *Nutrition and Physical Degeneration*, it often changes their lives because, not only does it describe how healthy people look, feel, and eat, it also shows in painful detail what happens to those people when they abandon their native eating patterns and adopt modern foodstuffs. The pictures Price took of natives and moderns on what Price disdainfully called *the displacing foods of modern commerce* are horrifying and stand in stark contrast to the pictures next to them of healthy, smiling natives. Nutrition writer and Price enthusiast Sally Fallon explains:

> "His photographs capture the suffering caused by these foodstuffs—chiefly rampant tooth decay. Even more startling, they show the change in facial development that occurred with modernization. Parents who had changed their diets gave birth to children who no longer exhibited the tribal patterns. Their faces were more narrow, their teeth crowded, their nostrils pinched. These faces do not beam with optimism, like those of their healthy ancestors. The photographs of Dr. Weston Price demonstrate with great clarity that the 'displacing foods of modern commerce' do not provide sufficient nutrients to allow the body to reach its full genetic potential—neither the complete development of the bones in the body and the head, nor the fullest expressions of the various systems that allow humankind to function at optimal levels—immune system, nervous system, digestion, and reproduction."

And what were the offending foods that these unfortunate people consumed? Why everything we find on our grocer's shelves: sugar, white flour, jams, jellies, cookies, condensed milk, canned vegetables, pastries, refined grain products, margarine, and vegetable oils. Price noted in several places that where modern foods had displaced traditional ones, suicide rates from dental caries were high. As most of us know, dental pain can be excruciating. With no drugs to ease their pain, and no dentist around to pull the dying tooth, people took their own lives to escape the torture. White Europeans who lived in Africa and ate these same foods had to leave periodically for health reasons. Children born there had to be sent away several times during their youth in order to survive. Such was the effect of modern foods on these people. Native Africans, of course, had no such problems as long as they stayed on their native diets.

As noted earlier, the major infectious disease at Price's time was tuberculosis, the White Scourge. Price took several photographs of children, usually the children of either Europeans or natives who had adopted the modern foods before their children were born. These pictures are disturbing in their depictions of suffering. Some of the children were too sick to be moved to better lighting for photographing. Others had pus visibly draining from their lymph glands and abscessed teeth. Invariably, parents and children who had adopted modern foods were highly susceptible to tuberculosis and other degenerative diseases.

The native Hawaiians are a tragic example of this shift. Price did visit the Hawaiian islands on his journeys. He noted that Hawaiians who ate their traditional diet of coconut, fish, shellfish, taro, sweet potatoes, and fresh fruits were healthy and strong. Today, however, the health of native Hawaiians is frightening. Obesity and diabetes are rampant. Because canned meats with nitrates in them are popular there, rates of stomach cancer are high (nitrates convert into carcinogens in the stomach—vitamin C halts the conversion). Hawaiians today eat their fair share of sugar, soft drinks, vegetable oils, macaroni salad, white flour, and white rice. Coconut is sometimes eaten, but usually as part of a sugary snack. High blood pressure and heart attacks are common. Rates of Alzheimer's are elevated as well. Such is the effect of processed foods on a beautiful race of people.

In the last decade or so, however, a diet was proposed called the Hawaii Diet. Though it is a little low in fat for my tastes, it advocates a full return to traditional eating patterns: fish, taro, sweet potatoes, fresh fruit and vegetables, and, occasionally, pork (wild boar and feral pig, are native to the islands). Specifically avoided are white rice, sugar, *Spam*, and processed foods in general. The change is dramatic: people lose weight, they have more energy, and their health problems dissipate or become more manageable. Their teeth invariably improve as well. Price noticed this pattern also. If a native abandoned his ancestral eating habits in favor of modern foods, ill health and dental caries followed. If that same person switched back to the original eating pattern, however, health returned, and the progression of dental decay stopped and reversed itself. This is perhaps the most uplifting aspect of Price's work: one can always reverse the trend; there is always hope.

Price accurately and ominously predicted that, as Western man consumed more refined sugar and substituted vegetable oils for animal fats, disease would increase, and reproduction would be more difficult. Today, some 25% of Western couples are infertile, and rates of cancer, diabetes, and heart disease have skyrocketed. Price was truly a modern Cassandra of Troy—prophesying the truth, but with no one listening.

A Return To Sanity

For many decades, Price's work has been buried and forgotten. Due to the efforts of the Price-Pottenger Nutrition Foundation, however, and the re-publication of Price's book for the public, that is fortunately starting to change. Several prominent nutritional doctors have traced their philosophical heritages back to Weston Price and his work. Abram Hoffer, founder and developer of orthomolecular psychiatry, Jonathan Wright, noted author, Alan Gaby, medical columnist, Melvyn Werbach, nutritional author, and other medical doctors all sing the praises of this ingenious dentist. Nutritional anthropologist H. Leon Abrams, associate professor emeritus at the University System of Georgia and author of over 200 papers and 8 books, points to Price as *"a giant, ahead of his time with a message relevant to us all."*

Price's conclusions and recommendations were shocking for his time. He advocated a return to breast feeding when such a practice was discouraged by Western medicine. He urged parents to give their children cod liver oil every day. He considered fresh butter to be the supreme health food. He warned against pesticides, herbicides, preservatives, colorings, refined sugars, vegetable oils–in short, all the things that modern nutrition and agriculture have embraced and promoted the last few decades. Price believed that margarine was a demonic creation. Let me tell you, with recommendations like these, he was really unpopular! But the result of his research speaks for itself.

Knowing that his data flatly contradict virtually everything that *politically correct* nutrition holds, it is common to find his work belittled. If Price's studies are accurate, then the low-fat school must go the way of all flesh: into the graveyard. It is typical, therefore, for critics to say things like Price only superficially examined the peoples he encountered and made simplistic conclusions about their health. Price is also accused of ignoring the nutritional deficiencies of the peoples he studied, as well as their high rates of infant mortality.

Its asserted as well that the modern foods that Price argued were these people's downfall were actually *wholesome,* but the primitive peoples overconsumed too much of them and didn't *balance* their diets correctly, hence their high rates of disease after adopting modern food stuffs. Critics also claim that malnourished people usually don't have dental problems, so it is immaterial that the natives Price photographed had perfect teeth, or that the modernized ones had poor ones. It is truly amazing how far some *experts* will go to defend the processed food industry and shaky nutritional hypotheses! Even a cursory look at Price's book will tell any rational person that Price did not *superficially examine* the people he studied. The detail about native customs, eating habits, and history of the various areas argues against any accusations of superficiality.

Additionally, Price was a physician with many years of experience; it is ludicrous to claim that he would make a *superficial examination* and reach *simplistic conclusions* about people's health. If there were nutritional deficiencies, he would have noted them, but no such descriptions exist for the simple reason that no such deficiencies existed. We know this to be true for, if we examine the modern descendants of Price's subjects, we find that they enjoy robust health and freedom from both dental caries and more chronic diseases, if they have not abandoned their native diets.

It is true that high infant mortality rates existed, but only *after* exposure to and adoption of the white European way of life. Further, if the foods of modern commerce were so wholesome, then they would have provided the nutrients to avert death, dental decay, and disease, regardless of how they were ingested. Claims of *unbalanced diets* of native foods is plain old doubletalk that does not stand the test of logic. The last claim about the dental condition not being related to the body's nutritional state is simply false. Numerous researchers have noted the clear and obvious connection between dental and bodily health. They all assert without hesitation that the health of the body is reflected quite accurately in the health of the teeth.

Dr. Price's Message

The obvious conclusion of Price's research is that for humanity to survive, it must eat better. And the foods it must eat must are whole, fresh, and unprocessed. More and more, people are beginning to see this and have been changing their eating patterns.

But for the majority, the continuation of negative dietary habits will inevitably lead to decreased vitality and unhealthy children; in short, the degeneration of the human race. In this world of survival of the fittest, we need to take every opportunity to bolster our position or we risk going the way of the dodo bird: into extinction. Besides, eating whole foods tastes good! The first happy lesson to be gleaned from traditional diets and Price's work is that good food can and should taste good. Its OK to saute' vegetables and meats with butter. Its OK to consume whole milk, meat with its fat, eggs, shrimp and lobster, and liver with onions and bacon. Its OK and healthy to eat home-made soups prepared from gelatin-rich bone broths and sauces made from drippings and cream.

Eating whole foods is good for the environment as well. The building blocks of a whole foods diet are pesticide-free plant foods raised on naturally enriched soils, and healthy animals that live free to graze and manure the paddocks of their farms, as opposed to standing in a cramped stall, never seeing sunlight, being fed soybeans and corn meal, and being shot up with steroids and antibiotics. Eating whole foods is better for the economy as well. Organic foods are usually raised by small farms. Each time you buy an organically raised plant or animal product, you are helping someone to earn a living. Isn't that preferable to giving your money to a multinational food company that mass produces its product, not caring about the health of the soil, the planet, the animals, or humans?

Finally, eating whole foods is healthier. We humans evolved eating certain food stuffs in certain ways. You did not see a caveman trimming the fat off of his meat—he ate the whole thing. You did not see a Swiss Alps villager eating low fat cheese — she ate the whole thing. You did not see Maori fishermen avoiding shellfish for fear of cholesterol—they ate the whole thing. Foods are packaged in ways that Nature intended: they contain all the nutrients within themselves for optimal assimilation by our bodies. Eating whole foods insures us the highest amount of nutrients food has to offer. Tampering with them is ill advised.

Francis Pottenger

Between the years 1932 and 1942, Francis Marion Pottenger, Jr. M.D., conducted a feeding experiment to determine the effects of heat-processed food on cats. His ten-year cat study was prompted by the high rate of mortality he was experiencing among his laboratory cats undergoing *adrenalectomies* for use in standardizing the hormone content of the ad renal extract he was making. Because there were no existent chemical procedures for standardizing biological extracts, manufacturers of such extracts necessarily had to use animals to determine their potency. As cats die without their adrenal glands, the dose of extract required to support their lives calibrated the level of the extract's potency. In his effort to maximize the preoperative health of his laboratory animals, Francis fed them a diet of market grade raw milk, cod liver oil and cooked meat scraps from the sanitarium. These scraps included the liver, tripe, sweetbreads, brains, heart and muscle. This diet was considered to be rich in all the important nutritive substances by the experts of the day, and the surgical technique used for the adrenalectomies was the most exacting known. Therefore, Francis was perplexed as to why his cats were poor operative risks. In seeking an explanation, he began noticing that the cats showed signs of deficiency. All showed a decrease in their reproductive capacity, and many of the kittens born in the laboratory had skeletal deformities and organ malfunctions.

As his neighbors in Monrovia kept donating an increasing number of cats to his laboratory, the demand for cooked meat scraps exceeded supply, and he placed an order at the local meat packing plant for raw meat scraps, again including the viscera, muscle and bone. These raw meat scraps were fed to a segregated group of cats each day and within a few months this group appeared in better health than the animals being fed cooked meat scraps. Their kittens appeared more vigorous, and most interestingly, their operative mortality decreased markedly. The contrast in the health of the cats fed raw meat and those fed cooked meat was so startling, it prompted Pottenger to undertake a controlled experiment.

What he had observed by chance, he wanted to repeat by design. He wanted to find answers to such questions as, "Why did the cats eating raw meat survive their operations more readily than those eating cooked meat? Why did the kittens of the raw meat fed cats appear more vigorous? Why did a diet based on cooked meat scraps apparently fail to provide the necessary nutritional elements for good health?" He felt the findings of a controlled feeding experiment might illumine new facts about optimal human nutrition. The cat study of Francis M. Pottenger, Jr., MD is unique. There is no similar experiment in the medical literature. The pathological and chemical findings were supervised by Francis in consultation with Alvin G. Foord, M.D., professor of pathology at the University of Southern California and pathologist at the Huntington Me morial Hospital in Pasadena. Accordingly, the studies met the most rigorous scientific standards of the day, and their protocol was observed consistently. Since the cat study is unique, its findings are frequently quoted–and misquoted–in order to justify the ideas of others. For example, one author of a popular selling book states that 200 cats died of arthritis; this, indeed, did not happen. Another author states that the cats were fed sprouts and survived in full health for four continuous generations. Again, no such experiment took place, and yet such misinformation has been traced over a dozen or more different articles and books.

A frequent criticism of The Pottenger cat study is that it was not properly controlled. Here it is necessary to ask, "By what standards?" Every one of the studies followed strictly defined protocol. All variables in the stock of the animals were reported and explained. Because some of the test procedures may seem crude forty years later, this in no way invalidates the fact that the procedures were meticulously controlled and that the results of the experiments were reported as observed.

Another criticism is that the cats were kept in an artificial environment unrelated to real living conditions. Such a criticism overlooks the experimental necessity of maintaining a controlled environment to provide valid findings. It also overlooks the evidence that, given specific living conditions, specific changes repeatedly occurred in the health of the cats under observation. Another frequent criticism is that the experimental work done on *cat nutrition* has no appropriate application to *human nutrition*. Francis M. Pottenger, Jr., never stated that a one-to-one comparison could be made between his findings in cat nutrition and human nutrition. He did say, "While no attempt will be made to correlate the changes in the animals studied with malformations found in humans, the similarity is so obvious that parallel pictures suggest themselves."

All too often, self-appointed authorities will state categorically that they do not believe other's observations and so seek to close the door on any further inquiry into these observations. They declare, "Because I do not believe the facts as presented, they are not so." It is far better for science if responsible individuals maintain an attitude of open inquiry and test the observations of others before forming rigid opinions. In the case of the cat study, human welfare might well be served if concerned researchers made every effort to discover whether valid correlation's can be made between cat nutrition and human nutrition.

It must be remembered that cats and humans both are mammals. It would be of great value to the field of nutrition to repeat the cat study within the parameters of present day technology and with the use of present day antibiotics. Most of the cats on deficient diets died from infections of the kidneys, lungs and bones. If these infections were eliminated as a cause of death by antibiotics, it would allow the cats to reveal their ultimate degenerative fates. As an extension to this experiment, it would be of interest to study the effects of vitamin and mineral supplementation in the diet of cooked-food-fed animals.

This section presents the observations made by Francis M. Pottenger, Jr., M.D., on the effects of deficient and optimum nutrition in cats and human beings as recorded in his articles and clinical records written between the years of 1932 and 1956. Nothing has been added or subtracted from his findings, and for the most part, the words describing his work are his own. Though some of the scientific interpretations have not withstood the test of time, the observations are valid. A careful and selective interpretation by an inquiring mind will readily differentiate this.

Important advances in medicine and dentistry have always sprung from the minds of independent and original thinkers–keen observers whose imagination, integrity and common sense give them the courage to question official dogma. Such a man was Dr. Francis M. Pottenger, Jr., MD. He was dedicated to the cause of preventing chronic illness and made significant contributions to the understanding of the role of nutrition in maintaining good health. His chance observation regarding the effect of foods on the mortality rate of cats led to his classical experiments in cat feeding. More than 900 cats were studied over ten years.

Dr. Pottenger found that only diets containing raw milk and raw meat produced optimal health. Cats on the all-raw diet had good bone structure and density, **wide palates with plenty of space for the teeth**, shiny fur, and freedom from parasites and disease. They reproduced with ease and were gentle and easy to handle. Cooking the meat or substituting *heat processed* milk for *raw* resulted in *heterogeneous reproduction* and *physical degeneration*, **increasing with each generation**. Kittens of third generation cats failed to survive six months. Vermin and parasites abounded. Skin diseases and allergies increased from an incidence of five percent in normal cats to over ninety percent in the third generation.

Bones became soft and pliable; calcium and phosphorus content diminished. The cats suffered from adverse personality changes. Females became more aggressive, while males became docile. The cats suffered from hypothyroidism and most of the degenerative diseases encountered in human medicine. **They died out completely by the fourth generation.**

The following diets were the basis of the study:

The Meat Study

Diet A (Adequate)
1/3 raw milk, cod liver oil
2/3 RAW meat
Diet B (Deficient)
2/3 COOKED meat
1/3 raw milk, cod liver oil

The Milk Study

Diet A (Adequate)
1/3 raw meat, cod liver oil
2/3 RAW milk
Diet B (Deficient)
1/3 raw meat, cod liver oil
2/3 PASTEURIZED milk
Diet C (Deficient)
1/3 raw meat, cod liver oil
2/3 EVAPORATED milk
Diet D (Deficient)
1/3 raw meat, cod liver oil
2/3 SWEETENED CONDENSED milk
Diet E (Deficient)
RAW METABOLIZED VITAMIN D milk only
E1: From cows on dry feed
E2: From cows on green feed

Degeneration proceeded more quickly on Diets C and D. Diet E1 produced unexpected results–rickets and early death of male kittens. The **changes in facial structure** and onset of degenerative disease that Pottenger observed in cats on deficient diets **paralleled the human degeneration** that Dr. Price found in tribes and villages that had abandoned traditional foods. Dr. Pottenger tried to return degenerating cats to health. He found that **it took four generations on raw meat and raw milk to bring the kittens of second-generation degenerating cats back to normal**. This experiment could not occur with third-generation degenerating cats because they could not give birth to viable offspring.

For further information Sally Fallon's organization: The Weston A. Price Foundation is an invaluable source of nutritional information and details on Dr. Price's work. It is located at:

The Weston A. Price Foundation
4200 Wisconsin Ave, N.W.
Washington, D.C. 20016.
(202) 333-HEAL
www.westonaprice.org

Biological Dentistry

Biological Dentistry

Biological dentistry is a multi-faceted integrative treatment approach focused on the oral cavity, and on the resultant effects of oral-disease and general dentistry on the overall health of the body. Biological dentistry's goal is to neutralize the harmful effects that dentistry and oral dysfunction has on the whole body. Not only are toxic materials and conditions removed from the mouth, the functional and structural components of the mouth that are both dependent and independent units of the body, are also restored, returning the oral cavity to its proper biomechanical role. The mouth is addressed in its entirety.

Teeth are individual units of bone-like material supported by surrounding structures, such as ligaments, gingival tissue, muscle and bone. All of these must be considered in the dental assessment. The removal of a toxic material is only one step in the process of restoring dental and physical health. A replacement material may be *biocompatible* at a certain level of health and *incompatible* at another. Health cannot be measured by approximations; a temporary solution to a dental problem may create further problems for the patient later on.

The oral cavity is a unique functional, structural and esthetic organization of several different kinds of tissue that are bordering and meticulously support the instrumentation of the dental orifice. The oral cavity includes the mandible and maxillary jawbones, which are parts of the cranium. The cervical and thoracic portions of the spinal column support the cranium, housing the brain which is comprised of 80 percent of the nervous system. The spine innervates the entire body with nerves that provide information processing. Throughout this complex system are muscles and fascia that support and provide further biochemical feedback, essential for the functioning of the body. Dentistry, therefore, has the capacity to influence, especially when energetic acupuncture meridian connections are considered. Each tooth, and its supporting structures, have *physical* as well as *energetic* connections to the whole body.

For instance, *mal-occlusion* (improper bite) can result in a physical malalignment of the spine, as well as a blockage of energetic pathways that can affect associated organs and glands. Therefore, careful regard must be taken when appraising and treating the teeth and any apparatus of the oral cavity.

There are several kinds of dentistry; the superior one addresses as many factors as possible at once and attempts to convey the least undesirable impact to the body on all levels. Ultimately, the superior dentistry is no dentistry, as this is an invasive advancement against health; however, once pathology has commenced, intercession is necessary. If ignored, the disease process will likely progress to severe and painful results. Dentistry is like building a house, the structure upon which the house is built needs to be solid, not damp and moldy, and must have good drainage.

Bone, which is the supporting base in the oral cavity, needs to be solid and free of voids and inflammation. Upon this is the *periodontium*, which must be flexible, have a good blood supply and be free of microorganisms. Attached within the periodontium are ligaments, performing as shock absorbers and providing foundational support for the teeth. Finally, the teeth are to be free of infection, toxic materials and trauma of any kind. A healthy lymphatic, blood and nerve supply sustains this entire functional structure.

If the bite is left too *high* or too *low* after tooth restoration, biomechanical stress will preclude the body's ability to adapt to the stress, causing adaptation mechanisms to progress into a disease process. Holistic dentistry must appreciate and embrace toxicology, pathology, biochemical and biomechanical mechanisms, hormonal balance, biocompatibility, meridians, proprioceptive integrity, proper occlusion, functional integrity, structural soundness and esthetics. Dentistry is multi-faceted, which has the potential to enhance, hinder or dismantle health, depending on the practitioner's and the patient's approach to health.

The patient should first accept that they are ultimately responsible and the practitioner is only there to expedite a return to health. If a patient presents with many signs and symptoms of disease and expects to be cured by the removal of a single offensive material, then let the practitioner beware. It is a rare occurrence when a single material is responsible for the ill health of an individual; it is usually a combination of many different factors including lifestyle choices, nutrition, environment, dentistry and medicine.

The disease process is a gradual one; to restore health one must often *ascend* the same pathway originally *descended* into ill health. This requires continuous auditing in order to find the cause of ill health.
The biological dentist, part *detective*, part *technician* and part *artisan*, necessitates an intuitive commencement into multiple levels of practice. Dentistry is partly interpretive; the practitioner assesses the patient's present state of health based on what is presented. However, there are no diagnostic absolutes, even with lab tests, electro-dermal screening tests and muscle testing, etc. These are only approximately safe parameters for the dentist to choose from. If there is a misinterpretation of materials, it is the patient who suffers. The same goes for an improper occlusion, extraction of too many teeth, and functional but structurally improper dentistry. Holistic treatment requires seeing the patient's *whole* picture, as the overall health of the individual is at stake.

Is the removal of an infected root canal-filled tooth more of a priority than the removal of mercury fillings? This can be a hard decision to make, as each individual responds uniquely to the insult of infection or mercury. Westernized allopathic medicine and dentistry have attempted standardization. However, since each individual is bio-chemically unique, there cannot be a "one-size-fits-all" application of the health care process.

Some individuals will respond more strongly, in a negative way, to the mercury than to the infection, and vice versa. Ideally, none of these should be present, but when they are, there must be prioritization when it comes to biological dentistry. If there is deep, infectious necrosis in the bone, then this must have priority in what dentistry shall be applied. To proceed otherwise, is to build upon a shaky foundation.

Furthermore, no foreign material is completely biocompatible. Only an intact, natural tooth is decidedly compatible with the patient's system. As alternative dentists, physicians and practitioners of varying fields, our ultimate goal is not to add to the toxic load of the body. But it is difficult because there are materials that are bio-hazardous to the body, that create chaotic energy vortices, that block energetic pathways and that mimic hormones. Some materials are too abrasive to opposing teeth and others do not last long enough to be worthy of placement.

Many alternative practitioners believe only in composites, some in porcelains, and some in high noble gold. When given the choice, even after the patient takes a serum compatibility blood test, the dentist will often choose the non-reactive materials they like and are accustomed to from the list provided.
Long-term health should be the highest priority. Is it of any benefit to refill a deep amalgam filling with biocompatible filling material when it might create more trauma, leading to more intervention, which might result in extraction, and which in turn lead to the possible danger of it becoming an infected necrotic cavitation? This all must be assessed. The more teeth that are removed, the more difficult it becomes to balance the mandible and maxillary as a well functioning structural whole.

An imbalance has the potential to throw off the cranio-cervical relationships, possibly leading to TMJ problems, migraines, muscle spasms, fatigue, postural problems, depression, etc. If more than ten teeth are extracted, the proprioceptive biofeedback mechanism of the entire body can be disrupted, causing systemic calamity as the body is then no longer in a state of homeostatic equilibrium.

Teeth are small pearl-like objects, requiring exacting care and respect. A multi-dimensional, multi-faceted approach in caring for the teeth needs to be taken. Simply substituting one material for another, although a good starting point, is not comprehensive enough for optimal health. A very important component to remember is that *xenoestrogens* from environmental pollution are exceedingly stressful to the body. A patient should ideally work with a reputable alternative practitioner in conjunction with the biological/holistic dentist. This will facilitate both the dental work and any medical treatment. Backtracking is sometimes necessary, as the return to health, although not exactly sequential, is progressive.

There are cases of individuals responding remarkably well to the removal of toxic dental materials; but there is the rare individual who is outright allergic to a material. The majority of patients become immunologically sensitive to a dental material with the passage of time. This, in combination with environmental and nutritional toxins, weakens the immunity. A weakened immune system will not be able to tolerate many dental materials. However, as the body is purged of both dental and environmental toxic materials and as infections are removed, occlusions are corrected, the vertical dimension restored, cavitations removed and gum disease

treated, a stabilizing effect will occur in the patient. Then *homeopathic* and *isopathic* treatments can be effective, chiropractic adjustments can hold and orthomolecular, quantum and whole food therapy can hit the targeted areas.
The patient is then primed to return to full health, as the body is again responsive and receptive to further treatment with whole body modalities that enhance endocrine and organ function.

Biological dentistry is a delicate art with major health ramifications at issue. The implication that there is only one thing causing ill health—lacks ultimate humility on the part of the dentist and the patient. As can be seen, dentistry is health care of the entire body; the impact of treatment extends far beyond the teeth.

High-Speed Drilling

High-Speed Drilling

Every medical discipline has its inherent capacity to cause iatrogenic damage, but the dental turbine or rotor, should be considered as a sort of time bomb. Its devastating effects have been completely underestimated by most dentists. The industry has propagated the ergonomic benefits of these high-speed drills, constantly developing more function; and without long-term clinical, histological or pathological monitoring of the effects of turbines in general, the entire dental profession, including universities, has adopted these diabolical machines.

The turbine does not grind down in the manner of slower machines, but rather breaks up the enamel prisms by impact, not only on the edges of cavities and preparations, but also far down into the enamel supposed to remain intact. This has been proven by samples recorded through electron microscope. The cracks thus caused not only allow bacterial toxins, but also the bacteria themselves and macromolecules to pass and penetrate into the dentine, encouraging caries. But the major change is caused in and on the dentine itself.

Many dental practitioners are of the opinion that **the pulp receives too much heat** due to friction when turbines are used in treatment. Additional abundant cooling would avoid such a burden. Due to the high rotation speed, both a *congestion* and *negative pressure* occur on the dentine, and a dry (water-less) zone is formed at the very point of drilling or grinding/milling. After 5-20 seconds of milling or grinding with turbines, there is an increase in pulp temperature by 12 degrees C. or about 22 degrees F., **causing irreversible damage** in 60% of the pulps examined for this effect. One kind of damage which is not produced thermally, but which equally spells doom to the pulp is damage from negative pressure.

As a result of the high rotation speed, turbulence is produced around the burs, which produces a very high negative pressure over the dentinal tubules. This amounts to as much as a 10 mm water column per 100,000 revolutions. This negative pressure does not increase in linear, but in exponential fashion. As a result of this state, the *peritubular dentine linings*, the cylindrical ***odontoblastic processes*****, are damaged** or sometimes torn out. Even **odontoblast cores may be partially sucked into the tubules**. The metabolic processes in the enamel and dentine regions are disrupted decisively.

Approximately 5 million *dentinal tubules* per square centimeter (12 million per square inch) are located in the crown area of the pulp. This number decreases down toward the root apex, although it still contains approximately 1.4 million at the cement limit. One single dentinal tubule has a diameter of 1.3 to 4.5 microns. When the drilling or grinding bur is withdrawn, so that the negative pressure ceases, the empty and now open tubules can be filled in a retrograde manner by bacteria and grinding debris, as reported in electron microscope studies. The denatured protein of the destroyed odontoblastic processes and cores can be broken down proteolytically by these bacteria.

Bacterial toxins, capsular antigens and proteolytically broken down protein matter from the dentine tubules act as antigens and result in permanent, auto-aggressive processes and finally in chronic irritation of the pulp. The pulp tissues with damaged odontoblasts then have no chance of survival. They then become the potential focus of infection. Dentists are in no position to differentiate macroscopically whether they are still working in the enamel or are already in the dentine. Even if the bur only contacts the dentine at one single point, the suction effect on the dentinal tubules has then already been produced, causing irreversible damage to the pulp.

The application of conventional methods of pulp testing on teeth treated with turbines in this way merely produces changed sensitivity values. Not until measuring with an electro-acupuncture stimulation current test can the damage be established in an exact manner. Responses to cold or heat stimuli or to electric currents—i.e., via the usual clinical "vitality tests"—provide no evidence for the functionality of the pulp's resistance as an organ. Histological examinations on extracted teeth which had been previously been "treated" with turbines have provided supporting evidence.

When you consider how many dentists apply their turbines day by day without hesitation on millions of patients, you can understand why we consider it a "time-bomb." By means of this machinery, dentists are knowingly or unknowingly damaging the health of their patients, to a criminal degree. When considering the tooth/body connection, it can be surmised that a connection exists between the turbine era and the recent precipitous rise in chronic illness. Turbines have been in use for grinding at least in 99% of dental practices for about 20 years already.

It is a known fact that a chronic disease requires a longer time to develop. If one considers that pulp tissues die at a relatively slow rate and do not always immediately constitute a secondary source to the patient, they must, however, finally result in a breakdown of the local defense mechanism. This fact must at least be given some consideration. It is a belief of many aware ethical biological dentists that the high speed turbines, as presently used in dental practices, must be withdrawn from circulation at least in order to avoid damage, of the kind described, being inflated in the future. Physiological and histological examinations have shown that the upper rotary speed limit is 20,000 rpm.

Hydrokinetic Technology

Hydrokinetic energy is produced by firing laser energy into a spray of atomized water. The water is energized and then is capable of cutting a wide range of human tissue including enamel (the hardest substance in the body), bone, cartilage and soft tissue. Hydrokinetic cutting does not transmit heat to the target tissue whereas other modalities of cutting, such as a high speed dental drill, laser power and electro-cautery, create heat when cutting tissue. As everyone knows, heat causes pain. Hydrokinetic energy can perform numerous dental procedures **with little or no pain, virtually eliminating the need for anesthesia in most cases.**

With lasers being the dominant instrument of choice in eye surgery, dermatology, surgery and other medical fields, it was only a matter of time before they became the instruments of choice in dentistry. The process is the removal of tissues with YSGG laser-energized water droplets. Hydrokinetic energy is produced by combining a spray of atomized water with laser energy. The resulting Hydrokinetic energy gently and precisely removes a wide range of human tissue including tooth enamel (the hardest substance in the body), and soft tissue (gum tissue) **with no heat and no pain in most cases.**

The *Waterlase* works because of its patented Hydrokinetic energy, which is produced by emitting laser energy into a spray of atomized water. The water is energized and is then capable of cutting a wide range of human tissue including enamel (the hardest substance in the human body), bone, cartilage and soft tissue. The Biolase *Waterlase* uses a unique crystal made from yttrium, scandium, gallium and garnet that is "doped" (laser lingo which means "mixed with") with erbium and chromium to create laser energy of a clinically superior wavelength of 2,780 nanometers.

When combined with water, this wavelength produces Hydrokinetic energy with important 21st Century benefits for both the dentist and their patients that include: **Most procedures can be done without anesthesia, without needles or patient trauma;** Quickly cuts all parts of the tooth including enamel, dentin and caries; **Effectively performs numerous soft tissue procedures with little or no bleeding.**

The Benefits of the Hydrokinetic Laser

Heat and vibration are the causes of most of the pain associated with the drill. Since Hydrokinetic cutting does not transmit heat or vibration, most dental procedures can be performed with no pain, virtually eliminating the need for anesthesia in most cases.

The laser's pinpoint accuracy is precise enough that **your dentist can leave behind as much healthy tooth structure as possible,** allowing you to keep your own teeth longer.

Effectively performs numerous soft tissue (gums) procedures **with little or no bleeding.** The laser gives your dentist a new high-tech tool for many procedures that previously required referral to a specialist. Now you can have them performed during your scheduled appointment.

Avoids many common problems of the high speed drill, including cracks in the teeth from the vibration and rapid turning of the drill burs which can weaken your teeth, creating future problems. **The laser sterilizes as it cuts, leaving less chance for bacterial contamination.**

The *Waterlase* prepares your teeth in a way that maximizes the bonding of tooth colored fillings, allowing them to last longer.

Waterlase vs. Drill

The high speed dental drill may cause a smear layer, a layer of dead organic material. The *Waterlase* creates cuts with no smear layer, providing a better surface for bonding, and allowing your filling to last longer. In October, 1998, the Food and Drug Administration cleared the Waterlase YSGG laser for cutting hard dental tissue including enamel, dentin and caries.

Mercury

"How is it that mercury is not safe for food additives and Over the Counter drug products, but it is safe in our vaccines and dental amalgams?"--Represenative Dan Burton (R-IN)

"The evidence tells me very succinctly that there is a chronic low-dose exposure to a toxic heavy metal that 80-85 per cent of the industrialised world have implanted in their teeth, and it's a situation of timed-release poisoning."--Dr Murray Vimy, research scientist and former World Health Organization consultant"

..there is no safe level of mercury, and no one has actually shown that there is a safe level. I would say mercury is a very toxic substance...-- Dr Lars Friberg, Former Chief Adviser to the World Health Organization on Mercury safety.

Mercury

Mercury is the only metal that is liquid at room temperature. Its elemental symbol is Hg, which is derived from the Greek word *hydrargyrias*, meaning "water silver." Mercury is found in *organic* and *inorganic* forms. The inorganic form can be further divided into *elemental mercury* and *mercuric salts*. Organic mercury can be found in long and short *alkyl* and *aryl* compounds. **Mercury in any form is toxic.** The difference lies in how it is absorbed, the clinical signs and symptoms, and the response to treatment modalities. Mercury poisoning can result from vapor *inhalation, ingestion, injection*, or *absorption* through the skin.

The use of mercury in medicine predates its use in dentistry by centuries. Mercury has been found in Egyptian tombs, indicating it was used as early as 1500 BC. As early as 500 B.C. there is evidence that India was using mercury as a drug. However, Arabian physicians first studied mercury as a drug and introduced the use of a mercurial ointment in the 10th century. It was towards the end of the 18th century that mercury found its way into medical practice in the U.S. as a prescription item. In the late 18th century, antisyphlitic agents contained mercury. For centuries, mercury was an essential part of many different medicines, such as diuretics, antibacterial agents, antiseptics, and laxatives.

Mercury poisoning usually is misdiagnosed because of the insidious onset, nonspecific signs and symptoms, and lack of knowledge within the medical profession. In medicine, mercury is used in dental amalgams and various antiseptic agents. Mercury is found in many industries such as battery, thermometer, and barometer manufacturing. Mercury can be found in fungicides used in the agricultural industry. Before 1990, paints contained mercury as an antimildew agent.. On July 7, 1999, a joint statement by the American Academy of Pediatrics and the US Public Health Service was issued alerting clinicians and the public of *thimerosal*, an *ethylmercury*-containing preservative **used in vaccines**.

Elemental mercury is found in liquid form, which easily vaporizes at room temperature and is well absorbed through inhalation. Its lipid (fat)-soluble property allows for easy passage through the alveoli into the bloodstream and red blood cells. Once inhaled, elemental mercury is mostly converted to an inorganic *divalent* or *mercuric* form by *catalase* in the red blood cells.

This inorganic form has similar properties to organic mercury. Small amounts of non-oxidized elemental mercury continue to persist and account for CNS toxicity. Elemental mercury, as a vapor, which escapes from fillings, penetrates the blood-brain-barrier and enters the CNS, where it's ionized and trapped, attributing to its significant toxic effects. It is not well absorbed by the GI tract and, when ingested, is only mildly toxic. Inorganic mercury is highly toxic and corrosive and is the most destructive form, but its destruction is **limited to** where it's located. It doesn't have the ability to move through tissues like other forms. It gains access orally or dermally and is absorbed at a rate of 10% of that ingested. It has a nonuniform mode of distribution, secondary to poor fat solubility, and accumulates mostly in the kidney, causing renal damage.

Although poor lipid solubility characteristics limit CNS penetration, slow elimination and chronic exposure allow for significant CNS accumulation of mercuric ions and subsequent toxicity. Chronic dermal exposure to inorganic mercury also may lead to toxicity. Excretion of inorganic mercury, as with organic mercury, is mostly through feces. Renal excretion of mercury is considered insufficient and attributes to its chronic exposure and accumulation within the brain, causing CNS effects. Organic mercury can be found in 3 forms, *aryl* and short and long chain *alkyl* compounds. This is **100 times more toxic** than the ionic or vapor forms. Bacteria in the mouth, stomach and intestines, or in the blood, through a process called *methylation,* converts mercury vapor and ionic mercury into deadly *methylmercury*.

Organic mercurials are absorbed more completely from the GI tract than inorganic salts are; this is because of intrinsic properties, such as lipid solubility and mild corrosiveness (although much less corrosive than inorganic mercury). Once absorbed, the aryl and long chain alkyl compounds are converted to their inorganic forms and possess similar toxic properties to inorganic mercury. The short chain alkyl mercurials are readily absorbed in the GI tract (90-95%) and remain stable in their initial forms. Alkyl organic mercury has high lipid solubility and is distributed uniformly through the body, accumulating in the brain, kidney, liver, hair, and skin. Organic mercurials also cross the blood brain barrier and placenta and penetrate red blood cells, attributing to neurological symptoms, teratogenic effects, and high blood-to-plasma ratios.

Today, members of the American Dental Association (a trade association and political lobbying arm of dentistry) who even talk against mercury, run not just the possibility of expulsion, but of having the ADA pressure state regulatory agencies to remove the license of any dentist who mentions that mercury might be toxic. The ADA even calls it "unethical and unprofessional conduct" to inform patients of the potential dangers of **the most hazardous metal known to mankind**. For decades the ADA has claimed that mercury is tightly bound within amalgam and cannot possible get out. Chemists and toxicologists, on the other hand, point out that not only does mercury escape, but it's release is greatly enhanced by chewing and heat. The World Health Organization has published research which shows that **between 3-17 micrograms of mercury is released into the body every day simply by chewing pressure on dental mercury fillings**.

Of this amount, **between 74% and 90% is absorbed** and combines with body tissues. Scientists point out that industrial meters held over a filling for 10 seconds after chewing can register levels higher that the EPA allows us to be exposed to for a few hours a day. Fillings, of course, emit mercury vapor 24-hours a day. Fish and other environmental pollutants provide only 0.5-2 micrograms of mercury. **There is no known safe limit of mercury ingestion**. Mercury accumulates within your body, as humans do not have a good mechanism for eliminating it. Yielding to scientific pressures, the ADA now admits that mercury is indeed released from amalgam fillings even after placement, but state that it is perfectly safe and still support the use of amalgam fillings. They claim their use is safe, based on over 150 years of use, and that no scientific evidence shows mercury exposure from dental fillings causes any known disease.

Scientific evidence of the toxicity of mercury is abundantly supplied in any scientific fields related to biology. This includes *immunology, pharmacology, toxicology, endocrinology, genetics*, and *birth defects*, etc. It does not include *dentistry*. There is no scientific evidence showing amalgam's safety and mixed dental amalgam has never had FDA research or approval. If it were to be classified as a *class II medical device* and made to undergo the rigorous testing needed to prove safety, it would never pass. The ADA does admit there is a potential hazard for dental office personnel with the handling of dental amalgam and recommend that dentists use a "no-touch" technique, because dentists and their staff might become contaminated.

They admit that the "scrap" amalgam, the excess amalgam left over after filling a tooth, also **constitutes a hazardous threat** because of continuous vapor release.

Mercury is associated with 258 different symptoms, and copper, also found in amalgam, with over 100. The severe toxicity of methylmercury is attributed to its ability to **pierce any cell membrane in the body and cross all barriers**, even the placental and blood-brain barriers. After crossing these barriers, *methylmercury* is converted back into the highly destructive *ionic* form and **destroys all cell components in its path**. The transportation mechanism into cells is its primary damaging component. Its conversion to ionic form then deposits the "killer" form of mercury in areas it could never penetrate in the ionic form. By this mechanism, methylmercury is credited with initiating **degeneration and atrophy of the sensory cerebral cortex, paresthesia,** (numbness and tingling), **autism, behavioral and emotional aberations,** as well as **hearing and visual impairment**.

In crossing the placenta, it can **inhibit fetal brain development** and bring on **cerebral palsy** or **psychomotor retardation** in the latter stages of development. Other symptoms of mercury toxicity include: anorexia, depression, fatigue, insomnia, arthritis, multiple sclerosis, moodiness, irritability, memory loss, nausea, diarrhea, gum disease, swollen glands, headaches, and many others. Mercury amalgams have set us up for most of the health problems we see today. Toxic metals interfere with the normal energy patterns in acupuncture channels, setting up interference patterns in the meridians. The body, in trying to protect itself against mercury, creates a problem of yeast infection.

One of the natural absorbers of heavy metals is *Candida albicans*. The body attracts yeast into the intestines to act as a natural sponge for the mercury. Heavy metals such as mercury act as *free radicals*, which are highly reactive, charged particles that damage body tissues. Free radicals prevent nutrients from entering the cells and wastes from leaving and block enzymes necessary for the body's detoxification processes. Mercury can bind to the DNA of cells, as well as to the cell membranes, distoring them and interfering with normal cell functions. The immune system no longer recognizes the target as part of the body and will attack it. Once mercury reaches its destination tissue, it has many ways in which it may express its toxicity in many ways.

1. Altered cell membrane permeability
2. Alteration of tertiary structure
3. Alteration of enzyme function
4. Interference in nerve impulses
5. Alteration of the genetic code
6. Inhibition of DNA repair
7. Interference with endocrine function
8. Contribution to autoimmune disease
9. Digestion and absorption alteration
10. Contribution to the development of antibiotic resistance

Millions of U.S. citizens are being exposed to mercury levels that exceed established health standards. Occupational exposure to mercury is a hazard for dental personnel. **The only defense for its use comes from the total support of organized dentistry.** Science, in over 12,000 scientific studies, has not been able to determine one constructive purpose served by the presence of this toxic metal in the human body. **No amount of exposure to mercury vapor can be considered harmless.** Once it has leached from the dental fillings and infiltrated the body, mercury becomes a neurotoxin. **Mercury is more neurotoxic than arsenic and far more neurotoxic than lead.** Mercury has been used quite extensively by the medical profession in anti-fungal preparations, diuretics, antiseptics, brain scans (radioactive mercury), etc. *Merthiolate* and *Mercurochrome,* which were very common "first-aid" items in most households and are still used extensively in hospitals, **contain mercury**.

Nerve endings in the peripheral nervous system constantly scan their environment, engulfing foreign particles and bringing them across the cell membrane for inspection. These substances may then travel all the way up from the foot to the spinal cord to be presented to the nerve cells there. As it travels up the *axon*, mercury destroys a substance called *tubulin*, used as insulation for *neurofibrils* in the *microtubules*, effectively destroying the nerves. Within 24 hours of injecting a minute dose of mercury into a muscle anywhere in the body of test animals, it is detectable in the spinal cord and brain. The mercury is also found in the kidneys, lungs, bloodstream, connective tissue, adrenals and other endocrine glands. In the brain, it tends to congregate in the hypothalamus, which regulates the autonomic nervous system, and in the *limbic* system, believed to be the seat of emotions.

The most devastating effect of mercury in the nervous system is that it interferes with energy production inside each cell. Nerve cells are impaired in their ability to *detoxify* and *nurture* themselves. The cell becomes toxic and dies, or lives in a state of chronic malnutrition. It is common for heavy metals to migrate to and acumulate in nerve *ganglia* (nerve relay stations). As a heavy metal (which means heavier than water), mercury tends to accumulate in the lowest parts of the body, such as the floor of the mouth, the pelvic floor, and the feet. Pelvic symptoms, in both men and women, are very commonly caused by metal toxicity of the *Frankenhauser's ganglion*. This can account for premature ejaculaton and an enlarged prostate in men, and endometriosis, pelvic pain, and hormonal dysfunction in women. *Neural therapy* cleans up this area through the painless injection of the Frankenhauser's ganglion (just above the pubic bone) with a local anesthetic. This opens up most of the ionic channels in the cell wall; the cell is then able to excrete much of its toxic components. This spurs the body to dump large amounts of mercury into the urine.

Mercury is in many of the foods we eat and it is also contained in a great many **over-the-counter drugs** and **cosmetics**; e.g. mascara, **contact lens solution**, **hemorrhoid preparations**, etc. Thus, sensitization to mercury can come from a number of sources. The escape of mercury vapor from amalgam is the **primary source** through which mercury gains access to the body. **Mercury vapor is absorbed through the mucous membranes of the mouth and by direct inhalation into the lungs**. The stomach and intestinal tract also absorb swallowed mercury, freshly formed from the highly reactive vapor in the mouth. All of these portals of entry allow mercury relatively direct access to the bloodstream, where binding to hemoglobin can take place. **The majority of the mercury in the blood is contained within the red blood cells.** Many of those dentists who have inquired into mercury toxicity have lost their licenses or been put on probation for challenging the safety of mercury. The dental industry is scared of legal responsibility for continuing to say that mercury is safe, when all the scientific evidence says otherwise. It is only logical that they would do everything they can to protect the financial interests of the dentists, the manufacturers, and the insurance industry.

If everyone who had come down with *MS, lupus, arthritis, epilepsy, leukemia, ALS, diabetes*, etc., could relate their disease to dental procedures, the ensuing legal battle would be for more money than exists.

A dentist can't legally throw amalgam material or extracted amalgam filled teeth in the trash, bury them in the ground, or put them in a landfill, but the ADA and the EPA say it's okay to put it in people's mouths. In 1976, the U.S. Congress requested that the FDA "classify" dental amalgam fillings. The *Federal Register* recorded another such request in 1980. Multiple requests have been made over the years, yet there is still no classification of dental amalgam. The FDA has steadily refused to classify amalgam. The government agencies have been defending the use of mercury. Consider for a moment the national consequences if mercury in fillings were reported to be dangerous. The offending parties (dentists, the ADA, dental manufacturers and distributors), if found guilty, would be liable.

Mercury Vapor

Silver mercury fillings are not stable. These fillings emit mercury vapor at a rate of 2.8 micrograms per cubic meter of air breathed in the resting state, and their emission rate accelerates dramatically (as high as 49 mgs) after minimal mechanical, chemical, and temperature stimulations. It is also very volatile. This means that "metallic" mercury gives off *mercury vapor* when agitated, compressed or exposed to increases in temperature. **Mercury vapor**–which is colorless, tasteless and odorless–**if inhaled into the lungs, passes into your bloodstream for distribution to all body tissues**. It is at this point that *biotransformation* begins. Some of the mercury vapor remains unchanged, and some of it is *oxidized*. (This means to remove a pair of hydrogen atoms and to combine with oxygen. Chemically it means the increase of a positive electrical charge and the decrease of the negative charge, which in effect *ionizes* the vapor). **The unchanged portion exists dissolved in the blood fats**. The toxic effects are produced by that portion that is oxidized into mercuric ions which occurs mainly in the red blood cells.

Several researchers, beginning with Jernelov in 1969, have demonstrated the microbial conversion or *methylation* of mercury by various microorganisms. This was demonstrated in the laboratory as well as inside the bodies of animals. In 1975, Edwards and McBride demonstrated the methylation of mercuric chloride in human feces. It was also in 1975 that Rowland, Grasso and Davies determined that most strains of *staphylococci*, *streptococci*, yeasts and *escherichiacoli* found in the human intestine (these are bacteria and yeasts of different forms and shapes normally present in the human gut) were capable of methylating mercury.

It was in 1983 that Heintze and his associates made the startling discovery that **saliva can also methylate mercury** being released from the amalgam fillings. Confirmation of the escape of mercury vapor and ions from amalgam dental fillings is provided by The World Health Organization (WHO) Environmental Health Criteria 118 document (EHC 118) on inorganic mercury. It clearly states that **the largest estimated average daily intake and retention of mercury and mercury compounds in the general population, is from dental amalgams**, not from food or air. **Mercury vapor inhaled into the lungs is absorbed almost 100 percent and immediately passes into the bloodstream.** It takes approximately **four minutes** before mercury is converted or oxidized into an ionic state from its elemental vapor state. While in its elemental form, **mercury vapor is lipid** (fat) **soluble** and **readily passes through the blood-brain barrier** or the **placental membrane**.

It can also accumulate in other organs and tissues of the body. The estimated average daily intake of mercury from dental amalgams is 3.8 - 21 micrograms per day. Two-thirds of the body burden of mercury is derived from the mercury vapor released from amalgams. **The static, unstimulated release of mercury vapor from amalgam fillings**, which goes on 24 hours a day, 365 days a year, **is a major contributor to total mercury body burden.** Large amounts of mercury vapor are released during chewing. After only ten minutes of gum chewing, there is an average increase in mercury release of **15.6 times more than during the resting state** in test subjects. That converts to a 1,560% increase in mercury release.

Mercury Vapor Analyzer

The *Jerome 431-X* Mercury Vapor Analyzer uses a patented gold film sensor for the detection and measurement of toxic mercury vapor in the air, including the air in your mouth. It is a portable hand-held unit, weighing only seven pounds that can easily be carried to locations where there is a concern about mercury. It is the same unit used for chemical toxicology testing by OSHA and the EPA to monitor industrial hygiene, mercury spill cleanups and mercury exclusion testing. It is also suitable for monitoring mercury concentrations in a dental office during a daily routine. The simple push-button operation allows users to measure mercury levels in just seconds. The detection range is from 0.000 to 0.999 mg/m^3 Hg.

The gold film sensor is inherently stable and selective to mercury, eliminating interference common to ultraviolet analyzers, such as water vapor and hydrocarbons. When the sample cycle is activated, the internal pump in the 431-X draws a precise volume of air over the sensor. Mercury in the sample is adsorbed and integrated by the sensor, registering it as proportional change in electrical resistance. The instrument computes the concentration of mercury in milligrams or nanograms per cubic meter, and displays the final result in the LCD readout.

The 431-X includes features not available in older Jerome models. When attached to either a data logger or computer, the analyzer automatically regenerates the sensor when it becomes saturated and then resumes sampling. An improved film regeneration circuit makes the sensor last even longer. It operates up to six hours on a fully charged ni-cad battery.

This analyzer can easily be used to measure mercury vapor concentration on a patient before and after chewing a piece of gum for 5 minutes. Chewing, or tooth grinding, increases the heat between teeth and, thus, enhances the release of mercury from amalgams.

This is an insightful eye-opener for those skeptical dentists who still refute the possibility of mercury leaking out of dental amalgams and their own health and their patients' health being in jeopardy by their refusal to acknowledge something that is clearly visible with this machine. Some reported measurements of dental patients' oral mercury vapor have been twice the OSHA standard of 50 μg/cubic meters which would place them in violation of the OSHA standard based on an employee's 8-hour work exposure for a 40-hour work period seven days a week. Once measurements are taken, you will realize that the most toxic spaces may not be at one of the EPA's superfund sites, but simply right under your nose.

Mercury Ingestion

Mercury readily mixes with food and is swallowed with it. The body uptake from inorganic mercury, **swallowed with saliva**, can be as much as **hundreds of micrograms per day** for individuals with a large number of amalgam fillings. Urinary excretion is a common indicator of mercury toxicity, even though **fecal excretion of mercury is twenty times greater than the corresponding urinary excretion.** There is a statistical correlation between the mercury concentration in saliva and the number of amalgam fillings.

The United States government has determined and ruled that the continual exposure to mercury from amalgam fillings is not without risk to patients. **We are concerned over picograms and micrograms of mercury in apples and are looking the other way when milligrams, one million times more, are being implanted directly into a child's mouth.** There is a phenomenon that occurs in the mouth that can contribute to the release of mercury, and is called *corrosion.* Corrosion is similar to "rust" and means that surface particles of the filling material are being chemically broken down and released into the oral cavity.

Mercury vapor is released when you chew or grind. Additionally, **minute rusted particles of the amalgam are being abraded and taken up by your food or saliva and swallowed**. Intestinal enzymes and bacteria to produce methylmercury, an even more toxic form than elemental mercury, may act upon these minute particles of mercury filling. Conventional amalgam was routinely placed until 1976, when the new state-of-the-art amalgams (50% mercury and 30% copper) were introduced. They **emit up to 50 times more mercury** than the earlier, conventional amalgam fillings. That means that every new high-copper amalgam filling placed today has the effective **toxic equivalent of fifty of the older amalgam fillings**. If other fillings are in the mouth, such as gold crowns, nickel crowns, and removable bridges or braces, the mercury emission further increases from the amalgam. This is due to the electrical current generated by the presence of dissimilar metals in an electrolyte such as saliva. Heat will reliably increase the rate of escape of mercury vapor from amalgam fillings. Vapor detectors, held above amalgams, revealed an **increase from 3 micrograms to over 500 micrograms** ten seconds after a hot drink was swallowed.

Blood-Brain Barrier

The *blood-brain barrier* is a normal mechanism that is supposed to restrict the entry of substances into the brain. The transfer of substances such as nutrients, waste products, oxygen and carbon dioxide, hormones, and poisons in and out of the cells of the body is accomplished through the smallest of blood vessels, the capillaries. The capillaries of the brain have a special structural design to provide extra protection for the critical brain cells. Unlike capillaries elsewhere in the body, the cells lining the brain capillaries are overlapped and less porous. This special structure prevents many substances from passing into or out of the brain that would easily pass to and from other body cells.

Substances that can dissolve in fats readily penetrate the membranes of cells, as these membranes have large amounts of fat-containing molecules. Elemental mercury vapor and methylmercury are fat-soluble and therefore easily penetrate cell membranes, including those of the placenta and the blood-brain barrier. This barrier does, however, selectively allow passage of certain smaller water-soluble substances necessary to the brain, such as glucose and essential amino acids. Mercury vapor has no electrical charge (non-ionic) and is fat-soluble, which accounts for its extremely potent toxicity in the elemental vapor form. The oxidation of mercury vapor occurs in the blood and in the body cells. Ionic mercury is the harmful form of mercury because it is chemically active and can readily combine with tissues, exerting its toxic influence in that manner.

Elemental mercury vapor, after entering the bloodstream, is oxidized through the *mercurous* into the *mercuric ion*. These reactions requires several minutes for completion; because of this delay, elemental mercury stays in the blood long enough to reach all tissues and organs. In its elemental form, mercury easily penetrates the blood-brain barrier and infiltrates nerve cells, where final oxidation proceeds. By easily overcoming the *blood-brain* and *placental* barriers, elemental mercury is particularly dangerous during long-term or chronic exposures, representing a potentially serious hazard in many occupations. Once mercury has penetrated the blood-brain barrier, its oxidation to the *ionic* form is completed. This ionic mercury now has an electrical charge and is no longer fat-soluble. Ionic mercury is **very active chemically** and **readily combines with body substances**, thereby exerting its toxic effect.

This ionic mercury can no longer easily penetrate the blood-brain barrier and is very resistant to removal from the brain. **Mercury is retained in brain tissue for extremely long periods of time.** Autopsy studies have demonstrated a definite correlation between levels of mercury found in the brain and the number and surfaces of dental amalgam fillings present. When mercury ions are absorbed into the bloodstream, even in minute amounts (less than 1.0 parts per million), they are **capable of impairing the blood-brain system within 4-6 hours**, allowing passage of normally barred plasma solutes into the brain from the blood, that otherwise would be denied entry. Mercury will not only damage the brain but it will also **increase exposure of the brain to other harmful substances in the blood**. The blood-brain barrier is also an active site for the regulation of the uptake of metabolites from the blood to the nervous system.

The impairment of the blood-brain barrier, together with the possible inhibition of certain associated enzymes by the mercury, is probably responsible for the great reduction of the uptake of amino acids and other metabolites by the nervous system after mercury administration. Amino acids are the building blocks of proteins which are the structural materials used to construct the cells of the body, along with physiological materials such as enzymes and hormones. There is no scientific evidence that brain cells can be regenerated. This is why mercury damage to the brain is **permanent and irreversible**. Since mercury vapor readily traverses the placental membrane, the oxidation of mercury vapor in the fetal blood or at the fetal blood-brain barrier itself no doubt results in **damage to the fetal blood-brain barrier.** But the damage to the fetal blood-brain barrier may be even more important, **preventing the uptake of vital amino acids** for the construction of the irreplaceable brain cells.

There is absolutely no doubt that **exposure to methylmercury in pregnant women presents a serious threat to the fetus**. A number of studies have described the effects on infants of prenatal exposure to methylmercury, while the exposed pregnant mothers exhibited little or no observable signs or symptoms from exposure. The neurological effects on these infants were as severe as cerebral palsy and even death, but less easily recognizable symptoms were more common, such as **delayed mental development**, **delayed speech development**, **delayed motor development**, and **learning deficits**. The major influence of mercury vapor on the fetus is not the promotion of birth defects; but rather the **toxic effect on the body cells**, particularly those of the brain. In spite of the wealth of information strongly demonstrating the potential risk of elemental mercury vapor to the unborn child, the scientific community has not yet seen fit to responsibly investigate this awesome question.

Fertility

Mercury has been shown to pass the placental membrane in pregnant women and cause permanent damage to the brain of a developing baby. A special relationship regarding mercury distribution exists between the mother and the fetus. **Much higher levels of methylmercury have been reported in cord blood versus that contained in maternal blood.** In animal experiments it has also been shown that there is a much higher accumulation of mercury in the fetal brain tissue than in the maternal brain tissue. Mercury exposure leads to hormone and immune disturbances that can reduce fertility.

Reduced fertility among dental assistants with occupational exposure to mercury is a common problem. Many of the female fertility cycle events are related to *posterior pituitary* activity, so amalgam is another factor that can disturb fertility as well as functions unrelated to pregnancy. Estrogen function can also be influenced by amalgam. Blood serum phosphorus is a guideline to endocrine balance. If the phosphorus is below 3.5 mg%, there is an endocrine disturbance, somewhat related to the degree of drop below 3.5. The most effective hormones in balancing the phosphorus level are the sex hormones. All males and all females produce both estrogen and testosterone. The males produce more *testosterone* and the females more **estrogen**, but there is a balance between the two in both sexes. Small doses of **both hormones** are used in **both sexes** to balance the serum phosphorus.

The menstrual and reproductive cycles are controlled by a very complex feedback mechanism between the *ovaries, hypothalamus*, and the *pituitary*. In the case of *follicle stimulating hormone* (FSH), there is a negative feedback relationship with *estradiol* at all times. When estrogen levels are *low*, the release of *leutinizing hormone* (LH) is *increased*, and when estrogen levels are *high*, LH is *decreased*. This ebb and flow controls the hormonal function leading to ovulation and the mid-cycle surge of both LH and FSH and the reduction of LH and FSH at the *luteal* phase relate to a feedback relationship with progesterone.

Progesterone is not secreted by the ovary until just before ovulation. This, in turn, provokes ovulation–progesterone secretion, which undergoes a tremendous increase. The high levels of progesterone and estrogen associated with the luteal phase combine to suppress FSH and LH during the corpus luteum phase. **Mercury inhibits release of FSH from the pituitary** by damaging membranes of cells in the anterior pituitary.

Chronic inhalation of mercury vapor from amalgam fillings for twenty years or more can result in accumulation of pathologic quantities of mercury in the brain and other critical organs and tissues. Human autopsy studies of accident victims have shown a positive correlation between the numbers of mercury amalgam dental fillings and the concentration of mercury in the brain. The onset of clinically observable signs or symptoms of mercury toxicity may take as long as 20-30 years to appear, depending on a person's biochemical individuality. Lubricated condoms and birth control creams or gels have mercury as the primary spermicide.

It is not required that the word mercury appear on the label, as it is assumed that everyone knows mercury is in there. **The uterus is a collection center for mercury.** Hal Huggins reported that more than **90%** of the imbalances, created by sex hormone disturbances were **corrected within a few weeks of amalgam remova**l. His patients noted differences in fertility, less pain during periods, relief from endometriosis, and a trend toward optimization of the days of menstrual flow. PMS is one of the most common symptoms to change after amalgam removal. *Amenorrhea*, or the complete absence of a menstrual flow, responds to amalgam removal. This is usually in women in their twenties or thirties. Even in women who have gone through a sort of premature menopause in their early forties, the periods may start up again for a couple of years. This has resulted in surprise pregnancies. Women should avoid pregnancy for at least six months after amalgam removal.

The Placenta

The circulatory systems of the mother and fetus are separated by a very thin membrane in the placenta. The purpose of this membrane is to ensure that there is no actual mixing of maternal blood with the fetal blood. This placental membrane was formerly called the *placental barrier*. Its function was assumed to be one of protecting the fetus from possible damage from any of the potentially toxic drugs or substances that might be present in the mother's blood. The *Thalidomide* disaster in 1961 demonstrated that the passage of toxic substances from mother to fetus did occur and could result in tragic birth defects and deformities. Mercury reduces the blood's ability to carry oxygen and, although fetal blood flow might be normal, the reduced oxygen content of the blood would parallel the hypoxic condition. Mercury may affect the balance or status of most of the body's essential nutrients. No scientific study has ever addressed the relationship between chronic mercury exposure and placental weight/birth weight. From the time of fertilization until birth, the offspring is dependent upon maternal sources for all nutrition.

There are four major areas that are considered to be critical or determinants in the outcome of fetal development: (1) the mother's nutritional status, (2) the structural and functional quality of the placenta, (3) the genetic makeup of the offspring, and (4) the presence of physical, chemical, or mechanical insults to mother and child during pregnancy. Mercury can also affect the satisfactory outcome of fetal development in all four of these areas.

A possibly contributory factor in cadmium and mercury fetotoxicity may be an effect on the *transmembrane transport* of nutrients, such as amino acids, across the placenta to the fetus. An inhibition of nutrient transport may cause fetal death, congenital malformations, or growth retardation. The toxic effects of cadmium and mercury may be found in the placenta where presence of these metals prevent the passage of required nutrients to the embryo/fetus. The placental membrane will stop many substances. However, it is made of fat molecules, and mercury vapor and methylmercury, being fat-soluble, will penetrate the membrane. The lack of knowledge concerning the mechanisms of mercury toxicity as they relate to the human reproductive cycle is compounded by the scarcity of scientific studies investigating the effects of mercury vapor. The majority of scientific studies on mercury have dealt with methylmercury or inorganic mercury. Very little attention has been paid to the threat posed by low-level chronic exposures to toxic metals.

A great deal of the available scientific data was derived from observation of acute exposures where a large single injection of the toxic metal being investigated was administered and the results examined. While there is no barrier preventing the transfer of mercury, there is a slight barrier to the transfer of lead, and the greatest barrier is to the transfer of cadmium. Mercury is mercury once it reaches the body's cells, and **mercury vapor enters the body and its cells far more readily than most other forms of mercury**. Researchers have found that the placental transfer of mercury varies with the chemical form of mercury; that is, *methylmercury* is more readily transferable than *mercuric nitrate*.

The mercury concentrations in the placenta and the infant's hair are directly related to the infant's body burden of mercury. Total mercury and methylmercury, cadmium, and iron were *higher* in cord blood than in maternal blood, whereas copper and zinc were *lower*. Significant positive correlations were observed between maternal and cord blood with regard to total mercury and methylmercury, lead, cadmium, and manganese content. Significant correlations were also observed between many pairs of metals, particularly in the umbilical cord and its blood. These results suggest a more serious and complicated influence of heavy metals on *infants* than on their *mothers*. The presence of **selenium** in the placenta can modify and greatly reduce the transplacental passage of mercury to the embryo/fetus.

Environmental chemicals taken into the body may considerably increase the fetal body burden of mercury and its concentration in certain tissues, like the liver or thyroid, after mercury vapor inhalation. **Most scientists and researchers are ignoring elemental mercury vapor in their research** and in their recommendations for critical future research areas. These researchers either do not know or have forgotten that, once in the blood, elemental mercury vapor remains in its elemental form for minutes, during which time it can penetrate most tissues easily. It is this capability that permits it to also readily move through the placenta to the embryo or fetus, as does organic mercury. Most of the published research has assumed that the only exposure to elemental mercury vapor is from a minute amount contained in the atmosphere. Most research therefore has only focused on probable exposure from dietary mercury, which is usually in the form of organic methylmercury. A glaring omission has been made by not considering the exposure to elemental mercury vapor from mercury amalgam dental fillings.

Mercury In Vaccines

Approximately 100 years ago, children were on the receiving end of one vaccine, smallpox. Approximately 40 years ago there were five vaccines being promoted: diphtheria, pertussis, tetanus, polio and smallpox. Usually the child received eight shots of one kind or another by age two. A detailed count reveals that **kids now get 52 vaccines via 15 shots by age 16 months,** if parents stand still for the shots recommended by AMA medicine. Included is the preventive pediatrics pneumonia shot. Vaccines contain Thimerosal (mercury), MSG, aluminum, formaldehyde, sucrose and phenoxyethanol (antifreeze).

Thimerosal is nearly 50 percent mercury. In turn, **mercury is a neurotoxin with an EPA safe level of .01 microgram per 1 kilogram bodyweight per day**. Vaccines contain 12.5 to 25 micrograms of mercury. **A visit to the clinic can inject 50 to 62.5 micrograms of mercury into the bloodstream.** This is if the 10-dose vials were properly shaken each time they were used. If not, the recipient of the last couple of doses receives vastly larger quantities of mercury that precipitated to the bottom of the vial. Communicable Disease Centers has now revealed a trend linking autism to mercury-based vaccines. Thimerosal is a registered pesticide allowed into trade channels under the auspices of the EPA.

A child usually gets a hepatitis-B shot on the day of birth. It contains 12 micrograms of mercury, or 30 times the safe level. Four months later, the average American child receives the DTap-HiB combined vaccine. This one contains 50 micrograms of mercury, 60 times the safe level. At 6 months of age, Hep-B and Polio vaccines are given the "protected" child. The mercury load is 62.5 micrograms, or 78 times the safe level. It isn't over yet. At 15 months of age, the same child receives an additional 50 micrograms of mercury housed in shots, or 41 times the safe level. These data are recited here because even low levels of mercury have been associated with neurological disorders, including attention deficit disorder, autism and under-developed speech. Add to this the accumulated toxic load of mercury from the mother's amalgam dental fillings the child received in utero through the placental blood, and after birth through breastfeeding and they will have an incredibly high level of mercury in the first few months of life and it then builds up from that time on from the various sources of exposure in our environment, especially from amalgam.

Chronic Fatigue

The formation of hemoglobin can be impaired by the presence of mercury, which shows up as increased amounts of porphyrin, a building block of hemoglobin, in the urine. Porphyrin is a layered molecule with the first layer consisting of eight *carboxyl groups*. When enzymes cut off the carboxyl fragments, what is left is a core molecule known as *heme*. Heme has two energy functions involving its attachment to *globin* to form *hemoglobin*, used to transport oxygen, and it can also undergo a transformation down a chemical cascade of enzymes called the *cytochrome oxidase system* where the molecules of *adenosine triphosphate* (ATP) are formed in the *Kreb's cycle* within the *mitochondria* of cells. Mercury appears to create interference in porphyrin metabolism; the result being an identifiable increase in the urine of porphyrin breakdown products in lieu of energy forms.

In serious chronic fatigue conditions, the excretion is as high as 2100 micrograms. The levels of hemoglobin in chronic fatigue patients can run below normal. Readings below 12 grams clearly indicate inadequate blood levels of hemoglobin. But, many with chronic fatigue have normal or even high levels of hemoglobin. Often these people are referred to psychiatrists under the assumption that they are suffering from mental/emotional stress disorders. The oxygen binding sites in hemoglobin are a favorite of mercury.

When enough mercury combines with the hemoglobin, the body experiences chronic fatigue due to lack of oxygen transport, and may create **more red blood cells** in compensation. This would show up as normal or high hemoglobin readings. Since the body cannot block the daily mercury doses released from amalgams, it will typically make more red blood cells to compensate for this daily contamination. Physicians can easily make the mistake of thinking that they couldn't possibly be hypoxic or anemic with normal hemoglobin. Once mercury is bound to hemoglobin, it will typically stay there for the lifetime of the red blood cell, which is approximately 120 days. Since one molecule of hemoglobin has four oxygen-binding sites, then one atom of mercury will drop the oxygen-carrying capacity of that hemoglobin molecule by 25% after binding. If two atoms of mercury attach, that hemoglobin molecule will have a 50% reduction of its oxygen-carrying capacity. After amalgam removal, the oxygen saturation in venous blood **rises dramatically**.

Digestion

Through a process called *pleomorphism*, similar to *metamorphosis* in which a worm becomes a butterfly, many bacteria alter themselves in response to their immediate environment and become **different bacteria**. These changes in body function lead to differences in their personal biological wastes, which is the cause of many problems. As the stomach environment changes with the addition of new and different foods, some bacteria can undergo a pleomorphic change to accommodate the digestive needs of the new food. By the time a child is two years old, and their teeth have erupted, there may be as many as 400 variations of bacteria in the gastrointestinal tract, and the child is ready for the basic challenges of digestion. When mercury enters the digestive tract, it has an effect on the bacteria that reside there. Mercury readily mixes with the foods and is swallowed with it, then contacting the friendly bacteria.

Bacteria and Yeast

When people have mercury amalgams or just has elevated mercury in their body, the friendly bacteria (probiotics) will convert the mercury into methyl mercury, which is at least **100 times more toxic** than ordinary mercury. Research shows that oral bacteria, yeast and probiotics all methylate mercury, so you should minimize any contact between the bacteria and your mercury. The methylation of mercury could explain some of the adverse reactions reported by parents and patients who have begun detox with massive doses of probiotics to correct dysbiosis.

Dysbiosis is a pressing problem, but the production of large amounts of methyl mercury is much worse. Methyl mercury exacerbates damage to the nervous system and even further promotes dysbiosis by further compromising the intestinal immune system. One theory holds that the body deliberately builds up the population of candia as a coping strategy to deal with the heavy metal poisoning. The body actually fosters the presence of candida in a heavy metal toxic patient because the cell walls of the candida binds up the mercury and other toxic metals, providing a measure of relief. If the candida cell walls are destroyed, **the cell walls release their toxic metals back into the system**, causing symptoms. This release of heavy metals is possibly one explantion of *Herxheimer's reaction*, in which the patient feels more ill, and even more toxic, after the candida is attacked and killed. By using *NDF* (*Nanocolloidal Detox Factors*), an oral detox supplement, containing cell wall broken probiotics, the *bacteriocins* from the probiotics drive pathogenic bacteria and yeast away from their territory without breaking their cell walls. This *competitive exclusion effect* is safer than breaking the cells of the candida.

Mercury may kill the bacteria, but the ones that are stronger undergo *pleomorphic* change and become more resistant to mercury. These altered intestinal bacteria almost digest your food properly, but not quite. The resultant almost digested proteins are absorbed into the bloodstream. But, while almost the right shape and form, they do not fool the immune system. The immune system sees these undigested proteins as *foreign* protein and immediately sets up an **antigen/antibody reaction,** creating an **allergic reaction**. This is often how food allergies are created. Mercury can turn every meal into an **immune challenge** instead of the nutritional boost it is supposed to be. Altered bacteria also encourage the rotting of proteins (called putrefaction).

Putrefaction of proteins results in the production of more toxins interfering with the actual absorptive mechanism from the intestinal lining. As a result of these injuries, the selective absorption of the intestinal tract is impaired, allowing seepage of partially processed foods through the lining into the body itself. The lymphatic drainage system picks these up and places them in the blood. *Leaky gut syndrome* is one of the labels applied to this situation. There is another connection with root canal filled teeth and digestive problems. The common denominator appears to be toxic immune damage from toxins found in the periodontal ligament surrounding the root canal tooth.

These toxins are formed within the root structure of the tooth itself, regardless of what is used to fill the root canal. Once formed, they migrate to the outside of the root, to the interphase between bone and teeth. When one bites down, as during chewing, a few molecules of the toxins are forced up the root surface into the mouth. From the mouth, toxins are mixed with saliva and foods and swallowed into the stomach and intestinal tract. These toxins are unaffected by acids and enzymes in the stomach. There is nothing known in biochemistry or toxicology that is as toxic per volume as root canal generated toxins. It only takes microminute amounts of these *acute dentally associated* toxins only a minute or two to **inactivate many of the body's most critical enzymes.** The first layer of cells in the intestine in contact with the food is called the *epithelium*. These epithelial cells contain *glycolytic* enzymes that are critical in the production of *trypsin*, *chymotrypsin*, and *pepsin*–digestive enzymes.

As toxins from root canal teeth are released into the saliva, they mix with other components of the saliva, one of which will be mercury if there are any silver mercury amalgam filings in the teeth. In addition to root canal toxins, several other toxic chemicals are produced simultaneously in the periodontal ligament space. Among these are *hydrogen sulfide* and *methyl mercaptan*. As this team of chemicals is exposed to mercury, an immediate reaction occurs between them and a new "dual" toxin is formed that can easily enter the epithelial cells of the intestinal tract, inhibiting the production of trypsin, chymotrypsin, and pepsin that are necessary for complete digestion. This leads to chronic constipation, etc. The most significant factor to good digestion is thorough chewing of food, but chewing can trigger the release of these vicious toxins—and if you don't chew your food well, it will ferment and putrefy.

Diarrhea

Another reaction of mercury in the gut can be diarrhea. Diarrhea is an effective response by the body to rid the G.I. tract of harmful or toxic substances that may have been ingested. After an average of eight years from the time the body begins to fight the presence of mercury seriously, there is the onset of an alternating pattern of diarrhea and constipation, eventually settling into **chronic constipation**. This chronic constipation leads to parasites, causing the patient to be even sicker. Parasites rob these patients of essential nutrients, and supply their own toxic by-products as well, taking energy from the immune cells, liver and kidneys.

Leukemia

There is a significant cause and effect relationship between mercury amalgam fillings and the white blood cell count. A normal unchallenged, white cell count will run between five and ten thousand cells per cubic milliliter. Amalgam removal is often followed by **drops in the high levels of white blood cells** seen in leukemia-diagnosed persons. Even the presence of one or two amalgams would increase the white cell level to 7,000 or 8,000. Some researchers, like Hal Huggins, believe that leukemia might be the result of a valiant attempt on the part of a super-healthy immune system to rid the body of a challenge that the system considers extremely bad. Sometimes, the day after having fillings removed, the white count will drop over 10,000 to a more healthy level.

Diabetes

Insulin, the molecule of question in diabetes, has three sulfur-binding sites. Should mercury attach to one of these, there will be an interference with normal biological function. In diabetics, the daily requirements for insulin usually drop to less than half of what they had been before dental revision. It's important to monitor blood sugar changes after revision, as insulin overdose can occur. **Elevated insulin will supress the activity of white blood cells.**

Alzheimer's Disease

There is conclusive scientific research showing **a direct correlation between the numbers and surfaces of amalgam fillings and the mercury content of brain tissue.** Autopsy studies show **high levels of mercury in the brain tissue of Alzheimer's victims**. Chronic inhalation of low-level **mercury vapor can inhibit *polymerization* of brain *tubulin*** essential for formation of *microtubules*.

Hormones

The affinity of mercury for the pituitary gland was first identified by Stock in 1940. Autopsy studies in 1975 revealed that, contrary to accepted belief that the kidney was the prime accumulator of inorganic mercury, **the thyroid and pituitary retain and accumulate more inorganic mercury than the kidneys**. It has been well documented that mercury is an endocrine system disrupting chemical in animals and people, disrupting function of the pituitary gland, thyroid gland, enzyme production processes, and many hormonal functions at low levels of exposure.

People with high mercury levels have **more hormonal disturbances, immune disturbances, recurring fungal infections, hair loss and allergies**. Very few periodontists or dentists recognize amalgam mercury as an etiological (causing) factor in the development of periodontal disease. Hormones that are most often affected by mercury are *thyroid, insulin, estrogen, testosterone*, both *anterior* and *posterior pituitary*, and *adrenaline*. Most hormones have binding sights capable of connecting to metabolic cofactors, but mercury can bind here, too. Mercury frequently has a **stronger affinity** for these binding sites than the normal activators; even though the hormone is present in the bloodstream, it may not be able to act as it is supposed to act.

Mercury (especially mercury vapor or organic mercury) rapidly crosses the *blood-brain barrier* and is stored preferentially in the **pituitary gland, thyroid gland, hypothalamus**, and **occipital cortex** in direct proportion to the number and extent of dental amalgam surfaces. Mercury, through its affects on the endocrine system, is documented to cause other **reproductive problems** including *infertility, low sperm counts, abnormal sperm, endometritis, PMS*, adverse effects on reproduction, etc.

In general, immune activation from toxins such as heavy metals, resulting in *cytokine* release and abnormalities of the *hypothalamus-pituitary-adrenal axis,* can cause changes in the brain, fatigue, and severe psychological symptoms such as depression, profound fatigue, muscular-skeletal pain, sleep disturbances, gastrointestinal and neurological problems as are seen in *CFS, fibromyalgia*, and *autoimmune thyroiditis*. Symptoms usually improve significantly after amalgam removal. A direct mechanism involving mercury's **inhibition of hormones and cellular enzymatic processes** by binding with the *hydroxyl radical* (SH) in amino acids, appears to be a major part of the connection to allergic/immune reactive/autoimmune conditions such as autism/ADHD, schizophrenia, lupus, scleroderma, eczema, psoriasis and allergies.

Mercury inhibits the activity of *dipeptyl peptidase* (DPP IV) which is required in the digestion of the milk protein *casein* as well as *xanthine oxidase*. Studies involving a large sample of *autistic* and *schizophrenic* patients found that over 90% of those tested had high levels of the **neurotoxic** milk protein *beta-casomorphine-7* in their blood and urine and defective enzymatic processes for digesting milk protein. Elimination of milk products from the diet improves the condition.

ADHD populations have high levels of mercury and recover after mercury detoxification. As mercury levels are reduced, the protein binding is reduced and improvement in the enzymatic process occurs. Additional cellular level enzymatic effects of mercury binding with proteins include blockage of *sulfur oxidation processes,* enzymatic processes involving vitamins B_6 and B_{12}, effects on *cytochrome-C* energy processes, along with mercury's effects on levels of calcium, magnesium, zinc, and lithium.

Thyroid

Organic mercury causes severe damage to both the endocrine and neural systems. Studies have documented that mercury causes hypothyroidism, damage of thyroid RNA, autoimmune thyroiditis (inflammation of the thyroid), and impairment of conversion of thyroid *T4* hormone to the active *T3* form. Large percentages of women have elevated levels of *antithyroglobulin* (anti-TG) or *antithyroid peroxidase* antibody (anti-TP). Slight imbalances of thyroid hormones in expectant mothers can cause **permanent neuropsychiatric damage in the developing fetus**. Hypothyroidism is a well-documented cause of mental retardation. Maternal hypothyroidism appears to play a role in at least 15% of children whose IQs are more than 1 standard deviation *below* the mean, **millions of children**. Studies have also established a clear association between the presence of *thyroid antibodies* and **spontaneous abortions**. Hypothyroidism is a risk factor in spontaneous abortions and **infertility**.

In pregnant women who suffer from hypothyroidism, there is a **four-times greater risk for miscarriage** during the second trimester than in those who don't. **Women with untreated thyroid deficiency are four-times more likely to have a child with a developmental disability and lower I.Q.** Mercury blocks thyroid hormone *production* by occupying iodine-binding sites and inhibiting hormone *action* even when the measured thyroid levels appears to be in the proper range. There are several aspects of iodine deficiency and hypothyroidism-related effects on fetal and perinatal brain development that can be aggravated or otherwise affected by the presence of mercury. Mercury has the ability to reduce cerebellar brain weight through significant reductions in total cell populaton of the cerebellum. Reductions of total body weight at birth are related to maternal exposure to mercury. Lead and mercury also have a direct effect on neuronal development leading to learning deficits. These are the same type of birth defects produced by maternal iodine deficiency and hypothyroidism.

Mercury can have a negative effect on both iodine and thyroid status. A pregnant woman with a mouthful of mercury amalgam fillings has a much greater chance of experiencing some degree of hypothyroidism and/or iodine deficiency during pregnancy than one without amalgam fillings. Both the *pituitary* and the *thyroid* display an **affinity for accumulating mercury**. The enzymatic effects of mercury intoxication can be overcome by the administration of the thyroid hormone *thyroxine*. Through a feedback loop, the pituitary releases thyrotropin-releasing hormone, which in effect tells the thyroid how much thyroxine hormone to release into the blood. Mercury first *stimulates* and then *suppresses* the thyroid function. Chronic intake of mercury for more than ninety days results in signs of mercury poisoning, together with decreased uptake of iodine and depression of thyroid hormonal secretion.

The *thyroid* and *hypothalamus* regulate body temperature and many metabolic processes including enzymatic processes that, when inhibited, result in higher dental decay. Mercury damage thus commonly results in poor body temperature control, in addition to many problems caused by hormonal imbalances such as **depression**. Such hormonal secretions are affected at levels of mercury exposure much *lower* than the acute toxicity effects normally tested. Mercury also damages the blood brain barrier and facilitates penetration of the brain by other toxic metals and substances. Hypothyroidism is also a major factor in **cardiovascular disease**.

The thyroid gland has four binding sites for iodine. When mercury attaches to one of these sites, the hormone activity is altered. There is a relationship between thyroid function and the nutritional status of folate, vitamin B_{12}, and methionine. There is also a strong association between lowered zinc intake, lowered basal metabolic rate, lowered thyroid hormones and lowered protein utilization.

Mercury affects the nutritional status of folate, vitamin B_{12}, methionine, and zinc, as well as protein. The thyroid is **one of the important glands influencing dental decay**. There is a fluid flow from the pulp chamber, through the dentin, through the enamel and into the mouth in people who have no dental decay. Thyroid is part of the endocrine function that controls the direction of this fluid flow. Low thyroid hormone production allows this fluid flow to run in the opposite direction—from the mouth, into the enamel, dentin, and pulp chamber

This fluid brings bacteria and debris from the mouth with it, leading to dental decay. **When the teeth are susceptible to decay, the whole body is susceptible to degenerative disease.** The thyroid is involved with maintenance of proper body temperature. Most mercury toxic patients have lower than optimum body temperatures.

The most toxic persons may have temperatures as low as 96.2. When the amalgam fillings are removed, there is a trend for the temperature to approach 98.6, sometimes within 24 hours of removing all of the amalgams. The thyroid gland is controlled by the pituitary gland. When the thyroid is influenced by mercury, there is a high incidence of unexplained **depression** and **anxiety**. A person may have adequate levels of T_3 and T_4 hormones, but if the hormones are contaminated, the person is functionally thyroid deficient. Thyroid imbalances cause chronic conditions such as clogged arteries and chronic heart failure. People who test hypothyroid usually have significantly higher *homocysteine* and *cholesterol*, which are documented risk factors in heart disease.

Fifty percent of those also had high levels of homocysteine, and 90% were either *hyperhomocystemic* or *hypercholesterolemic*. The major regulator of adrenocortical growth and secretion activity is the pituitary hormone ACTH. ACTH attaches to receptors on the surface of the adrenal cortical cell and activates an enzymatic action that ultimately produces *cyclic adenosine monophosphate* (cAMP). cAMP, in turn, serves as a cofactor in activating key enzymes in the adrenal cortex. The adrenal cortex is able to synthesize cholesterol and to also take it up from circulation.

All steroid hormones produced by the adrenal glands are derived from cholesterol through a series of enzymatic actions, which are all stimulated initially by ACTH. Steroid biosynthesis involves the conversion of *cholesterol* to *pregnenolone*, which is then enzymatically transformed into the major biologically active *corticosteroids*. cAMP is produced from *adenosine triphosphate* (ATP) by the action of *adenylate cyclase*. Adenylate cyclase activity in the brain is inhibited by micromolar concentrations of lead, mercury, and cadmium. One of the key biochemical steps in the conversion of adrenal pregnenolone to cortisol and aldosterone involves an enzyme identified as *21-hydroxylase*.

Mercury causes a defect in adrenal steroid biosynthesis by inhibiting the activity of 21a-hydroxylase. The consequences of this inhibition include **lowered** plasma levels of corticosterone and **elevated** concentrations of progesterone and *dehydroepiandrosterone* (DHEA). DHEA is an adrenal male hormone. Because patients with 21-hydroxylase deficiencies are incapable of synthesizing cortisol with normal efficiency, there's a compensatory rise in ACTH leading to **adrenal hyperplasia** and excessive excretion of *17a-hydroxyprogesterone*, which, without the enzyme 21-hydroxylase, cannot be converted to *cortisol*.

The inhibition of the 21-hydroxylase system may be the mechanism behind the mercury-induced adrenal hyperplasia. Adrenal hyperplasia can stress the adrenal glands by their accelerated activity to produce steroids to the point that production begins to diminish and the glands will atrophy. The result is a **subnormal production of corticosteroids**. Both lead and mercury can precipitate pathophysiological changes along the *hypothalamus-pituitary-adrenal and gonadal axis* that may seriously affect reproductive function, organs, and tissues. Leukocyte production, distribution, and function are markedly altered by glucocorticosteroid administration. In Addison's disease (hypofunction of adrenal glands), *neutrophilia* occurs 4-6 hours after administration of a single dose of *hydrocortisone, prednisone*, or *dexamethasone*. Neutrophilia is an increase in the number of neutrophils in the blood. Neutrophils are also called *polymorphonuclear leukocytes* (PMNs). Mercury not only causes a suppression of *adrenocorticosteroids* that would normally have stimulated an increase of PMNs, but at the same time also affect the ability of existing PMNs to perform immune function by inhibiting a metabolic reaction that destroys foreign substances.

Posterior Pituitary Gland

The pituitary gland controls many of the body's endocrine system functions and secretes hormones that control most bodily processes, including the immune system and reproductive systems. One study found mercury levels in the pituitary gland ranged from 6.3 to 77 ppb, while another found the mean levels to be 30 ppb, levels found to be *neurotoxic* (toxic to nerves) and *cytotoxic* (kills cells). Amalgam fillings, nickel and gold crowns are major factors in *reducing* pituitary function. The *posterior pituitary* hormone joins forces with the *thyroid* in influencing emotions. Posterior pituitary hormone is really two hormones, *oxytocin* and *vasopressin*.

High blood pressure is related to the function of the posterior pituitary hormone *vasopressin*. It is a short trip for mercury vapor to leave a filling, and travel into the sinus, and then travel an inch through very porous, spongy tissues to the pituitary gland. Mercury is detected in **less than a minute** after placing amalgam in teeth of test animals.

Suicide

Part of the reason for depression is related to mercury's effect of reducing the development of posterior pituitary hormone (*oxytocin*). Low levels of pituitary function are associated with depression and suicidal thoughts, and appear to be a major factor in suicide of teenagers and other vulnerable groups. **As a profession, dentists rank highest in suicide.** Autopsy studies in Sweden showed that the pituitary glands of dentists held **800 times more mercury** than people who were not in dentistry. Suicidal thoughts are not limited to dental personnel though.

Suicide is close to the number-one cause of death in teenagers. Braces increase the electrical and toxic load people are carrying if they have amalgam in their mouths. Amalgam can create suicidal tendencies by itself, but the addition of braces, nickel crowns, or even gold crowns evidently increases the exit rate of mercury, and the glands *react*—or actually *stop reacting*. Suicidal tendencies tend to disappear within a few days of supplemental *oxytocin extract*, along with dental metal removal. Menstrual cycle problems, also normalize and fertility increases and endometriosis symptoms subside.

Frequent Urination

The center that controls the need to get up several times each night to urinate is the posterior pituitary gland. There is a certain amount of solid material that must be disposed of daily in the urine. If the concentration of these solids is high (yield a specific gravity of 1.022 to 1.025) then the proper volume of urine will be excreted in a day. Should the concentration be half that, or yielding a specific gravity of 1.012 for instance, then it will take double the amount of urine to rid yourself of the same amount of solid. In other words, the solids remain the same. If the concentration of the urine is reduced, the total volume of urine is increased substantially. This ability of the kidney is controlled by the posterior pituitary.

Adrenal Glands

Mercury accumulates in the adrenal glands and disrupts adrenal gland function. During stress, the adrenal glands increase in size as a normal reaction in order to produce more *steroids* (hormones). Both physical and physiological stress will stimulate the adrenal glands. The outer shell of the adrenal gland is called the *cortex,* and the inner core of the gland is called the *medulla*. The cortex produces three types of steroids called *glucocorticoids*. *Cortisone* is a corticoid essential to life and functions to maintain stress reactions. Mineral corticoids, such as *aldosterone*, regulate the balance of blood electrolytes and also cause the kidneys to *retain* sodium and *excrete* potassium and hydrogen. Mineral corticoids are also involved in *gluconeogenesis*, which is the process whereby your body converts *glycogen* to *glucose* (blood sugar).

Small amounts of corticoid sex hormones, both male and female, are also produced by the adrenal cortex. Two primary nutrients for the adrenal glands are *pantothenic acid* and *vitamin C*. A deficiency of pantothenic acid can lead to **adrenal exhaustion** (chronic fatigue) and ultimately to destruction of the adrenal glands. A deficiency of pantothenic acid also causes a progressive fall in the level of adrenal hormones produced. One of the largest tissue stores of vitamin C is the adrenals; it is exceeded only by the level of vitamin C in the pituitary. Physical and mental stress increase the excretion of *adrenocorticotropic hormone* (ACTH) from the pituitary, which is the hormone that tells the adrenals to increase their activity. The increased adrenal activity, in turn, depletes both vitamin C and pantothenic acid from the glands.

Humans cannot produce vitamin C. They therefor attempt to replenish the needs of the adrenals by taking the vitamin from other storage locations in the body. If your overall ascorbate status is low, there may be an insufficient amount available to satisfy the needs of the adrenals. Under this condition, normal adrenal hormone response may become inadequate, leading to an inadequate immune function. **Mercury builds up in the pituitary gland and depletes the adrenals of both pantothenic acid and vitamin C.** Stress and the presence of mercury will have a very negative effect on the adrenal production of critical steroids. The ability of the adrenal gland to produce steroids is called *steroidogenesis* and is dependent upon reactions mediated by the enzyme *cytochrome P-450*. Cytochrome P-450 reacts with cholesterol to produce *pregnenolone*, which is then converted to *progesterone*.

Cytochrome P-450 can then convert progesterone to *deoxycorticosterone* which is then converted to *corticosterone* or *aldosterone* by other enzymes in the adrenals. These adrenal functions are also affected by metal ions.

Still today, the ADA and other governmental agencies tell us that the mercury in your *mouth*, or from *vaccinations*, is perfectly safe. Scientists say this is a ridiculous statement that is in violation of science and common sense.

Sulfur & Mercury

Transsulfuration Pathways

Methionine

(ATP/Mg)

SAM (S-adenosylmethionine)

SAH (S-adenosylhomocysteine)

Homocysteine

(B_6; Mg)

Cysteine

Cysteine-sulfinic acid

B-sulfinylpyruvic acid

Toxic sulfite molecule

(Mo)

Essential sulfate molecule

Protein synthesis

Polyamines

Methyl group
creatine
choline
carnitine

Taurine

Pyruvic acid

Provides natural sulfur for detox pathways in the liver, specifically those that bind heavy metals, such as lead, mercury and cadmium.

SAM is an important methyl donor for vital substances, including neurotransmitters, *phosphatidylcholine*, and *phosphatidylserine*.

Homocysteine is recycled to methionine in the presence of B_{12}, folic acid, and methyl donors (choline or betaine)

B_6 & magnesium help convert homocysteine to cysteine

Molybdenum (Mo) is an essential trace mineral necessary to convert the toxic *sulfite* molecule to the essential sulfate molecule.

Sulfur & Mercury

Mercury, in its various forms, has a great affinity for certain minerals, as well as protein and non-protein molecules in the body. Mercurials have a great attraction to the *sulfhydryls* or *thiols*. The mercury atom or molecule will tend to bind with any molecule present that has sulfur or a sulfur-hydrogen combination in its structure. This process of combining with a metal to form a complex in which the metallic ion is sequestered and firmly bound is called *chelation*. A thiol is any organic compound containing a *univalent radical* called a sulfhydryl and identified by the symbol -SH (sulfur-hydrogen). A thiol can attract one atom of mercury in the ionized form and have it combine with itself. Because it is a radical, it can enter into or leave this combination without any change. **Mercury and lead both have a great affinity for sulfur** and sulfhydryls and are capable of affecting the transsulfuration pathways in the body.

The primary sulfur-containing protein amino acids in the body are *cystine, cysteine, methionine*, and *taurine*. There is also a sulfur-containing tripeptide (having three amino acids) called *glutathione* that is composed of *glutamic acid, cysteine*, and *glycine*. Sulfur exists in a reduced form (-SH) in *cysteine* and in an oxidized form (-S-S) as the double molecule *cystine*. Whenever mercury binds to one of these sulfur-containing molecules, it **reduces the molecule's availability for normal metabolic functions.**

Sulfur is **present in all proteins**, which makes it universally available throughout the body for binding with mercury. Some of the important biochemical sulfur-containing compounds of the body besides glutathione are *insulin, prolactin, growth hormone*, and *vasopressin*, and science has not yet investigated the effect of mercury upon them. Mercury has a particularly high affinity for thiol groups and progressively less for other groups in the following sequence: *sulfur, amides, amines, carbon*, and *phosphate*. Because of this, mercury has the potential of binding to proteins throughout the body. Mercury compounds are formed by the binding of mercury to the biological binders *albumin* or *cysteine.*

The principal biological reaction of mercury is with thiols to form mercury *mercaptides*. The sulfur groups are often referred to as *mercaptans* because of their marked affinity for mercury. Mercaptan is defined as any compound containing reduced **sulfur bound to carbon**.

When a metal, such as **mercury, replaces the hydrogen ion of the reduced sulfur**, the resulting compound is called a *mercaptide*. Mercury can form at least three compounds with cysteine in which all or a part of the mercury is bound firmly as a mercaptide. Mercury may cause damage, especially to the placenta, by inactivation of sulfhydryl groups in cellular enzymes. Mercury interacts with *sulfhydryl* groups and *disulfide* bonds, as a result of which specific membrane transport is blocked and selective permeability of the membrane is altered. Mercury also combines readily with *phosphate* and *heterocyclic base groups* of DNA. It also combines with other *ligands*: *amide, amine, carboxyl* and *phosphoryl* groups.

Homocysteine

Homocysteine is a natural substance made by the body. Homocysteine functions at a metabolic crossroad that can affect all the *methyl* and *sulfur* group metabolism of key enzymes, hormones, and vital nutrients. Many people lack the ability to break it down completely, and high homocysteine levels usually occur due to the inability to clear homocysteine because of faulty methionine pathways (mercury and lead toxicity). The result is a buildup of homocysteine in the system.

When it is not completely broken down, homocysteine becomes a very dangerous substance that can exert harmful effects and increase disease-causing oxidation. When it is broken down completely, it can furnish necessary substances for other beneficial reactions in the body (methyl and sulfur groups). These necessary substances provide the fuel for vital processes like liver detoxification, adrenal gland support, neurotransmitter synthesis, and **joint** cartilage and bone regeneration. Homocysteine is a very dangerous substance that is harmful to the arteries, which makes it a risk factor for heart disease if it is not broken down completely.

Homocysteine can cause clotting, increase harmful oxidation, and can injure the blood vessel wall (especially if already weakened by x-rays), allowing cholesterol and fat to infiltrate into the wall and cause what is known as a *foam cell*. This foam cell swells and protrudes into the space of the artery and obstructs the blood flow, potentially resulting in a **heart attack**. The artery is usually damaged and cholesterol is oxidized before infiltration into an artery and creation of a foam cell can occur, and homocysteine can damage the artery, oxidize the cholesterol, and decrease circulation, all of which increase the risk of heart disease.

The first correlation between homocysteine and disease involved cardiovascular disease, but since then, toxic effects have been revealed on other organ systems, including the liver, adrenals, joints, nerves, and general system blood vessels (inclusive of placental tearing). Neuropsychiatric conditions have also been traced to homocysteine problems, and a correctly functioning pathway is vital to neurotransmitter synthesis. Other conditions which have been linked to high homocysteine levels include *neural tube defects, multiple sclerosis, rheumatoid arthritis, spontaneous abortion, placental abruption, renal failure, osteoporosis*, and *type II diabetes*.

Homocysteine is not toxic when the pathway is functioning properly. Synergistic nutrients facilitate the homocysteine pathway, preventing toxic levels of homocysteine from accumulating, and make it possible for a functioning pathway to provide necessary methyl groups and sulfur groups for a myriad of biochemical reactions, especially those needed for detoxification and joint and cartilage repair. Nutrients which *facilitate* the methionine pathway and *reduce* homocysteine include *betaine, dimethylglycine*, and *vitamins* B_6, B_{12}, *folic acid, niacinamide, choline, betaine, dimethylglycine, magnesium*, and *molybdenum*.

Homocysteine is recycled to *methionine* in the presence of **B_{12}, folic acid**, and methyl donors such as **choline** or **betaine** (trimethylglycine). **B_6** (pyridoxyl-5-phosphate is the active form) and **magnesium** help convert *homocysteine* to *cysteine*. **Molybdenum** is an essential trace mineral necessary to convert the toxic *sulfite* molecule to the important *sulfate* molecule needed for many biochemical reactions. **Niacinamide**, a B vitamin, can increase the activity of two crucial enzymes needed to facilitate conversion of homocysteine to non-toxic substances.

Niacinamide is also necessary for steroid hormone synthesis (*cortisol, estrogen, progesterone, testosterone, DHEA*), and when chronic stress on the adrenals favors cortisol production, a limitation in niacinamide and/or precursors allows cortisol to be made at the expense of other steroid hormones (such as DHEA). This results in increasingly large ratios of *cortisol* to *DHEA*, leading to tissue **insensitivity to insulin**. All the excess cortisol will need to be *conjugated* (detoxed in the liver), and this happens largely through sulfur-dependent detoxification pathways in the liver.

For this, the homocysteine path has to be functioning to provide the sulfur groups for liver detoxification. Providing these sulfur groups can take some of the stress off the adrenals when cortisol is excessive. Zinc, selenium and magnesium are all minerals which are important cofactors in enzyme reactions of the homocysteine pathway. Zinc and selenium are cofactors for antioxidant enzymes. Magnesium is needed to convert methionine to SAM (*S-adenosylmethionine*) for the end reaction which converts the toxic *sulfite* to the essential *sulfate*, and for glucose metabolism (glucose is a substrate for *glucuronic acid, hyaluronic acid, N-acetyl-glucosamine*, and *chondroitin sulfate*–all building blocks for cartilage and joint repair). Chronic mercury inhalation from mercury fillings, with its great affinity to bind to methionine and cysteine can **decrease the availability of these amino acids** and affect the metabolism of both vitamin B_{12} and folic acid.

Mercury can inhibit or modify how the body uses ATP, zinc, selenium, rubidium, vitamins A and C, and calcium. Cancer cells have altered sodium and calcium transport and reduced oxygen transport through the cell membrane. The oxygen deficiency within the cell reduces or eliminates the ability of the cell to oxidize *glucose* to *carbon dioxide*, which in turn, results in the conversion of *glucose* to *lactic acid*, lowering cellular pH into the acid range. These combined effects radically change cell metabolism and ultimately DNA replication. Mercury can alter sodium and calcium transport and also reduce the amount of oxygen transported. Mercury competes with calcium for cellular binding sites and, through this mechanism, can *decrease* cellular calcium or *increase* extracellular calcium. Mercury binds avidly to rubidium and selenium. Decreases in available selenium can also reduce available *GSH-Px* (glutathione peroxidase), which, in turn, causes a proliferation of free radical cellular damage. Mercury, at extremely low levels, can inhibit the *respiratory burst* of killer-cell leukocytes, reducing their effectiveness in controlling cancer cell proliferation.

Cysteine and Cystine

Cysteine (sis-tee-in) is a unique amino acid, largely by virtue of its sulfhydryl group. It is an important constituent of proteins, being largely responsible for their molecular configuration, either by forming disulfide bonds with other cysteine molecules incorporated into the same protein or by forming disulfide bonds with free cysteine. It can link together a number of separate proteins or polypeptides by forming disulfide bonds between cysteine residues in different molecules. Cysteine is made from two other amino acids, *methionine* and *serine*. Methionine furnishes the sulfur atom and serine furnishes the carbon skeleton in the synthesis of cysteine. Cysteine is produced by enzymatic or acid hydrolysis of proteins. *Cysteine* can be oxidized to *cystine* (sis-tin), which is rather insoluble in water. Sometimes it can be found in the urine and in the bladder in a crystal form where it will form *cystine calculus* (stones) in the kidneys or bladder. Cystine is the main sulfur-containing compound of the protein molecule. Upon reduction, cystine produces two molecules of cysteine. Heavy metals catalyze the oxidation of *cysteine* to *cystine* and also react with cysteine to form *mercaptides*. Cysteine is very soluble in water and therefore can be easily eliminated via the urine.

However, *cysteine* can be oxidized to *cystine*, which can then present the potential of stone problems. If an adequate supply of vitamin C is available, it will help keep cysteine in its reduced and soluble form, thereby preventing the formation of stones. The ratio of vitamin C to cysteine should be three-to-one. *Cystathionase*, an enzyme that is necessary to change *cystathionine* into *cysteine,* and which is present in humans postnatally, is not present in human fetal liver or brain. Cysteine is not considered an *essential* amino acid in *adults*. Cysteine is an essential amino acid for the human *fetus*, and for prematurely born and full term infants for a short period after birth. Its concentration in maternal plasma is greater than or equal to that in fetal plasma. Cystathionine, which is present in human brain in large concentrations, may not be needed until some time after birth.

Methionine

Methionine is one of the *essential* amino acids required in the diet, whereas cysteine is considered to be *non-essential*. Eighty to 90% of the daily requirement can be replaced by cystine. The ability for one sulfur to replace another is called *transsulfuration* and represents an important route for either *cysteine* or *cystine*. Plasma levels of *taurine, serine, methionine*, and *threonine* have been found to be significantly lower in patients with essential hypertension (high blood pressure). The levels of these four amino acids, as well as total sulfur amino acids, correlated inversely with systolic blood pressure. Individuals with mercury amalgam dental fillings could have low plasma sulfur amino acids, leading to high blood pressure. Mercury has been shown to affect methionine use.

Taurine

Taurine is a sulfur-containing amino acid that the body makes from cysteine. Methionine is a precursor for cysteine and taurine biosynthesis. There are two primary bile acids needed to break down fats; one of them, *taurocholic acid*, **cannot be produced without taurine**. Taurine is concentrated in the brain where it functions as a neurotransmitter and/or as a modulator of neurotransmission, preventing excess electrical activity, such as that occurring during epileptic episodes. Taurine plays a major role in the transport regulation of blood electrolytes (calcium and potassium) and may affect in the cardiovascular system. Excretion in pregnant women falls dramatically starting at week-9 of pregnancy.

Reserves of taurine are increased for use during the latter phases of pregnancy. Concentrations are higher in the fetal liver and brain and some believe that it plays a role in brain development and also functions as a growth modulator. Both mercury and lead have a great affinity for the sulfur atom. Mercury can serously interfere in the transsulfuration pathway at many different locations, ultimately leading to a deficiency or reduction in available taurine.

Glutathione

Glutathione is present in almost all cells in the body in rather high concentrations. Glutathione serves as a storage and transport form of cysteine and also as a respiratory carrier of oxygen, both extremely important metabolic functions. Within the cell itself, it has some very important metabolic functions such as protecting the cells against damage that can be caused by free radicals and hydrogen peroxide. In the liver, glutathione is a reservoir of cysteine which is utilized for protein synthesis.

Glutathione can also replace cysteine derived from methionine, thus exerting a methionine sparing action. Vitamins C and E are two key nutrients that go through this recycling process. Once they have performed their function as an antioxidant, scavenging free radicals, they are reduced to an inactive state and must be regenerated to their original form. This process requires an adequate supply of reduced glutathione. *Reduced glutathione* (GSH) is present in red blood cells where it is functionally associated with the enzyme *glucose-6-phosphate dehydrogenase* (G6PD) and the coenzyme *reduced nicotinamide-adenine dinucleotide phosphate* (NADPH). Both G6PD and NADPH are needed to maintain red blood cell integrity.

Glutathione also plays a part in how our immune systems function. When the supply of glutathione is low, or has been depleted, this can inhibit the activation of lymphocytes, and may also have a bearing on the response of *cytotoxic T-lymphocytes*. The ability of mercury to affect the available supply of glutathione also affects these same lymphocyte functions. Mercury also inactivates G6PD, which results in altered red blood cell membrane permeability and blocking of active glucose transport into cells. Mercury itself increases red blood cell membrane permeability. The altered membrane permeability, in turn, disrupts a large number of essential membrane functions, ultimately leading to cell death. *Glutathione peroxidase* (GSH-Px) activity in the liver, kidneys, testes, and erythrocytes is significantly depressed by silver and mercuric chloride.

Glutathione peroxidase protects the human brain. When polyunsaturated fatty acids, which are located primarily in the brain, are oxidized, organic *hydroperoxides* are formed that can only be reduced by GSH-Px. Alterations in GSH-Px activity and tissue damage caused by peroxide accumulation is of significance in the development of senility and degenerative neurological diseases. One of the primary ways the body gets rid of metal compounds is through a pathway that goes from the *liver* into the *bile* where they are then transported to the *small intestine* and excreted in the feces. Inorganic mercury is complexed with glutathione in the bile, suggesting that glutathione status is a major consideration in the biliary secretion of mercury. This same pathway is affected by a mercury induced reduction of available **taurine** needed to produce bile acid *(taurocholic acid)*.

When the microflora of the intestine have been reduced through stress, poor diet, use of antibiotics and other drugs, fecal content of mercury is greatly reduced. Instead of being excreted in the feces, the mercury gets recirculated back to the liver. The person who is under stress, eating a poor diet, and/or taking antibiotics will tend to maintain a higher body burden of mercury derived from dietary sources–especially if they are eating fish.

Mercury And The Heart

Mercury and the Heart

Mercury is a potent metabolic poison; it harms any living cell or process. Although mercury is found in many forms, they all have the same effect once they get in the body and reach the cells. The toxic potential of the various forms depends on their ability to enter the body. The most toxic forms of mercury, namely *mercury vapor* and *methylmercury*, **easily enter the body and penetrate its cells**. Inhaled mercury vapor travels rapidly to **heart tissue**. This type of mercury exposure presents a significantly greater risk to the heart than does mercury consumed in fish (organic mercury) or medications (inorganic mercury).

For more than 70 years, scientific evidence, has demonstrated **widespread cardiovascular effects** from *inorganic mercury* and *mercury vapor*. Studies have revealed that subjects with amalgam fillings experience **significant mercury exposure** to the tissues of the cardiovascular system and have markedly higher blood pressure, lower heart rate, lower hemoglobin levels, and lower percentages of red blood cells. They also have a greater incidence of impaired cardiac electrical and neurotransmitter function, pathological changes in heart muscle tissue, damage to blood vessels and heart valves, arrhythmias, constriction of coronary arteries, chest pains, rapid heart beat, anemia, increased potential for blood clots, fatigue, tire easily, and are tired in the morning.

These studies have demonstrated how **mercury poisoning from inhaled mercury vapor** from *dental amalgam fillings* affects the cardiovascular system. Damage by mercury occurs when it attaches to or enters the cells of the body; no matter what form the mercury is in when it enters the body. *Ethylmercury* and *methylmercury* are very toxic forms of mercury because they **easily enter the body and its cells**. *Mercury vapor* is also very toxic for the same reason. Medical knowledge about cardiovascular disease was minimal prior to the 20th century. In the mid-19th century, the effect of occupational exposure to mercury in workers in mirror factories and the use of mercury in the treatment of syphilis was being practiced.

In 1861, it was reported that the activity of the involuntary muscles are affected. Together with a **weakness of the voluntary muscles**, there was an **impairment of the heart**. The pulse was slower, with **greater lability**; resting heart rate was 60-70 beats/minute, but at the slightest agitation, the rate rapidly rose to 80-100. Sometimes **pronounced tachycardia** occurred.

In the 1930s, it was recognized that mercury causes damage to the heart and blood vessels. It was then discovered that mercury poisoning has a paralyzing influence of heart and circulation, followed by a **reduction in blood pressure** and **death**. In 1938, researchers found **serious vascular damage** from mercury exposure.The analysis of cardiovascular disease depends upon sophisticated testing and sophisticated research, neither of which was available until the 20th century. Until recently, the cardiovascular effects of exposure to mercury were not recognized. Medical scientific researchers investigated mercury accumulation in cardiovascular tissue of humans and animals in controlled experiments in the 1950s. The animals exposed to mercury vapor had much higher levels of mercury in the *heart* and *brain*, as well as larger amounts in the *thyroid, adrenals, spinal ganglia and nerves*, *testes*, and *ovaries*. Exposure to mercury vapor results in larger accumulation of mercury in the heart than does inorganic mercury.

The mercury levels in the heart were **three to four times** those found in the brain of exposed animals, after only one hour of exposure. In humans, exposure to mercury vapor results in a *high* and *rapid* **accumulation of mercury in heart tissue**. Levels of inorganic mercury, methylmercury, and total mercury accumulation, were measured and high levels of mercury were found in heart tissue, about the same amounts as were found in the brain. It was also found that the levels of inorganic mercury in the heart *increased* with age, while the levels of methylmercury *decreased*. In human autopsy studies, high levels of mercury were found in the pituitary glands of dental personnel and those with amalgams.

Mercury absorbed from dental amalgam is rapidly **taken up by the heart tissue, in greater amounts and more rapidly than that which is absorbed into the brain**. Mercury specifically derived from dental amalgam fillings also influences heart function by accumulating in the brain, pituitary, thyroid, and adrenals, and are also target organs after exposure to mercury vapor. Among the earliest widespread indications of the cardiovascular effects of mercury were in victims of *Acrodynia*, a disease syndrome known to be caused by mercury, and was diagnosed primarily in children who were being exposed to various mercury compounds, mostly a *mercurous chloride* compound called *Calomel*, which was commonly used as a teething powder and to combat "diaper rash."

In 1952, it was found that *Calomel* (mercurous chloride) enhanced the influence of *epinephrine* (adrenaline) in constricting arteries and caus ing high blood pressure and tachychardia in children. Science has proven mercury's toxic action on a wide range of tissues, including those in the cardiovascular system. Researchers have found that **mercury affects several aspects of cardiac function**, including the ability of heart muscle to contract, the electrical conduction activity in the heart, and the function of regulators of cardiac activity. **Mercury toxic subjects exhibited an increased occurrence of rapid heart beat, irregular pulse, chest pains, heart palpitations,** and **high blood pressure**.

Mercury blocks the action of *acetylcholine*, the neurotransmitter that passes the nerve impulse from the *vagus* nerve to the *heart muscle*. Both acetylcholine and the nerve receptors in the heart muscle contain *thiol* (sulfur/hydrogen) proteins. When mercury attaches to the thiol protein in the heart muscle receptors and in the acetylcholine, **the heart muscle can't receive the vagus nerve electrical impulse for contraction**. Mercury accumulates in the heart muscle and heart valves, causing damage by attaching to thiol (SH-) proteins. This damage is indicated by EKG and confirmed by histologic study. **The damage is found in the coronary arteries and capillaries supplying blood to the heart tissue and in the heart muscle itself.**

Mercury has a high affinity for and readily binds to *selenium* and to the *thiol* or *sulfhydryl* (sulfur/hydrogen combination) sites in living tissues. The *higher* the attraction between chemicals or elements, the *stronger* they bond to each other, and the *harder* it is to separate them. The thiol combination is extremely common in the human body. It occurs as part of certain amino acids, which are building blocks of proteins. Since these amino acids are used to build *cells, hormones*, and *enzymes*, the occurrence of the thiol combination in the body is not only *common* but extremely *important*, as normal function is altered. There are several thiol sites in the *hemoglobin* molecule in the red blood cells used to transport oxygen throughout the body. Mercury accumulates in red blood cells in humans and other animals. When this mercury attaches to the thiol sites, the hemoglobin can't carry as much oxygen as it could. This results in decreased availability of oxygen (hypoxia) that is needed by all body cells and explains one way that mercury toxicity can cause **chronic fatigue** symptoms. This same interference occurs wherever thiols occur in the body, including the cardiovascular system.
Mercury and other thiol toxins affect many aspects of cardiac activity, including *nerve regulation* (especially the *vagus* nerve) and *chemicals*,

the *electrical activity* of the heart, and the *contractibility* of the heart muscle. Acetylcholine is the neurotransmitter for the vagus nerve. Receptors to receive the nerve impulses from the acetylcholine are located in the heart muscle. **The active portion of acetylcholine receptors in the heart tissue is a thiol protein.** When mercury attaches to the thiol portion of the protein, the **vagus nerve impulse is prevented from reaching the heart tissue** and the heart ceases to respond to impulses from nerves at these mercury-blocked sites. There are numerous vagus nerve receptor sites in heart tissue.

The effect on heart function depends on the number of sites blocked by mercury. Another important influence of mercury on the heart function is its adverse affect on the ability of the heart muscle to contract. This is because of the ability of mercury to attach to thiol proteins, this time in the heart muscle itself. Heart muscle consists of two major proteins, *actin* and *myosin*. The function of muscle tissue depends on the interaction between these two proteins and their combination to form *actomyosin*, resulting *in* tissue contraction. The connection of these two proteins occurs at thiol sites in the myosin molecule. If mercury attaches to those thiol sites, the muscle tissue will not be able to function.

With mercury vapor intoxication, there is a **decreased activity** of *respiratory enzymes* and *sarcoplasmic ATPase*. Cell respiration consists of a series of chemical reactions that provide the needed energy for cell functions. Cell respiratory enzymes are very sensitive to mercury; it alters or inhibits their function by removing the hydrogen atom from the thiol group.

Mercury affects heart function by influencing the hormones from the pituitary gland (*pituitrin*). Pituitrin contains several active hormones that have a profound and important influence of the body, including one that affects the constriction of arteries. Chronic mercury exposure affects cardiovascular functioning by **interfering with cardiovascular regulating hormones** (*dopamine, epinephrine*, and *norepinephrine*). In test animals, mercury exposure increases the force of heart muscle contraction, causing high blood pressure, by **blocking the passage of calcium ions** into the heart muscle cells. Low concentrations of various mercury **compounds accelerate blood coagulation** (clotting) process. Unborn babies are highly exposed and susceptible from their mothers' dental amalgam fillings. Prenatal exposure to mercury produces **marked**

toxicity to babies, including a high incidence of abnormal hearts, characterized by dilation with a thinning and weakening of the heart walls. **Inhaled *mercury vapor* penetrates the placental membrane far more thoroughly than does *inorganic* mercury**, thereby significantly increasing the potential for fetal damage. The integrity and proper function of living cells depends on the ability of certain materials to pass into and out of the cells. The cell membrane contains numerous thiol sites. Mercury binds to these sites and prevents the passage of certain materials into and out of the cells.

Mercury blocks the enzyme in the cell membrane that actively passes **calcium** in and out of the muscle cells by attaching to the thiol part of the enzyme. Calcium is necessary for the proper function of heart muscle. **Hypertension** is caused by mercury preventing the passage of calcium into the heart muscle cells, thereby **increasing the force of contraction**. It takes time for chronic mercury exposure to cause enough damage to manifest as clinically detectable dysfunction. This is characteristic of heart disease. It takes the body 30-70 days to eliminate half of each dose of mercury. If a person is only exposed to very small doses of mercury vapor, but is exposed many times each day, the mercury slowly builds up in body tissues. Some time may elapse before enough mercury accumulates in heart tissue to cause observable symptoms.

Abnormalities and Impairments of Heavy Metals

Abnormalities and Impairments of Heavy Metals

Psychiatric Disturbances

Social deficits, social withdrawal–*mercury*
Repetitive, perseverative, stereotyped behaviors, OCD-typical behaviors–*mercury*
Depression, mood swings, flat affect, impaired facial recognition–*arsenic, copper, lead, mercury*
Schizoid tendencies, hallucinations, delirium–*mercury*
Irritability, aggressive behaviors, temper tantrums–*lead, mercury*

Suicidal behaviors–*copper, mercury*
Sleep difficulties/ disturbances–*lead, mercury, thallium*
Chronic fatigue (CFS), weakness, malaise–*aluminum, arsenic, cadmium, copper, lead, mercury, thallium*
Anorexia, symptoms reflecting eating disorders, loss of appetite/ weight–*arsenic, lead, mercury*
Anxiety, nervous tendencies–*thallium*
Attentional problems (ADHD), lacks eye contact, impaired visual fixation–*lead, mercury*

Speech and Language Deficits

Speech disorders–*aluminum, mercury*
Loss of speech, developmental problems with language–*mercury*

Speech comprehension deficits–*mercury*
Dysarthria, articulation problems, slurred speech, unintelligible speech–*mercury*

Cognitive Impairments

Mental retardation, borderline intelligence–*arsenic, lead, mercury*
Uneven performance on IQ scores, low IQ scores–*copper, lead*
Poor concentration, attention deficits (ADHD), response inhibition–*aluminum, lead*
Poor memory (short term, verbal, and auditory)–*aluminum, lead*
Difficulties understanding abstract ideas, difficulty carrying out complex commands–*x metals*
Dementia, pre-senile and senile dementia–*aluminum*

Stupor–*aluminum, arsenic*
Impaired reaction time, lower performance on timed tests–*lead*

Sensory Abnormalities
Abnormal Sensations in the mouth and extremities–*arsenic*
Hearing loss, difficulty hearing–*arsenic, lead, mercury*
Abnormal touch sensations; diminished touch sensations, aversion to touch–*arsenic*
Blurred vision, sensitivity to light–*arsenic, mercury*

Motor Disorders
Choreiform movements, myoclonal jerks, unusual postures–*copper, mercury*
Difficulty walking, swallowing, talking–*copper, mercury*
Flapping, circling, rocking, toe walking–*mercury*
Problems with intentional movements or imitation–*mercury*
Abnormal gait/posture; incoordination, loss of balance, problems sitting, lying, crawling, and walking–*mercury*
Decreased locomotor activity–*aluminum, arsenic*
Convulsions, seizure–*aluminum , arsenic, copper, lead, mercury, thallium*

Other Physical Disturbances
Hypotonia or hypertonia, decreased muscular strength–*x metals*

Rashes, contact dermatitis, eczema, itchy/irritating skin–*aluminum, arsenic, copper, mercury*
Muscle pain, headache, acrodynia, colic–*arsenic, copper, lead, thallium*
Alopecia (hair loss)–*thallium*

Physiological Impairment
Brain and Central Nervous System
Neurofibrillary tangles–*aluminum*
Neuritis, retrobulbar neuritis, neuropathy–*aluminum, arsenic, thallium*
Encephalopathy–*aluminum, arsenic, lead, thallium*
Cerebrovascular disease–*x metals*
Alterations in nerve conduction velocity–*lead*
Alterations in the spinal chord–*thallium*

Accumulates in CNS structures–*aluminum, mercury*
Abnormal EEGs–*arsenic, lead*
Autonomic disturbances–*copper, lead, mercury, thallium*

Peripheral Nervous System

Peripheral neuropathy–*arsenic, mercury*
Alterations in peripheral nerves–*arsenic*
Loss of feeling/ numbness in the extremities, paresthesia–*arsenic, mercury, thallium*

Gastrointestinal Tract

Nausea, vomiting, diarrhea, loss of appetite–*arsenic, copper, mercury, thallium*
Abdominal pain, stomach cramps, burning of the throat and mouth–*arsenic, copper, lead, mercury, thallium*
Esophagitis, gastroenteritis, colitis–*arsenic, mercury, thallium*
Cancers (colon, pancreatic, stomach, or rectal)–*arsenic*

Renal and Hepatic Impairment

Hepatotoxicity, Liver dysfunction, damage–*arsenic, copper, thallium*
Cirrhosis of the liver; hepatitis–*copper*
Kidney disease, kidney failure–*arsenic, lead, mercury*
Renal toxicity, tubular proteinosis–*arsenic, copper, lead*
Kidney Damage, histological alterations–*arsenic, lead*

Cardiovascular System

Blood vessel damage–*arsenic*
Anemia, decreased red blood cell count–*arsenic, copper, lead*
Hypertension, increased heart rate (tachycardia)–*arsenic, copper, lead, thallium*
Electrocardiac disorders, Peripheral vascular disease, cardiovascular disease, vascular collapse–*arsenic, lead*

Respiratory System

Pulmonary Fibrosis–*aluminum, arsenic*
Pulmonary edema–*x metals*
Pneumonia, laryngitis, pharyngitis, bronchitis–*aluminum, arsenic, mercury*
Restrictive airway disorders, asthmatic conditions, pneumoconisis–*arsenic, aluminum*

Respiratory tract cancers–*arsenic*
Nasal ulcers, perforation of the nasal septum–*x metals*

Immune System

Increased incidences of asthma, autoimmune-like symptoms, & allergies–*x metals*
Inhibition of lymphocytes, T-cells, monocytes–*x metals*
Immunosuppression–*lead*
Decreased white blood cell count–*arsenic, thallium*

Reproductive System

Genital abnormalities–*aluminum, thallium*
Disturbances in menstrual cycle, menstrual pains–*copper, mercury*

Birth defects, premature births, Spontaneous abortion–*arsenic, lead, mercury*
Reproductive dysfunction–*arsenic, aluminum, cadmium, lead*

Amalgam Fillings

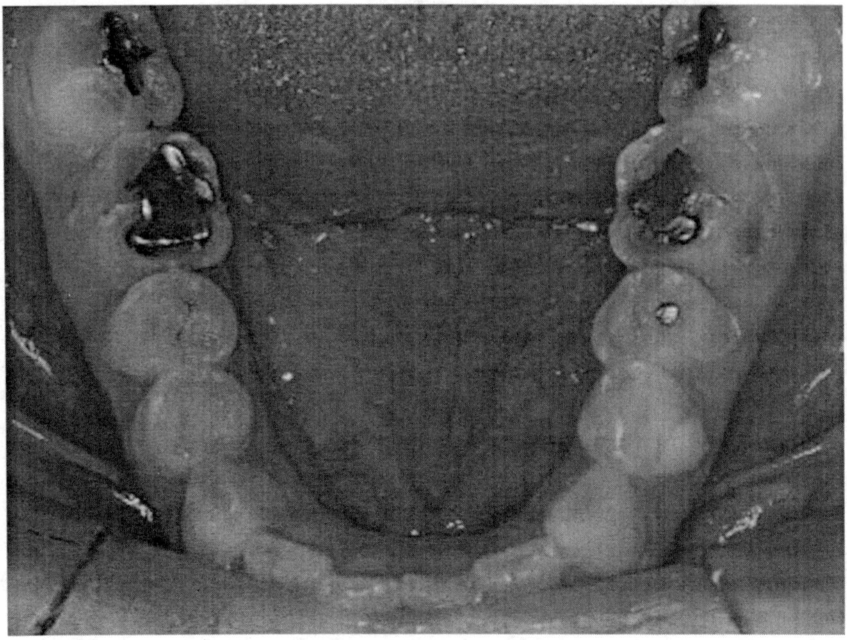

Amalgam Fillings

...if they have as few as 4 amalgam fillings present in their mouth, the average person's saliva is so high in mercury they cannot legally spit into the toilet. Their saliva exceeds the EPA maximum legal municipal discharge standard for mercury..--David Kennedy D.D.S.

Amalgam Fillings

Each year, more than 100 million amalgam fillings are placed in the U.S. alone. In this country, **approximately 150,000,000 people have amalgam fillings.** The average life of an amalgam filling is 5.5 to 11.5 years. Since amalgam has been used for more than 150 years, literally **billions of amalgam fillings have been used to restore decayed teeth.** Amalgam fillings contain approximately **50% mercury, 30% copper, 14% each of tin and silver, and 1% zinc**. All five metals in amalgam fillings are toxic. These metals react with each other and form sixteen more *corrosion products*, all of which are toxic.

After implantation in your teeth, and for an indefinite period of time, silver mercury fillings outgas detectable amounts of mercury vapor, in the range of **1 to 50 micrograms of mercury per cubic meter of air**. An adult breathes about 1/2 liter of air per breath, breathing over 17,000 times each day. As long as you have mercury dental fillings, you inhale mercury vapor **24 hours a day, 365 days a year.** The body's tissues, especially brain, kidneys, jaw, lungs, gastrointestinal tract, and liver, absorb and store mercury. Mercury toxicity has destructive effects on kidney function and contributes to cardiovascular disease, neuropsychological dysfunction, reproductive disorders, birth defects, and more. Like other heavy metals, and x-rays, **mercury causes damage to the lining of arteries**.

Only **one microgram of mercury is enough to destroy any type of cell in the body**, especially nerve tissue. Mercury releases from 20 to 150 micrograms per day depending on the conditions and the type of amalgam. The state-of-the-art *high-copper amalgams* release **50 times more mercury** in a given time than the older *conventional* amalgams. If one microgram is absorbed, **it will take 70 days to several months to eliminate half of it**. Meanwhile, the next day you absorb another microgram, and 69-and-a-half 70^{th}s of the original one microgram will still be there. On day three you absorb another microgram, and you still have $69/70^{th}$s from the first day, and 69 and-a-half 70^{th}s from the second day, so you can see that even with the fastest elimination, excretion is negligible compared to intake if you have amalgam in your mouth. **You will still increase your total body burden of mercury daily.**

Not all of the mercury escaping from a filling stays in the vapor form, especially if it is on the surface of a filling registering a negative electrical charge. In the electrical environment on the surface of a filling, mercury vapor is rapidly converted into the highly toxic *methylmercury*. The chemical product formed by the setting of the five metals is chemically reactive. A mercury vapor meter placed over a filling can detect toxic amounts of mercury vapor within ten seconds. **Fillings release mercury just sitting undisturbed in the mouth**, but there are several ways that we can cause our fillings to release increased amounts of mercury.

The action of **chewing foods increases the vapor release** due to *abrasion* as well as *compression* of the filling for **up to an hour and a half** after we stop chewing it. **Heat** from coffee or other hot beverages **increases the vapor release from the fillings**. When there are dissimilar metals in the mouth, and the mouth contains saliva, an electrolyte solution, you have a battery working twenty-four hours a day in your mouth, and *metals* and *metal oxides, sulfides*, and *sulfates* draining out of the fillings into your mouth; you can experience it as an unpleasant metallic taste. During detoxification, after removal of fillings, the body is dumping metals in the saliva, and the taste can persist for several weeks.

The *total* of the toxins is far greater than the *sum* of the toxins. With lead and mercury, for instance, a toxicity rating of *1* for each mercury and lead equals not *2*, but ***60*** when the two are combined. With *nickel, copper, beryllium, mercury, tin, silver, zinc, cobalt, chromium*, and *root canal toxins* in the mouth, **with just one crowned root canal and one amalgam filling—you can have a witches' brew of complex toxic reactions**, made even more complex if you include the *cements*.

The Controversy

On the other side of the problem we have the proponents who advocate continued use of amalgam fillings. The combined credentials and strength of this group is awesome. It includes the *National Institute of Dental Research, National Bureau of Standards, The American Dental Association* (ADA), *The Academy of General Dentistry* (AGD), most of the state dental societies, all of the teaching college and university dental schools and most of the medical doctors. Of the 100,000 plus practicing dentists in the U.S., there is only a small minority at this time (somewhere in the order of 2,000) that do not accept the ADA position on the use of amalgam in dentistry.

The type of material used to fill teeth has always presented problems of one kind or another to the dental profession. Manipulation of it to "fill" a small area in a toothalways presents difficulty to the dentist. Over the years it was a constant challenge to the ingenuity and inventiveness of the dental practitioner to eliminate the difficulties of working with single metals to make them more pliable and capable of being molded (plastic) so that they would then harden and have some permanence.

There are literally hundreds of scientific papers that show mercury can effect and cause some detectable damage to almost every component of the human body or comparable component of an animal body. However, there does not seem to be any way of proving or demonstrating in a human body that mercury is the sole cause of the detectable damage. To prove this in humans, we would have to be maintained in a totally sterile environment and not subjected to thousands of chemicals and pollutants in the course of our lifetime simply from the routine acts of eating and breathing.

There is a substantial flow of anecdotal evidence being reported by dentists and physicians who believe that the research to date has indicated with sufficient clarity that amalgams in teeth may be injurious to our health. These health practitioners have **recommended removal of amalgam fillings and replacement with new *composite* materials** that are basically non-toxic. **Where the patient has agreed to this type of reconstruction and the work was performed, there has usually been an abatement, amelioration or complete clearing of symptoms.**

Amalgam Removal

Dentists routinely remove amalgam fillings every day and replace them with other amalgam fillings. The ADA's own statistics are **that 75% of all restorations replaced are amalgam**. The average life of an amalgam filling is 5.5 to 11.5 years. **Most fillings are replaced because of decay under the filling, excessive corrosion, fracture, etc.** The procedure is so commonplace that the insurance companies will pay for replacement of an amalgam filling after only one year. The primary risk to a patient's health is the competence of the dentist, his/her ethics and integrity in taking the requisite precautions to protect their patients and staff. Newer materials are so much more flexible and advantageous to work with that, in many instances, teeth can be saved that would otherwise be lost if amalgam were the only material available.

There are special techniques usedby your dentist to remove amalgam fillings. If done properly, there is minimum exposure to increased levels of mercury vapor caused by the removal procedure. The correct protocol requires the use of high volumes of cold water both from the drill and separate irrigation by the assistant, who should also be simultaneously using high volume suction evacuation of the vapor and particles resulting from the removal procedure. The assistant should hold the high-volume evacuator next to the tooth being worked on until all of the cut filling and cavity have been cleaned out. It is the volatility of mercury that necessitates all the precautions and correct techniques. **Mercury vapor pressure doubles with every ten degree centigrade rise in temperature.** One acceptable procedure that minimizes extensive grinding involves sectioning the amalgam into chunks versus just grinding it out.

During amalgam removal, the dentist and assistant are at greater risk from exposure to mercury aerosol spray and vapor. They will be wearing special clothing, masks and surgical gloves. These actions protect them from excessive exposure to mercury during repeated removal operations. Some dentists utilize a *rubber dam* during the amalgam removal procedure. This is a square of latex rubber stretched on a frame. It isolates the tooth or teeth being worked on. The rubber dam prevents the patient from swallowing ground out amalgam particles and accidentally inhaling mercury fumes. The office and *operatory* should be well ventilated. Many mercury-free dentists are now installing central vacuuming systems in their offices. This provides an additional high vacuum suction source, drawing out mercury vapor and mercury aerosol generated during the removal process. Current information indicates that it is better to replace only a few amalgams at a time, with several weeks in between appointments.

Some individuals may experience reactions to the mercury released during the removal procedures. These are described as flu-like and can last from 1 to 7days. Symptoms may include fever, nausea, headaches, etc. *Sequential* removal requires the dentist to measure and chart the electrical current of each filling and to remove/and or replace the amalgam fillings based on the charted information starting with the highest negative readings. Most dentists around the world replace fillings by *quadrant*, thus removing the largest source of mercury first. If all available dentists worked at it full time, **it would take 10 years to completely remove the toxic metals from people's mouth**s.

Amalgam Replacement

The vast majority of individuals who have undergone amalgam replacement and the reduction of their mercury body burden have **experienced improvements in health that have ranged from minor to startlingly dramatic**. Dentistry has relied on and utilized potentially toxic metals in the oral environment because there were no acceptable alternatives available. But, today, there is a surplus of options available for consideration. The most common composite material used is called *white stuff.*

The white composite is all made with petroleum derivative resins and often with aluminum dioxide, which is quite toxic itself. Unlike aluminum trioxide or sand, aluminum dioxide **can have very strong reactions in the body**. The newer materials available on the market today are referred to *as bonded resin ceramics*, *composite resins* or just *composites*. Although there are several types available, their composition is essentially one of a quartz-filled *Bis-GMA resin*. The data produced by studies on these materials indicates a very high degree of biocompatibility when properly placed.

A key feature of composite plastics is their extremely large molecular size, which prevents penetration of body cells. However, **some composites contain elements such as aluminum**, which can be harmful if they're not bound to the material. The newer composites being used haven't been around long enough to be subjected to years of wear with longitudinal studies. However, there are several 5-7 year studies that indicate wear characteristics are as good, if not better, than amalgam. Some benefits of the composite materials are:

1) They do not contain mercury.
2) They are esthetically pleasing. When you smile, people do not see black, gray, or silver areas. All they see is what looks like natural tooth color.
3) They do not generate any electrical currents and therefore do not help to corrode any other metallic fillings or restorations you may have in your mouth.
4) There is less loss of your natural tooth structure because the dentist doesn't need extensive preparation for the new materials.
5) The end product using these materials can truly be called restorations rather than fillings.

Composite Materials

Which composite your dentist uses is very important. Many people seeking mercury removal are sensitive to other chemicals. Some chemicals may be in one composite and not another. helping to determine which composite or other dental material might be better for you is the purpose of *compatibility testing*. There are many methods including blood testing, kinesiology, electro acupuncture as per Voll (EAV), or electro-dermal screening. Individual dentists may use the most chemically inert filler for composite filling materials, which is quartz. Most new composites do not use quartz, but various glasses and ceramics that **contain heavy metals** which are added so the fillings show up on x-rays, making it easier for dentists to tell the difference between the tooth, filling, and possible new decay.

The heavy metals added are barium, strontium, and zirconium, the most common being barium. Barium does leach out of the fillings and is associeated with breast cancer. In the mouth, everything leaches. If you really wish to be metal-free, then the composite you use must be metal-free. **There aren't too many composites without heavy metals** because dentists want them to show up on x-rays. They're used to seeing the mercury fillings on x-rays and it's more comfortable for them to see the composites the same way. The goal of the ADA and manufacturers is to have a composite that handles just like mercury fillings so dentists can switch effortlessly. **Amalgam doesn't restore anything.**

Composites are bonded to remaining tooth structure, are thermally insulating, and, with the bases and bonding agents used to place the composite, there is much more protection for the pulp and enamel structure of the tooth. In fact, tooth strength increases, and the tooth can be restored to up to 98% of its predecayed state. Today, there is a much wider selection of materials available in dentistry that can be used as suitable alternatives to the metal. For example, there are products available that are heat and pressure cured, which imparts different structural and finishing properties to the final product. These types of materials are excellent for metal free crowns and for cosmetic dentistry applications such as thin laminates that can be bonded to teeth to cover bad stains, or to cover *diastemas* (spaces between teeth). There are also porcelain laminates and veneers being used for cosmetic applications; and there are metal-free ceramic and/or glass crowns available.

There is now a metal-free partial denture material available. These *flouropolymer thermoplastic* materials are chemically inert and possess remarkable stability. We have in our mouths (1) oxygen, which can cause metal to give up electrons by a process called *oxidation* (just like on your car when it starts to rust); (2) strong and weak acids from our food and drinks, such as coffee, tea, colas and citrus juices that can cause a chemical action to occur in the metals. (3) Heat and temperature differences caused by friction and from chewing as well as from the hot and cold food and drinks that we ingest.

All of these are capable of exciting or generating activity in metal. Where do we stand when we have metal in our teeth like amalgam, or gold or chromium or aluminum, etc.? What we have, is a potential electrical generating plant. Everything needed for electrons to flow from point to point is present. We also have tissue composed of millions of cells that all have some of the electrolytes around them or inside of them. We also have nerves that, for this over-simplified description, can act as transmission lines carrying electric charges to other parts of the body. When an amalgam filling is placed in a tooth, it is subjected to all the chemicals we put in our mouths (which are part of our normal intake of food and drink), and also to some of those produced by our own bodies. The acid or alkaline status of our saliva will vary with our food intake and individual body chemistry.

All of this starts corroding or rusting away that amalgam as soon as it is installed. That's one reason why you periodically have to have amalgam fillings replaced when they become loose and fall out. Besides the chemical corrosion in our mouths, we also have the corrosion that can be caused by the electrical activity previously discussed. We have both of these factors increasing the corrosion of the amalgam, which, in the process, is **releasing metal ions into our saliva**. This corrosion may also reduce the strength of the filling and cause increased marginal breakdown of the amalgam. There are processes by which mercury (and other metals) is **continually being released as vapor and abraded particles**. Electrogalvanic activity associated with metal in the mouth is not a new discovery or phenomenon. Dr. Henry S. Chase of St. Louis and Dr. S.B. Palmer of Syracuse N.Y. first discussed it in scientific literature in 1878. There have been a tremendous number of studies published since that date, all confirming the electrical discharge phenomenon associated with metals in the mouth.

Oral Galvanism

Oral Galvanism

When two different metals are placed in saliva, an electric current called a *galvanic* current is generated by the escape of metal ions into the saliva. It is called *oral galvanism* and literally means that your oral cavity is like a small car battery or miniature electrical generator. All living tissue has an electrical potential. Calcified tissues of the bone and teeth maintain a resting potential. Cellular activity is mainly responsible for the bio-electrical potential in the bone. When metabolism ceases, the potential also ceases. The addition of metals has been shown to increase this electrical potential. When two different metals are placed in saliva, an electric current called a *galvanic* current is generated by the escape of metal ions into the saliva.

Years ago, dentists would not mix metals; they knew that bimetal electrical charges (galvanism) can develop between mercury silver fillings and gold alloy crowns or inlays. Gold crowns and inlays are not pure gold, but an alloy of different metals making the god hard enough to withstand the forces of chewing. It's the mix of various metals, along with mercury silver fillings, that produce this bimetal current. Moreover, the galvanic current produces pathological changes in tooth pulp tissue, indicating that the battery effect of amalgams can affect the health of the tooth.

Electrical charges are created by the action of acids on metals. When acids attack mercury in fillings, a negative charge is created as mercury ions are released into the air and saliva. From there the ions can be absorbed into the body through the lungs or even directly into oral tissues. The *negatively* charged ions can also be attracted to *positively* charged metals, such as gold. Mercury will readily plate gold so that any gold that is in the mouth at the same time as mercury, will have mercury ions on its surface. Another electrical effects occurs when a gold crown is placed over a mercury filling. About half of all crowns have old mercury fillings under them. **This creates an internal current that can cause the tooth to decay.** First reported in the scientific literature over 100 years ago, the existence of this current is common knowledge among any science student and certainly among all dentists.

Anyone who has metal fillings and has bitten into aluminum foil or touched a filling with a metal fork has experienced the discharge of the built-up electricity created by the galvanic current, resulting in a mini-jolt of electricity.

Amalgam fillings (normally having 4 or 5 different metals) **provide the dissimilar metals** and **your saliva provides the electrolytes** (saliva contains various elements such as calcium, magnesium, potassium and acid). **You have all the ingredients available in your mouth to create electrical currents**. Many people have a constant metallic taste, which is accepted as normal. Once all the metals are removed, the galvanic current and the metallic taste leave too. **These electrical currents can be measured** with a special amp meter, and they have two types of electrical charges, *positive* and *negative*. **For every microamp, there are three times ten to the 12th power ions leaving the restoration per second.** Animal studies support the movement of mercury and silver ions leaving amalgam fillings. These ions, that leave the mercury amalgam fillings, have been found in different issues and organs throughout the body.

The current flows from negative to positive. Mercury fillings are generally *negative* and gold is generally *positive*, but the current flow varies greatly because so many different metals are involved. **Amalgam, being electronegative is attracted to the positive calcium ions, which migrate together with the metallic ions of the amalgam, resulting in a separation between the amalgam fillings and the tooth. This process is followed by decay.** It is important to remove the most negatively-charged fillings first, because they are releasing the most mercury. *Amalgam tattoos* are the result of the transference of metallic ions into the gingival or gum tissue. These tattoos also carry an electrical current, and their effect on general health should be examined.

It has been reported in some dental journals that the electrical potential of the bacterial plaque may play a role in the decalcification of the tooth structures associated with the caries process. Voltages produced by bacterial mats vary depending on temperature and the strains of organisms. Mats of mixed cultures may produce up to 160 millivolts. A dramatic increase of up to 450 millivolts has occurred when the mat was flushed over by sugar.

According to Hal Huggins, DDS, it is necessary to measure every tooth for electrical activity so that the patient can start by removing the amalgam with the highest electrical reading. This protocol achieves the best results and makes sense, since highly electrical fillings can often cause surrounding teeth to have higher readings as well

Therefore, it is imperative that accurate measurements of all teeth are taken. Moreover, new measurements should be taken before each amalgam removal procedure, since prior removal may change the electrical readings of the rest of the fillings.

All metals have been identified or graded by their *electropotential* from strong to weak. The stronger the energy capability of the metal, the more electrons it can attract. The weaker the energy force of the metal, the easier it releases or gives up some of its electrons. This is because electrons are always negative and always move from the weaker to the stronger attraction. The galvanic current generated in the mouth can be quite strong, strong enough to sometimes cause small muscle bundles to contract or spasm, like the high school science experiment where a frog's leg is made to move using the electricity in a battery. The muscle contractions caused may create spasms in the lower jaw, leading to discomfort and pain in the *TMJ.*

Now we have an electrolyte in our mouths bathing all our teeth and tissues with a film of liquid having the capability to transport or conduct electrical current from point to point. Each tooth is "wired" to an acupuncture meridian energy channel, and when electricity is applied to this circuit, it can negatively affect the associated organs and glands. Amalgam, like most other metals, when exposed to moisture and oxygen will rust or oxidize. **The corrosion that results produces free electrical currents. When your miniature battery starts generating electrical current, the process of corroding of amalgam fillings is increased.** This increases both the amount of mercury vapor and abraded particles that can be released into the oral cavity. It can also facilitate the **release of free-mercury droplets from the filling.**

Some people are very susceptible to these internal electrical currents. The electrical currents forcing metal ions from amalgam fillings into cells and bones of the oral cavity, causing their transport into the brain via the *trigeminal* nerves or valveless venous pathways. **Gold and mercury fillings, placed opposite each other, can enhance electrolytic corrosion.** So, it could exacerbate corrosion and increase the release of mercury particles and vapor into the oral cavity. **Even standard dental textbooks have warned against this for years.** The silver in mercury fillings tarnishes just as silverware will tarnish and turn black.

As an example, when gold and aluminum are combined with milk as the electrolyte, a current of 65 *microamperes* is registered; if an equal quantity of saliva is added to the solution under similar conditions, the current registers 400; strong tea 110 and zinc chloride mouth wash 300 microamperes.

If a nerve happens to be close enough to a large metal restoration that is capable of generating 900 millivolts or more, and **the nerve only requires 400 to 450 millivolts to cause it to fire**, we have all the ingredients necessary to cause "pain." If the metal in the tooth discharges its electrical current to the nerve, it will cause the nerve to fire and cause a *nerve shock* which the sensory system will then register as pain (it would be almost the same as sticking a pin or needle into the jaw). The anatomic pathways pain may take from the upper jaw may explain why some changes can occur in reflexes, emotions, heart and lung functions.

These pathways permit the pain to travel the network of nerves of the brain stem to the hypothalmus and pituitary, which are the control centers for the autonomic nervous system and major endocrine glands that produce hormones. While the dental profession continues to ignore the dangers of mercury, the medical profession is becoming more aware and concerned about the harmful effects of mercury on the environment and human health. Scientific data clearly demonstrates that **dental amalgam is an unstable product**, that **mercury, even in small amounts, can damage the brain, heart, lungs, liver, kidneys, thyroid gland, pituitary gland, adrenal glands, blood cells, enzymes and hormones, and that it suppresses the body's immune system**.

One part per million (PPM) will alter cell membrane function. Cessation of cell growth or reproduction can occur at levels as low as 0.2 ppm. One ppm ionic mercury will substantially reduce the activity of *succinic dehydrogenase*, *ATPase*, and *alkaline phosphatase* in the brain. *Glioma* cells of the brain are destroyed at 0.2 ppm ionic mercury, and only 0.04 ppm of methylmercury. Even the most resistant parts of the central nervous system are destroyed at 2.5 ppm. Ten ppm ionic mercury will induce cancer-producing DNA-DNA *cross-links*. This amount can also cause genetic defects. Only 2 ppm of the inorganic form will inhibit the rejoining of single-strand breaks in DNA. The blood-brain barrier loses its protective selectivity at 1 ppm within hours of administration of either *ionic mercury* or *methylmercury*.

Oral Potential Meter II

The newly designed Pertec *Oral Potential Meter II* (OPM II) now allows practitioners and patients to see hidden problems for the first time—quickly recording, storing, and displaying electrical activity from metallic restorations in the oral cavity. Unfortunately, the practice of avoiding galvanism has long been forgotten. However, the OPM II now allows one to document this invisible electrical current and helps doctors and patients see the unwanted energy flow and hidden currents.

How Are the Measurements Taken?

The device has two small metal probes. One probe is placed on the filling or crown and the other on the gum just below the filling or crown. A measurement of electro-chemical potential difference of the restoration or crown is taken. The OPM II is equipped with a wireless infrared transmitter that can transmit measurements to a computer receiver. These electrical measurements provide various pieces of information. When a person has ideal health, the electrical readings are as low as possible. Any reading above 10 millivolts would require further investigation by a dentist. If there is a cavity, the OPM II would produce a high electrical reading. A high reading when measuring a crown could mean one of three things: (1) there is tooth decay beneath the crown; (2) there is a silver filling beneath the crown that is reacting with a dissimilar metal in the crown. In any case, a high electrical reading would indicate the necessity for further investigation by a dentist familiar with these concerns.

Functions and Uses of the OPM II

The OPM II performs two basic functions. The primary function is to detect caries susceptibility related to the migration of calcium ions from the enamel, with the metallic ions form the amalgam fillings. Measurable current from amalgam causes decalcification, as evidenced at the margin of the enamel in contact with the filling. The secondary function of the OPM II is to measure the micro amps of the metallic restoration that determines the number of ions of metal leaving the amalgam.

If a patient decides to remove his or her amalgam fillings and embark on a detoxification program using chelating agents to rid the body of mercury, it is imperative to ensure that no crowns with hidden silver fillings underneath them remain. It is not wise to purge mercury while there are still silver fillings in the mouth. Therefore, the necessary precautions, such as diagnostic testing with the *Oral Potential Meter*, must be taken.

Root Canals

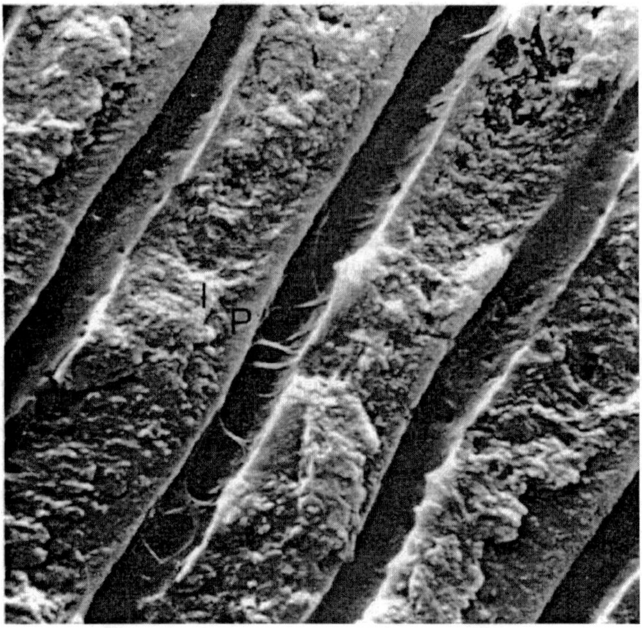

Dentin Tubules Cross-section (6000X)

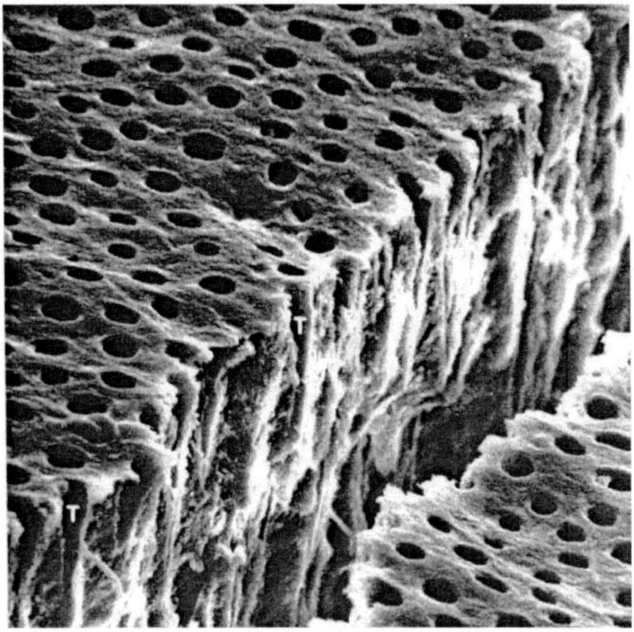

Dentin Tubules (1210X magnification)

Root Canals

Root canals are a part of dentistry called *endodontics*, which is concerned with the pathology of dental pulp and the area surrounding the root. A root canal is a procedure to allow a tooth that is painful or no longer viable because of nerve damage or death to remain in the mouth. Most dentists consider root canals an advance in dentistry--superior alternative to removal of a seriously compromised tooth. However a growing number of physicians, including dentists, believe that root canals can be the cause of, or at least contribute to, a long list of illnesses and degenerative diseases.

A "root canal" allows a patient to keep a dead tooth in his or her mouth. The fallacy with this concept is that the body doesn't like dead things in it and will try, sometimes desperately, to get rid of the dead thing. Notwithstanding, the fact that it may be "handy" to save a tooth for "dental convenience", it does not change the fact that root canal treatments can devastate the human immune system. Twenty million root canals are performed in the U.S. annually, and this number is estimated to double within a few years.

Conventional root canals have been controversial since the turn of the century, when formaldehyde was used to treat the nerve which inevitably killed it, and the bone around the tooth, as well. This treatment is still used by 20% of American dentists and is called the Sargenti method, but it is denounced by the ADA because it contains formaldehyde compounds and lead. The current formulas are said to have removed the lead, but tens of millions of root-canal treatments using the old formulas are still in people's mouths. While the normal dental profession has been striving to improve the technique, much research has shown that even modern root canals pose health hazards to the body. This is due to the delitirious effects of residual infections; from the seepage of toxic substances still used in the process; and from the interference of the flow of bioelectrical energy through acupuncture meridians associated with all the organs of the body.

All conventional root canals still employ toxic substances to sterilize the interior of the tooth, such as eugenol (oil of clove) and formocresol (formaldehyde-creosote). Most dentists also use gutta-percha to fill the canal. In the 1950s. Reinhold Voll, a German M.D., using an electro-acupuncture biofeedback system he had developed, discovered that each tooth in the mouth relates to a specific acupuncture meridian.

He found that if a tooth became infected or diseased, the organ on the same meridian would also become unhealthy. (Conversely, he found that a diseased organ could cause a problem with its corresponding tooth.)

When you have a root canal, or even a big filling, or crown or anything that is not compatible with the body, it sets up an interference field, blocking or altering the energy meridian passing through it. It will affect different parts along that meridian, different organ systems in the body. And usually will cause it to have a problem as well. If the tooth is removed, the energy does tend to pass through it. However, without the tooth in the bone, it is still altered. Without stimulation from a tooth, blood circulation and lymphatic drainage will be impaired, and the bone and tissue surrounding the extraction site can become diseased and die. Infections in the teeth, and toxins, have no place to go but down; down into the jaw bone and into the rest of the body, creating systemic pathologies.

"Root canals" cause:

Suppression of the immune system

The creation of an "interference field" on the meridian that the particular tooth is on (meridian - a channel of energy that flows between different tissues, organs and structures).

Production of the most toxic organic substance known to man.

Root-canal fillings can cause serious side effects. Dr. Weston price is recognized as the greatest researcher that the dental profession has ever produced. Dr. Price, after observing many patients with crippling degenerative diseases not responding to treatment, suspected infected root canal-filled teeth to be the cause. He then embarked on a 25-year-long study to see if his suspicions were correct. This study was done during the first 3 decades of the 20th century! However this information was not shared with us when we were dental students so we had a big void in our dental education where root canals are concerned.

The Procedure

After numbing the tooth, a hole is then drilled in the top of the tooth, just as if a filling were being placed. The hole is deepened until the internal canal (pulp chamber), containing the nerve, blood and lymph vessels, is reached. Then, little tiny files are used to remove the contents of the chamber (live, dead, or dying pieces of nerves and blood vessels).

The dentist now has access to the whole length of the root-canal. Front teeth are supposed to have one, but may have an additional one splitting off of the main canal about one-third of the way up from the apex. These will not show up on X-ray. Multi-rooted teeth, such as some bicuspids and most molars, have two or three roots. Each root has a primary canal and may have a secondary one as well. Lower molars frequently have two canals in one root that sort of blend into each other, forming what is called a ribbon canal. Curved canals present a problem, as the files used to cut out infected dentin are straight.

Sometimes a file will penetrate the tooth at the curve, and cut its way out of the tooth, missing the curve entirely. Toward the bottom 10 millimeters of the tooth, accessory canals may exit the tooth. Removing the dead tissue and bacteria from each of the canals presents the problem of not being able to see whether all the contents are removed. It's a dark tiny hole, down a long skinny root, and bacteria and debris are smaller. Knowing when to stop at the apex is another trick. X-ray films are shadows, and show an approximation of how long the root is, but they don't provide detail about the end of the root. Filling the canal to the x-ray end would actually overfill the canal. Overfilling is a condition most often apt to create infection, thus the presence of unwanted bacteria.

The now empty canal is widened. Next, a series of treatments is begun which clean and shape the root-canal, which kills the tooth. It is then flushed, treated with chemicals to kill bacteria, and eventually filled with one of a variety of materials, the most popular (93% in U.S.), is a substance called gutta-percha. Gutta-percha is a a rubbery, wax petroleum-based latex material, to which some people are allergic. First, the wax is mixed with chloroform to make it soft. Since gutta-percha does not show up on x-rays, heavy metals, including mercury and lead, are added, to make it radiopaque--sometimes up to 20% of its content. Other chemicals it may contain include formocreasol or para-chlorophenol. These substances can cause inflammation and infection, allergic reactions, and compromise the immune system.

Eugenol based cements are used to cement the gutta percha cones into the enlarged canals. Eugenol has an acid pH whereas the living tissues that surround the root have an alkaline pH. To kill the bacteria, caustic solutions are flushed into them, but the surface tension of the solutions is too high to allow it into the narrow dentin tubules.

Sodium hypochlorite (Clorox) and hydrogen peroxide mixtures are used to "sterilize" the inside of the main canals. Sodium hypochlorite and hydrogen peroxide both will injure tissue. These cause inflammation and infection, allergic reactions, and compromised immunity. Studies on thousands of teeth have demonstrated the presence of bacteria in 80% to 90% of the canals after they have been "sterilized."

Once the root-canal treatment is completed, the top of the tooth in which the hole was drilled is restored with either a filling or crown, depending upon the amount of tooth that remains. A patient is routinely told that a crown will be needed for strength because root-canal treated teeth become brittle and weak because of the inside, including the blood vessels and nerves, having been drilled out to do the treatment. It is quite possible that there will be little of the original tooth left above the gum line and that which is left will be weak. In many cases, a post is placed into the root-canal itself to hold the crown.

Compatibility

Conventional dental procedures do not take into account biocompatibility of the filling materials, potential injury to surrounding tissues due to the caustic nature of substances used and a high percentage of residual bacterial contamination. According to research by Dr. Boyd Haley of the University of Kentucky, at least 75% of root canal teeth have residual bacterial infections remaining in the dentinal tubules, of which there are 3-5 miles in length in each tooth. There is no drug, homeopathic remedy, vitamin or mineral that can effectively kill these tiny bacteria that live in the small tubules in the tooth.

Only the use of bio-frequencies (Rife technology) has the capability of pentrating the surrounding bone and root without any damage to tissues. Even then, there is no way to stop new bacteria from entering these tubules from the oral cavity again. These lingering infections produce the most toxic substances known to biochemistry and toxicology, that enter the blood stream and can affect any part of the body.

A dentist, Weston A. Price, brought this information to light in the 1940s. Unfortunately for patients and the dental profession, his scientific documentation and views were pushed aside. To date there is no acceptable conventional therapy to resolve this issue.

Focal Site of Infection

A tooth is an organ, just as any other organ or bone in the body. An abscessed or gangrenous tooth is not only a dead tooth, it is a dead organ. The problem arises because these teeth are dead and prone to infection can threaten to infect surrounding tissue, including the jawbone, possibly triggering cavitations. Today we know that the toxins made by the bacteria that live by the billions in root-canal teeth contain the most toxic organic substance known to man—thio-ethers. Thio-ethers are 1000 times more toxic than botulism toxin, which used to be considered the most toxic organic substance.

So, from a practical standpoint, one would be well-advised to worry less about anthrax and smallpox, and instead, focus on root canals which are much more likely to cause you personal harm. In addition to thio-ethers, other severe toxins from these root-canal bacteria include thio-ethanols and mercaptans which have been found in the tumors of women who have breast cancer, draining through the lymphatic system down the cervical chain of lymph nodes and ultimately in to the breast tissue. Besides being harbored in root canals, these dangerous bacteria also take up residence in cavitations which result from most extracted teeth (see "Cavitations"). Thus one can get a "double-whammy" from the root canals and the cavitations.

Dr. Weston Price

Based on a 25 year extensive study by respected researcher, Dr. Weston Price, scientific data suggests that root canal therapy is the cause of many systemic diseases and illnesses. Dr. Price devised a testing method which disclosed the presence of infection in a tooth which otherwise seemed to be healthy--that is, the implanting of the root canal filled tooth under the skin of a laboratory animal. He found that when the root-filled tooth of a patient with a degenerative disease was extracted and imbedded in an animal, that animal would develop the patient's disease. He did this in over 5000 animal studies and the results were consistent. In the beginning, Dr. Price did not know just where the infection was hiding in the tooth, only that a patient's illness was rapidly transferred from his root-filled tooth to laboratory animals in case after case.

Dr. Price was able to culture the bacteria in root-filled teeth and trap their toxins, reproducing a disease in a rabbit by implanting the extracted root-filled teeth and injecting the cultured material into the animal.

Dr. Price discovered a wide variety of degenerative diseases to be transferable to rabbits.This involved diseases or conditions such as endocarditis and other heart diseases, kidney and bladder diseases, arthritis, rheumatism, mental diseases, lung problems, stomach ulcers, ovarian diseases, phlebitis, osteomyelitis, and pregnancy complications. Those infections proved so devastating that most animals died with 3-12 days. When these same teeth were sterilized with steam heat and embedded in animals, no adverse health effects were experienced. Furthermore, a large percentage of people recovered from their illnesses after extraction of the root canal filled teeth used in the experiments. When sound, uninfected natural teeth were implanted in animals, no adverse health effects were experienced. This vitally important research was forced underground, and has remained virtually unknown since its 1923 publication.

Although root canal therapy is usually successful in eliminating pain and swelling associated with dead teeth, and in allowing those dead teeth to remain in the mouth to function, the side effects can be hazardous to overall health. It is estimated that only about 30% of the population has a healthy enough immune system to ward off the side effects. The problem is that root canal therapy cannot sterilize the inside of the tooth. As a result, the trapped bacteria mutate and migrate to infect the heart, kidneys, eyes, stomach, and countless other body tissues. This theory, called the focal infection theory, states that a person can have an infection someplace and that the bacteria involved can be transferred by way of the bloodstream to another gland or tissue and therein start a whole new infection. Modern experiences also support this theory. Dr. Issels, a German physician, recommends extraction of root canal teeth as part of his protocol for terminal cancer patients.

Over the last 40 years with 16,000 patients, he has observed a 24% total remission rate. Some transplant surgeons require root canal filled teeth be extracted before performing transplant surgery, because of the risk of focal infection to the new organ from the teeth. If a person has chronic health problems, existing root canal filled teeth or dead teeth should be suspected as a possible cause or influence. Estimates for 1996 ran as high as thirty-five million recipients of root canal therapy; however, most cannot describe the procedure beyond the basics. Root canal or endodontic therapy is performed primarily because of bacterial infection. Frequently pain is the motivating factor. Bacteria infiltrating through the dentin tubules under decay can set up housekeeping in the pulp chamber.

This is an ideal environment, being warm, with a constant supply of nutrients, and a waste removal system. Bacteria can wiggle into the dentin tubules (miles-long passageways that traverse the dentin of each tooth) and multiply in accordance with the available oxygen supply.

Since there are varying degrees of oxygen deprivation, each level of oxygen stimulates the bacteria to mutate into a slightly different bacterium; a whole plethora of critters can develop from just one bacterium. Over 150 different bacterial strains have been identified at the apex or within the pulp chamber of dead or dying teeth. All but five are classified as anaerobic, or those that thrive in the absence of oxygen. These bacteria produce toxic waste products. The toxins can either be picked up by the drainage system at the apex of the tooth, or flow down the dentin tubules into the periodontal ligament. At the ligament, they can slip into the fluids around the tooth and flow into the bloodstream. They may also be forced up the ligament space into the mouth when the person bites down or chews. Regardless of which direction the toxins go, they will be introduced to the innermost parts of the body.

The root canal treated tooth is a tooth that is typically still being used in normal chewing. While much of the nerve and blood supply has been removed or damaged by the procedure itself, the tooth still has its original attachment to the jawbone. The high pressures generated in chewing can be expected to physically push toxins out of the socket where they can eventually be picked up by the blood circulation.

Dentinal Tubules

A tooth is basically comprised of 3 layers. The enamel (what we see when we look at another person's teeth, the hard, white attractive outer layer of the tooth), the pulp (a tiny island of soft tissue at the center of the tooth - the same place in a tooth that a core would be in an apple - the so-called "nerve"), and the dentin. Dentin accounts for about 90% of the tooth. When looked at under a microscope, dentin has a very specific structure. It is made up of "millions" of incredibly tiny tubules that radiate outward from the pulp to the outer edge of the tooth.

If one could some how take each of one of these "millions" of tubules in a front tooth and lay them end to end, they would stretch for 3-5 miles. These dentinal tubules are like tiny pipes that radiate outward from the pulp to the outer surface of the tooth–kind of like spokes of a wheel.

The centers of these tubules are filled with living protoplasm. The protoplasm in these tubules has no blood supply so it depends on the blood vessels in the pulp for it's nourishment or sustenance.

Dentin tubules within the root of the tooth can harbor millions of bacteria. These tubules extend from the pulp chamber to the outer bounds of the tooth called the cementum. The periodontal ligament and the apex of the tooth still contain bacteria from the original infection. It is impossible to sterilize the tubules, the ligament, or the apex. Since 93% of root canal treated teeth in the U.S. are filled with gutta percha, and the purpose of filling the canal is to seal the canal from access by bacteria, several basic principles must be ignored to pronounce the canal "sealed."

First, the wax is mixed with chloroform to make it soft. The chloroform evaporates, creating 6.6% space that was occupied by the chloroform. Instruments used to condense the gutta percha are heated in order to soften the wax. When heated wax cools, it shrinks--up to 30% in the first week after placement. This allows a half-micron-sized bacterium to easily make it through the apex, up the root, and into the dentin tubules.

The relatively huge white blood cells cannot get into a dentin tubule. Antibiotics can't gain access either. And the periodontal ligament access is difficult if not impossible. Debris from filling the canal spills out the end of the root, forming a good culture medium for bacteria, while providing a barrier for entrance into the canal. Anaerobic bacteria (those living without oxygen), can inhibit phagocytosis of the white blood cells. Root canal bacterial waste products are the real problem. No white blood cell or antibiotic can destroy the chemicals that are produced by bacteria around the root canal treated tooth.

These chemicals kill the most important enzymes in our bodies at lower concentrations than the most toxic of known organic poisons. Disease can result when these are present at little more than the molecular level of concentration. Mercury at 1 to 5 micromolar concentrations will totally abolish the activity of tubulin without any noticeable effect on other brain proteins. Even one-half part per billion can destroy the most resistant enzymes. Inactivating these essential enzymes can lead to many hormonal neurological, autoimmune, and emotional diseases.

In the presence of these root canal poisons, tubulin and creatine kinase, two critical proteins involved in brain function, are inactivated within a few minutes. In a healthy person, the immune system will form pus, soreness, tenderness, and pain--to tell us dead teeth do not belong there. The dentist, anxious to protect his investment in the root canal, will usually prescribe broad-spectrum antibiotics in an effort to calm the situation. Antibiotics will eventually halt the inflammatory process around the root canal tooth, and the pain will subside, but there is no repair.

The doctor and patient are now lulled into the illusion that the root canal is successful, but the body undergoes further protective activities; if it cannot loosen up the tooth and exfoliate it, the body builds a wall around it and set up a quarantine, a dense layer of calcium, called *condensing osteitis* is laid down around the root, giving the x-ray appearance of healed bone. The bacteria cannot invade the body, nor can the white cells invade the tooth. Even though cells cannot cross the calcium barrier, nutrients can get through to nourish the isolated bacteria, and the toxins can flow into the body unimpeded, to set up disease. There is intense resistance from the dental profession to admit to the potential of root canal teeth being a primary source of "incurable" diseases today. The legal profession and insurance carriers aren't anxious to confront these problems. The root canal tooth can then start the usually silent process of ischemic osteonecrosis (cavitations) in the bone marrow, that can then spread and destroy the blood vessels and nerves supplying adjacent teeth.

Millions of people are ill, suffering from degenerative diseases for which the medical profession is at a loss regarding cause and treatment; the degenerative disease problem continues to bankrupt our people and country. Once a "root-canal" is done to a tooth, the pulp is gone (sacrificed) - which makes a root canal tooth a dead tooth - an expensive, dead tooth. Now the protoplasm in these miles and miles of dentinal tubules dies, and these tubules become a "dandy" place for bacteria to hang out. They have "free eats" on the dead, decaying protoplasm in the tubules.

These tubules are 1 to 1.3 microns in diameter--big enough to accommodate bacteria, but too small to allow entry of white blood cells (which are the body's principal way of controlling excessive bacterial populations). Now your root-canal tooth becomes a bacteria factory. The bacteria now are cloistered away from the body's defenses and thus have free reign to proliferate.

Existing inside the tooth, these bacteria have no access to air so they mutate into the anaerobic form--the kind that can live in the absence of air. When the bacteria mutate, their metabolism changes so that they give off waste products that are incredibly toxic. These toxins include thio-ethers, thio-ethanols, and mercaptans (see "Cavitations").

75% of Root Canaled Teeth Have Residual Bacterial Infections In the Dentinal Tubules

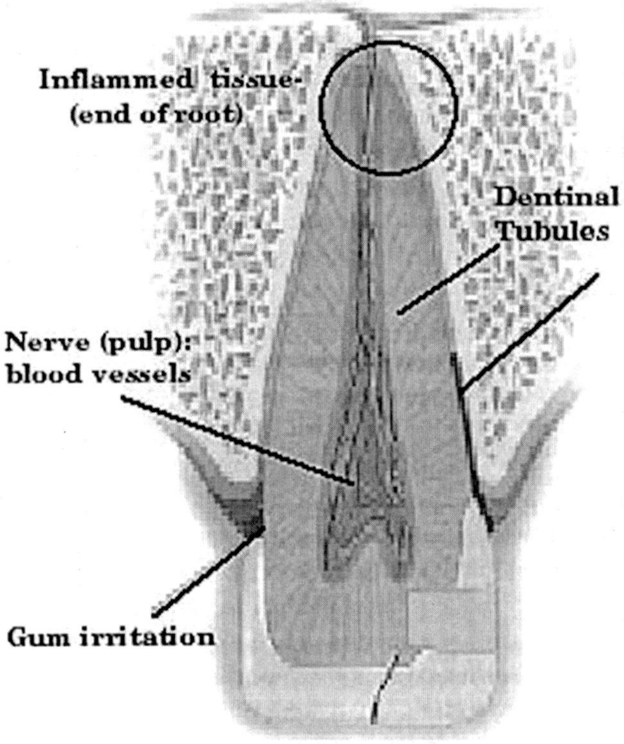

Cavitations

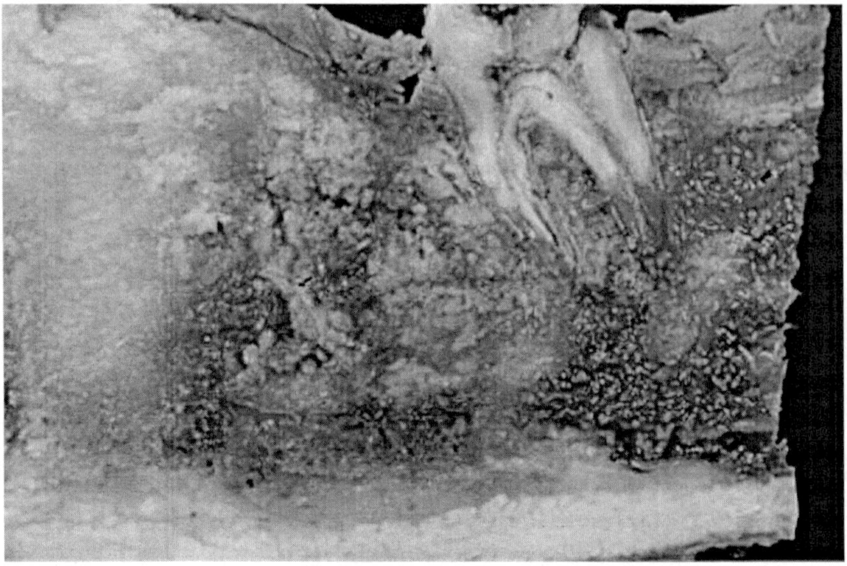

Cross-section of Jawbones Showing Osteonecrosis

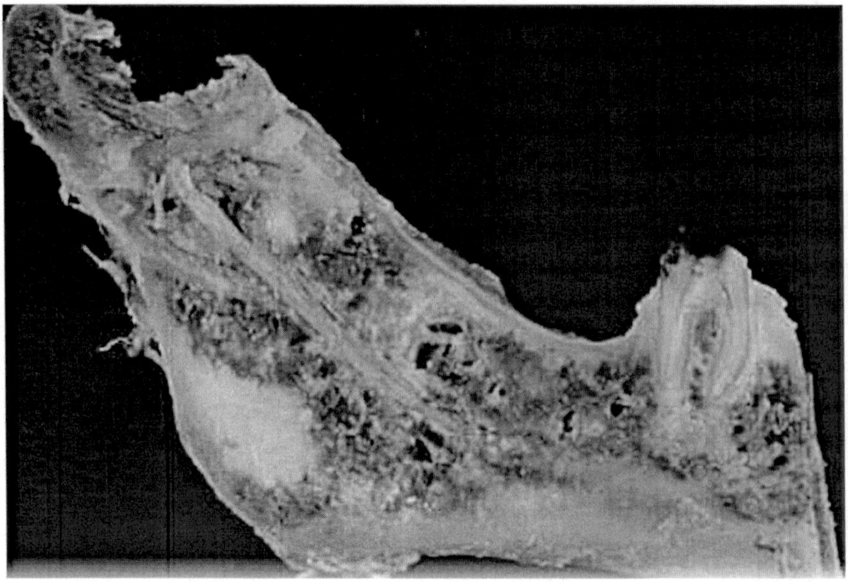

Cavitations

Recent work in the field of facial pain syndromes and *Neuralgia Inducing Cavitational Osteonecrosis* (NICO) has led to the realization that the jawbones are a frequent site of *Ischemic Osteonecrosis*, also known as *aseptic necrosis*, the same as is found in the femoral head or knee. As a result, many extraction sites that appear to have healed have actually not healed completely, and can trigger pain in other parts of the face, head and distant parts of the body.

Even though most of these sites actually present with no symptoms at all, pathological examination reveals a combination of dead bone and slowly growing anaerobic pathogens, with a soup of highly toxic waste products, where we would otherwise think there has been good healing. The incidence is alarmingly high. Researchers in the field have implicated such diverse factors as oral surgery techniques and clotting factors, both endogenous and microbial, in its pathogenesis.

This is a newly emerging disease entity, although the phenomenon of "bone caries" was known and written about in the days of G. V. Black. Criteria for case selection and therapeutic methods are in the early stages of development, as are methods for preventing routine extractions from becoming osteonecrotic lesions. But it's already clear that this is going to be a big issue in the future, and may ultimately force us to totally reevaluate our understanding of the relationship between the tooth and the bone.

A *cavitation* refers to a toxin-containing hole in the jawbone, often at the site of a previously extracted tooth. Cavitations have many scientific names such as *ischemic osteonecrosis, chronic non-superative osteomyelitis*, and *neuralgia inducing cavitational osteonecrosis* (NICO). This is not so much an *infection* in the bone, as a *necrosis* or gangrene (dead tissue) in the bone marrow, as a result of impaired blood flow (ischemia).

A cavitation often develops because of incomplete healing after routine extraction. The contents of cavitations are always **necrotic, dead or dying material**. The microscopic picture looks the same as gangrene! If a gangrenous extremity is not amputated, the rest of the body will sicken and die, due to a high concentration of anaerobic bacterial toxins.

Incomplete healing of a cavitationis promoted by a number of factors, including the following:

* Failure to completely remove the periodontal ligament lining the tooth socket that holds the tooth to the bone

* Physically large surgical excavations, such as with impacted wisdom teeth, where the resulting holes can be expected to be larger than usual and more new bone is required to fill the holes

* Failure to clean out the infected adjacent bone and periodontal ligaments seen in the extraction of root canal treated and abscessed teeth

* Failure to remove condensing osteitis, the reactive bone formation that attempts to wall off infection, usually involving the periodontal ligament as well

* Poor systemic healing support from a compromised immune system

* Poor nutrition and a weak thyroid gland.

* Failure to allow the formation of a complete blood clot at the excavation site; too early dislodgment of a clot after extraction; also bleeding

* Smoking

* Antibiotic therapy
* Chronic osteoporosis of the jawbone

* Systemic and adjacent toxicity from other dental toxins and other sources

* Pre-existing periodontal disease, in addition to any other factor that would also promote periodontal disease

One of the primary factors in cavitation formation seems to be that the initial extraction does not include the thorough removal of the periodontal ligament from the socket after the tooth is removed. Unfortunately, this inadequate socket cleaning is the routine procedure with most extractions.

Cavitation formation after tooth extraction is the rule and not the exception; yet, the condition is still largely unknown to most of dentistry, and underestimated by those who are aware of it. A cavitation can be expected to form when the socket lining separating the tooth from the bone is not thoroughly removed. A thorough removal of the ligament requires that a portion of the bony socket be removed as well.

One purpose of this ligament is to give a certain amount of natural shock absorption to the tooth. Without it, chewing would be much like riding on rims rather than tires. When the periodontal ligament is not thoroughly removed from the socket after the extraction, the surrounding bone receives no notification that the tooth is gone. The continued presence of any portion of the ligament gives the biological message to the surrounding jawbone that all is well, and no new bone growth is needed. Bone cells are not going to start new growth and then migrate through a barrier naturally designed to limit such growth. The jawbone determines that if the ligament is still there, the tooth must be there as well.

Since the periodontal ligament does not extend to the upper edge of the extraction site, new bone growth activity will not be inhibited at the top of the socket, and a characteristic **thin cap of bone will eventually extend over the extraction hole**. Larger cavitations often have only a cap of gingival, or gum tissue, over them. Even the thin overlying cap of bone does not form in these cases. In routine dental extraction, portions of the periodontal ligament will sometimes remain more strongly attached to the tooth than the bone and be removed along with the tooth. When partially removed in this fashion, the spotty absence of the ligament will permit equally spotty growth of bone, resulting in the wide variety of cavitation shapes and sizes.

Even when large wisdom teeth are removed surgically from impacted sites with extensive excavation, **cavitations are nearly always present**. When the excavated hole is large enough, cavitation formation can be anticipated, even if most, or all, of the periodontal ligament is removed, since so much more new bone growth is needed to completely fill the hole. Condensing osteitis must be completely removed to give the opportunity for complete healing. Solid, healthy bone must be reached to allow the normal regeneration of bone. When infection or necrosis remain throughout the socket and adjacent bone, with or without condensing osteitis, **healing will rarely ever be completed**.

Blood clot formation, with its gradual retraction over time as the surrounding tissue heals in, is nature's way of promoting proper healing throughout the body, not just in the mouth. When a nicely formed blood clot fills the socket, healing gets a good start. But when it is dislodged early, or adjacent periodontal disease or smoking causes too rapid a retraction, a dry socket is the result, and cavitation formation can then be anticipated. Preexisting diseases, such as osteoporosis with poor bone structure in the jawbone before the extraction, can clearly promote the formation of cavitations. Bleeding disorders, which would directly impair the formation of the important blood clot, can also be promoting factors. Periodontal disease can also serve to more easily infect the freshly extracted sites and bathe them in the toxins produced by the anaerobic bacteria trapped in the diseased gums.

The presence of local and systemic toxins will also impair the healing process anywhere in the body. The presence of toxins such as heavy metals will chronically disrupt the calcium/phosphorus balance in the body, promoting the continuous mobilization of calcium from the bone into the tissues and into the urine. Any healing bone needs *more* bioavailable calcium, not its *removal*. The procedure to clean a cavitation has often involved use of a blind approach, due to a lack of reliable diagnostic tools. Consequently, dentists have missed smaller and unusually located cavitations. Even a larger cavitation could be missed by the wrong angle of attack by failing to explore the one cusp site that had cavitated. Cavitations will also interconnect and form channels in the jawbone.

An explored channel might be counted as only one cavitation when it actually developed from more than one unhealed extraction site. Many smaller cavitations will never be found because the operator may not opt to explore a smaller area between the teeth on either side of the old extraction site. Larger cavitations can extend below the *mandibular nerve*. Such large cavitations allow the toxins more access to the rest of the body by utilizing the mandibular and other nerve channels. Most dentists seem to convince themselves that if a cavitation cannot be seen on x-ray, it must not be there. However, **a cavitation characteristically cannot be seen on x-ray**. While some cavitations can be clearly visualized on a panoramic x-ray, by those who are trained to identify them, the vast majority of cavitations, even large ones, will be completely missed on a careful examination of the x-rays.

Only a cavitation that has formed with additional calcification around a well-defined border will be visualized on X-ray. The cavitation officially forms when healing at the top is complete. The healing over on top allows the rapid development of an oxygen-deprived, or anaerobic, state in the hole. Native mouth bacteria produce highly toxic metabolic by-products when deprived of oxygen. Bacteria that are normally harmless to man when oxygen is present form a deadly toxin when oxygen is removed. An example of deadly toxins forming when oxygen is absent is the botulism toxin, resulting from vacuum-packed foods, sealed with bacteria present. Some toxins found at cavitation sites are up to 1,000 times more toxic than botulism in their effects on enzymes systems.

Antibiotics will not help the individual poisoned with botulism, nor will they help the cavitation patients, as the problem stems primarily from bacterial toxins, not bacteria.. Only a rapid neutralization of a large toxin dose will save the patient. Toxins in both cavitations and root canal filled teeth **rapidly kill vital human enzymes at the lowest imaginable concentrations**. **Cavitation toxicity tends to be cumulative.** The more cavitations you have, the more toxicity is present. Cavitations also may make other diseases worse. They will make it more difficult for a compromised immune system to ever completely recover. The immune system characteristically tolerates all stresses fairly well until it collapses relatively suddenly. It will compensate as long as possible, then very suddenly its defenses will no longer be effective. Cavitations might not be the cause of an illness, but they can easily be the factor that prevents recovery from it.

Sonic Imaging

There is a new technology that has been developed that can image the jawbone using unfocused ultrasound that provides a color-coded three dimensional representation of the density of the bone and shows loss of bone or ischemic dying bone tissue that is usually not seen on x-ray imaging. This technology, called a *Cavitat,* has been recently approved by the FDA and is now available. It has an incredibly high accuracy record in the findings of a correctly performed scan. This can be done chairside at a dental facility so equipped. Check out the Cavitat website at www.dentalhelp.org. They have references for dentists who have cavitat devices, as well as other educational materials, etc.

Treatment

Surgery is often necessary to properly and thoroughly clean out a cavitation site, for there is no other way to remove dead bone. The key to bone healing and regeneration is through removal of necrosis and support of the thyroid gland, especially by using detoxified iodine. Neither injections into the bone with homeopathic remedies or laser light treatments will work to stop the progressive necrosis. If necrotic tissue is not thoroughly removed, the necrosis will spread and cause more destruction to the bone, nerves and blood vessels. **This kills teeth in the process**, for they are cut off from their blood supply. After cleaning out the necrotic bone, healing can then take place and new bone cells will fill in the cavitations. Unfortunately, there are only a handful of dental surgeons today who do a proper job of thoroughly cleaning out the diseased bone tissue.

Dr. Wesley Shankland has written a very comprehensive book for individuals who suffer with TMJ and related disorders. ***TMJ: Its Many Faces***, 2nd Edition, published by Anadem Publishing, has drawn on Dr. Shankland's experience of over 23 years of treating patients from all over North America and around the world. These patients have seen, on average, six other health professionals prior to seeing Dr. Shankland.

While many of these patients have been told that their TMJ problem is a result of stress, Dr. Shankland has found that nearly 100% of these patients do have physiological and/or anatomical reasons for their pain. This book discusses how the patient can become actively involved in his or her treatment. Included are complete instructions and diagrams of exercises. Lifestyle changes are outlined and a chart of dietary modifications are contained within the book. An entire chapter is devoted to choosing and evaluating a TMJ doctor.

Beyond Amalgam
–The Hidden Health Hazard Posed by Jawbone Cavitations–

Susan Stockton is a recognized writer and researcher in the field of natural health and medicine. In this popular book, she draws from her own experience, as well as obscure but significant scientific research often overlooked by doctors and dentists. Stockton warns the reader about this hidden health hazard that is serious and prevalent enough to warrant the attention of any person who has ever had tooth extractions.

Her website is: www.healthcarealternatives.net

Implants

Implants

Dental implants are intimately involved in the toxicity of cavitations. A dental implant involves the direct insertion of a metal anchor to which a prosthetic tooth is later attached into the jawbone. Even if the procedure were done perfectly, other problems can occur because there is a major difference between a tooth and an implant. A tooth is attached to the bone by tiny ligaments, which act as shock absorbers, letting you sense the hardness of what you are chewing, while an implant is coated so that the bone attaches directly to it This makes the bite extremely critical. If it's too heavy the implant can be damaged or lost. If it's too light, you can't chew well.

Another major difference between an implant and a real tooth is that the gums are not attached to the implant but only "snug up" to the collar that surrounds the post where it comes through the gums. This leaves an opening from the mouth down the side of the post to the bone. Bacteria can make this trip easily, particularly if the oral hygiene is less than perfect. To make matters much worse, the collar is made of **nickel**, a carcinogenic metal or **titanium**, or other metals and, like all of these metals, **creates electrical current**, which is grounded into the bone like a lightining rod.

If a single missing tooth is being replaced with an implant, the crown that fits on the implant has to fit perfectly in the space between the other two teeth. If it is too tight, it will not go in. If it is too small, then **food will tend to pack between the teeth and the implant's crown**. This causes damage to the gums and will quickly damage the implant. Any foreign substance, however biocompatible it may be, can be expected to initiate some degree of **autoimmune reaction** when placed into the body. The dental implant is screwed or planted directly into the jawbone.

Removing dental implants is part of a total dental revision protocol. Sometimes a full cap of bone has already formed, and the cavitation is completely mature in its toxicity when the implant is inserted. There are several types of implants that have been used over the past few decades. There were *pin implants* at one time. These were oversized needles that were drilled into the bone and bound together with a hard plastic. They were quick to place and did not cause much trauma until later.

Stainless steel (a nickel alloy) was used in *blade implants*, then **sapphire** (another word for aluminum oxide) and today **titanium** is popular. There are various ways to place implants, and varying details about what constitutes success. According to Dr. Hal Huggins, anything that is implanted within the bone that is not your own bone will initiate an autoimmune process. The only difference is the speed at which the reaction will occur. Some may react within days, others may go for years before the reaction is noted. He observed this demonstrated once, when we did the dental treatment on a patient with multiple sclerosis. After all the root canals, nickel and amalgam were removed, she experienced a *spontaneous remission*. She was doing quite well, then her hometown dentist looked at her compatibility report, and found that she was not reactive to titanium. He placed three expensive implants, and waited for them to heal. Next he planned to cover them with bridges. Within 3 weeks her MS came back. She called for advice, and he told her to get the implants removed. "But I'm compatible with them." Yes, in the mouth, not in bone

She came back to see Dr. Huggins after healing had taken place, and he constructed partial dentures for her, using titanium. It is *immunocompatible* in the mouth, (the entire digestive tract is considered *outside* the body), where there is a barrier between the material and the *insides* of the body. But nothing is really compatible inside your body except your own tissue. This is upsetting to many people who would like to depend upon the super stability of an implant to place a crown, bridge, or clip onto an *overdenture*. Mechanically they prove to be a boon to the problems of missing teeth. From the biochemical standpoint however, one should know that if you have one placed, you are courting **autoimmune disease**. Which one? Pick one from your genetic host of possibilities. Where is your weak link?

Longevity

How long will an implant last? The dentists who place implants say that over 90% last 10 years or more. The question then has to be asked, "What happens next?" A second implant is rare because whatever causes the first to be lost would stop a new one from being placed. Basically, **you can only get one implant at each acceptable site**. If the patient was 35 when the implant was placed, he may only be 45 when it fails. If it lasted twenty years, he would only be 55.

No further treatment may be the only treatment possible. Some popular brands need to have the crown **removed every year** and a new "shock absorbing" insert placed in the implant. This adds over a hundred dollars in maintenance costs each year. The insert is held in place with a screw that has a tendency to get loose, but if over-tightened, its threads can be stripped. This is a disaster because the threads are in the actual implant and it may be difficult or impossible to repair. If this happens, it may be possible to re-thread it. If the repair fails, the implant must be removed altogether and replaced or abandoned and just left in the bone. Either of these options has many problems, such as contamination of the bone with metal fragments if the implant is cut out, or open access to the bone for oral bacteria if it is left. In addition, there are potential comfort problems trying to find a functional treatment when there is an abandoned implant underneath.

Dental Implant Complications

Infection

The mouth contains many potentially harmful bacteria that lurk in the gums tissues and any of these bacteria can possibly invade the area around an implant. The bone and gums surrounding a dental implant can get infected and cause a dental implant complication. This is most likely to happen when the dental implant is first placed into your jaw. The human mouth is a cesspool and even with the greatest care to avoid contamination, the tissues around a newly inserted dental implant can become infected.

Rejection

Your body does not want anything in it that is not you. A possible dental implant complication is when the body pushes a dental implant out because the dental implant is viewed as a foreign body. Rejection sometimes occurs with other surgeries such as a kidney or liver transplant. Our body protects itself by rejecting anything it does not believe belongs. One of the risks of kidney or heart transplants is that the patient's body can reject the new organ. Dental implant rejection is when this happens to a dental implant. Typically, the first thing that happens with dental implant rejection is that the bone and gums surrounding the dental implant gets inflamed, red and swollen. The patient's immune system attacks this tissue. As the support for the dental implant is lost, the area around the dental implant becomes painful and the dental implant gets loose. In most cases, the dental implant must then be removed.

Overload

Until the bone heals around a dental implant, the biting pressures should be reduced to protect the supporting bone while it builds up. Placing two or three teeth on one implant can cause overload, also. Nature designed teeth to have on tooth root for one crown. The same rule should apply for dental implants. Nobody likes to be overworked. Dental implant dentists say that a dental implant is overloaded when the dental implant has too much work to do. However, dental implant patients do not always want to pay for the best treatment available and dental implant dentists try hard to please their patients.

A dental implant patient can get by with less than one dental implant per missing tooth, but this is not ideal and leads to overworking the dental implants harder than the original natural teeth! In the long run, the money saved may not be worth it. In matters of health, it is always best to choose the best road, not the cheapest. Dental implants can also be overloaded by poorly designing the dental work on top of the dental implants or by poorly placing the dental implants.

Breakage/Failure

Dental implants are made of metal, usually titanium. Metal can bend and break. A dental implant complication is having the metal fixtures coming out of a dental implant break. Things break. There is only so much pressure that metal can take before it snaps and dental implants are made of metal. It is usually the dental implant post that breaks and causes the dental implant failure, not the dental implant. The constant crushing forces of a dental implant patient's bite can cause a tremendous amount of pressure to build up on the dental implant and the dental implant post which can then result in a dental implant failure.

It is very important to place a dental implant in the jaw bone so that it can best handle the forces put upon it. This is the first step in preventing a dental implant failure. The dental work on top of the dental implant must also be designed so that the dental work does not bend the dental implant post when the patient chews. Some dental implant patients grind their teeth constantly and this grinding applies a great deal of force to the dental implant post. When you bend a metal bar with a light force, the bar bends and then returns to its original shape when you let go. This is because the metal is elastic with light forces much like a rubber band. A rubber band can be stretched and it returned to its original force.

When more force is applied to the metal bar, the bar bends but does not return to its original shape. With heavy forces metal is not elastic. It is inelastic! When large sudden forces or constant heavy forces are applied to a metal bar, the metal bar can break. In a dental implant, this results in a dental implant failure. This is what happens when a metal dental implant post or a dental implant screw breaks.

Bone Loss

A patient can have bone loss around a natural tooth. This is called *periodontal disease.* A dental implant complication can be bone loss around the dental implant. Jaw bone supports a dental implant and the dental work connected on top of the dental implant. This bone must remain healthy after the dental implant is placed for the dental implant to last. Unfortunately, the bone surrounding a dental implant is sometimes lost. That's why regular dental x-rays taken of implants are required to monitor the surrounding bone. **X-rays cause cancer.**

There are several reasons for bone loss around a dental implant. If a dental implant patient does not keep the gums surrounding a dental implant clean, the gums can become inflamed. This inflammation can extend into the supporting bone and endanger the dental implant.

If a dental implant is overloaded, this can cause loss of the bone surrounding the dental implant. In most cases, the bone loss starts at the top of the bone (crest) and progresses around the dental implant to form a saucer type defect. In many cases bone loss around a dental implant can be bone grafted after the original reason for the bone loss is successfully treated. The dental work on top of the dental implant is removed to give the dental implant a rest and the gum tissue is carefully treated to restore its health. The same dental work can often be replaced but in some cases, new dental work must be made.

Inflammation

The bone and gums around a dental implant can become inflamed for many different reasons. Inflammation can be a dental implant complication. Inflammation is when a tissue gets red, swollen, and usually hurts. With dental implants, this inflammation can be caused by infection or trauma. Inflammation is bad and it causes lots and lots of special defensive cells to migrate to this inflamed area. Inflammation can lead to bone loss and with dental implants, bone loss is a really bad thing. The supporting bone holds the dental implant in the jaw.

In all cases, the dental implant dentist's objective is to eliminate inflammation. The way this is done is based on the cause of the inflammation around the dental implant. If it is due to infection, then antibiotics and cleaning out the infected area is done. Antibiotics weaken the immune system. If the inflammation is due to trauma, then the dental work on top of the dental implant may be removed or adjusted so it does not bite as hard.

Incision Line Opening

An incision is when a dentist makes a cut in the gums using a scalpel. An opening is then made into the underlying bone in order to place a dental implant. The two edges of the cut gums are then sewed together and this is called *suturing*. An important goal that every dental implant dentist has it to completely close the opening after the dental implant is placed. However, this is not always possible and incision line opening can occur.

Sometimes the dental implant incision line opens and there are several reasons that this incision line opens. The underlying reason is usually that the area of bone exposed was so large that the amount of gums pulled up off of the jaw bone was too large to keep its blood supply. All human tissues, especially gums, need blood to live and when the blood is cut off; the tissue has problems and can even die (*necrosis*).

If bone grafting was done and the dental implant dentist put too much bone grafting material in the dental implant surgical site, the gum tissue could have been pulled too tightly when the suturing was done. This tightness cuts off the blood.

Dental Mercury Disposal

Dental Mercury Disposal

Dental offices have been collectively identified as the major source of mercury pollution in wastewater, and they're not buying the excuse that amalgam is stable and doesn't break down. Regulatory action has begun in several jurisdictions. It's considered a hazardous material before it's used, and a hazardous waste after it's removed, but not when stored in people's mouths?

Mercury is a persistent, bioaccumulative toxin that poses a risk to human health, wildlife and the environment. While there has been considerable public debate about the potential health effects of mercury fillings, little attention has been focused thus far on the disposal of waste dental mercury. While mercury is a naturally occurring metallic element, human activities—including the use of dental fillings—contribute 70% of emissions into the environment. Levels of mercury in the environment have increased dramatically, with **a twenty-fold increase** over the past 270 years. Today, dentists are the third largest user of mercury in the U.S., consuming **over 40 metric tons of mercury annually** with most eventually released into the environment. In 1993, it was estimated that 150 million amalgam restorations were placed in the USA, weighing over 75 tons, by 175,000 U.S. dentists, and that there are 22 billion existing amalgam restorations that will eventually have to be removed, according to the A.D.A.

The name "mercury-free dentist" is misleading. The so-called mercury free dentist releases enough mercury in one day to contaminate a 22,000-acre lake to above acceptable discharge levels. The largest single source of dental mercury released into the environment comes from the removal of existing amalgams from patients during dental procedures (replacement fillings, crowns, extractions, etc). Extracted amalgam materials are either rinsed down the drain—usually to a municipal wastewater system (or septic system) where it can build up in sewage sludge—deposited in biomedical waste containers destined for waste incineration or autoclaves, or placed in the trash that is later disposed in municipal waste landfills or incinerators. It is estimated when an amalgam is prepared for a filling, 10% is leftover and is often simply discarded. The "over-pack" portion is either drawn into the dental clinic's waste vacuum system or is expelled by the patient into a chair side cuspidor. But the majority of dental mercury waste is discarded into wastewater systems.

Dental clinics remain largely unregulated for mercury disposal and extracted amalgam materials are often rinsed down the drain, usually to a municipal wastewater system or septic systems, deposited in biomedical waste containers destined for waste incineration, or placed in trash disposed in a municipal waste landfill or incinerator. The American Dental Association (ADA), as well as many state dental associations, have refrained from promoting, and oppose mercury reduction efforts. Following the lead of the ADA, the U.S. dental establishment has **consistently resisted efforts to reduce releases of mercury** and follow suit with the rest of the health care establishment.

The ADA refuses to encourage its members to assume responsibility for curtailing dental mercury pollution, opting instead to **obstruct initiative at the state and local levels**. Many countries, especially in Western Europe and Canada—and a small, but growing number of local and state governments in the U.S.—now recognize dental mercury waste as a serious environmental pollutant and are enacting both voluntary guidelines and stringent policies to curtail its release.

Studies by EPA and numerous municipalities document that most municipal wastewater treatment plants have high levels of mercury with significant contributions from dental clinics. Recently, the *Association of Metropolitan Sewerage Agencies* (AMSA) evaluated seven major municipal wastewater treatment plants (WWTPs) to determine and quantify sources of mercury coming into these facilities. AT all plants, dental uses were identified as "by far" the greatest contributors to the mercury-load, accounting on average for 40% of the load, more than three times the next largest source.

There is little debate that municipal wastewater treatment systems are not designed to treat hazardous waste or reduce mercury loadings to the environment. Consequently, all mercury in the influent wastewater remains unattenuated in municipal treatment plants, and either settles out in the *grit chamber* or residuals (*sludge*, or *biosolids*), or passes through the system to be discharged into a downstream lake, river or ocean along with the "treated" effluent. Moreover, conditions at certain points within the wastewater treatment process are perhaps favorable for promoting methylation of mercury within the wastewater or sludge. This has the effect of converting a portion of the influent mercury into its more toxic, organic form (methyl mercury), which is also highly soluble and able to pass through the facility to the receiving water body. Mercury amalgam particles that drop out of wastewater in the grit chamber (the initial coarse settling chamber at the front end of a treatment plant), are most commonly landfilled along with all other filtered materials. The residual sludge, which is the primary byproduct of the treatment process, is frequently incinerated. **Incineration releases the mercury directly into the atmosphere as mercury vapor**.

Studies indicate that as much as 95% of the mercury load to the treatment plants is released to the atmosphere during sludge incineration, with the balance discharged to a body of water or landfilled. When not landfilled or incinerated, *biosolids* are **used in fertilizers or other soil additives**. Agricultural sludge application can lead to mercury contaminated soil and groundwater, as well as direct volatilization to the atmosphere. Regulations for land application of sludge in the U.S. are far less restrictive for mercury and other heavy metals than many other countries. This practice has not been thoroughly studied and is further hindered by the fact that both state and federal agencies responsible for regulating sludge-spreading are also often responsible for promoting it.

Mercury In Traps, Drains, and Sewer Pipes

Following years of use, the plumbing in dental offices can become significantly laden with dental amalgam. Studies show that high levels of mercury are accumulating in sewer pipes from dental offices, presenting potential liability concerns to land owners. Amalgam particles trapped in dental office plumbing and drainage pipes have been found to provide a continuing source of dissolved mercury to wastewater over time. The slow dissolution of mercury amalgam in dental office plumbing, as well as the municipal sewer system, serves as a long-term source of mercury to the receiving facility and is eventually released in the environment.

Mercury In Septic Systems

Where no publicly operated treatment works exist, dental clinics frequently rely on septic systems for wastewater disposal. Similar to municipal treatment plants, the potential for methylation exists in the *anaerobic* environment of a septic tank, which can lead to the production and **discharge of methyl mercury** at private disposal fields. At these locations, the mercury path to the environment is more direct and the soils and groundwater surrounding the drain fields of these systems can become contaminated with mercury.

Significant levels of mercury contamination have been detected both within septic tanks as well as adjacent to, and downgradient from, disposal fields receiving wastewater from dental clinics. The drain fields of septic systems receiving dental wastewater have the potential to serve as point sources of **mercury contamination to the underlying and adjacent soils and groundwater**, and may potentially convey environmental liability on to the property owner, and/or wastewater generator.

Solid Waste

Mercury-bearing scrap amalgam is often discarded into the trash and leaves the dental office by solid waste hauler and is either landfilled or incinerated. The mercury in amalgam disposed in a landfill may break down over time and co-mingle with landfill leachate. Depending on the landfill, mercury may enter groundwater, contaminate underlying soils, volatilize into the *vapor phase* and dissipate to the atmosphere or, when landfill leachate is sent to a wastewater treatment plant, is taken up in sewage sludge that is either **re-landfilled** or **distributed**.

Also, formulation and release of methane gas from landfilled mercury may contribute to production of mercury emissions within the landfill.

Biomedical Waste Incineration/Sterilization

Waste dental mercury is often disposed into the biomedical waste container. A recent survey found that 25 to 30 percent of dentists place their contact amalgam wastes into biomedical "red bags" that are often incinerated. Medical waste is a special type of regulated waste due to the potential presence of bacteria and pathogens, which is separated and handled differently from other solid wastes. If any amalgam has come in contact with the mouth or has been removed from or with teeth, it is considered *contact amalgam* and is often discarded into biomedial waste.

So-called "red-bag" waste is often sent to a medical waste incinerator, where the mercury is vaporized into the atmosphere. Some handlers of biomedical waste sterilize it with high temperature and pressure steam in a process known as "autoclaving." Oftentimes, these facilities operate with **no emission controls or standards**, which result in **mercury vapor releases**, and discharge of effluent to the local wastewater system following sterilization. The residuals from this process are landfilled.

Recycling

A small but increasing number of dental clinics are beginning to have their mercury recycled. Where collection systems are in place, approximately 60% of all mercury-bearing amalgam waste is captured in coarse filters at chairside, and 95% or more of the mercury can be cost-effectively captured when an amalgam separator is added to the system. These programs are, in general, effective and require only a modest shift in practices, and add a very minor increase in operating expense. According to recent estimates, an amalgam separator unit capable of removing both particulates and dissolved mercury can be operated for between $47.95 - $100.00 per month.

Human Wastes

Amalgam has been determined to be the primary source of mercury in human waste. After releases from dental offices, human wastes are the **next greatest contributor of dental mercury to waste water treatment plants**. In addition, amalgam fillings are responsible for additional environmental releases of mercury at the end of life. Each **cremation** in the U.S. accounts for, on average, **one gram of mercury,** due to vaporization of mercury contained in dental amalgam fillings, being **released into the atmosphere.**

Solution

It costs less than $50.00 a month, about the cost of placing a single filling to remove and recycle mercury from amalgams. However, only a small percentage of dentists nationwide have taken the steps necessary to reduce use and release of this dangerous toxin. Clearly, the time has come for U.S. dental associations—as other health care industry associations are already doing—to embrace the fundamental credo of "first do no harm," by taking responsibility to reduce amalgam use and mercury pollution. Environmentally responsible dental clinics reduce the use of mercury where feasible, employ best management practices and operate amalgam separators to get the highest capture rates of dental mercury. This protects human health and the environment while requiring only a modest, compact, and available shift in clinical practices and expenses.

The *MAXIMUM Separation System* is a dental amalgam separator that removes dental amalgam, thus removing mercury from dental wastewater before it is discharged into the public sewer system and the environment.

A cost effective way for small and large dental offices and institutions to manage their amalgam waste is pollution reduction at the source with the use of the MAXIMUM Separation System. It has been certified to ISO 11143 standard.

It can be retrofitted into existing dental vacuum systems. It is located BEFORE the vacuum pump, thus removing the amalgam waste before it is agitated by the vacuum pump impellers. This decreases the release of mercury and reduces wear on the pump.

Heavy Metal Detoxification

Heavy Metal Detoxification

The most common source of heavy metal toxicity is dental amalgam fillings and other metal dental appliances. In 1989, the Environmental Protection Agency (EPA) declared that amalgams are a **hazardous substance** under the Superfund law. Scrap dental amalgam was declared a hazardous waste in 1988 by the EPA. Outside of your mouth it has to be: 1. Stored in unbreakable, tightly sealed containers away from heat. 2. It is not to be touched. 3. Stored under liquid glycerine or photographic fixer solution. So, once it is taken out of the mouth it is *toxic*, but when it is placed in the teeth it is labeled *nontoxic*. You can't legally throw it in the trash, bury it in the ground or put it in a landfill, but they say it's okay to put it in people's mouths!

It is **truth decay**! Lead, mercury and cadmium exert most of their toxicity by **destroying important proteins**, many of which are enzymes, hormones, or cell receptors. Mercury will attach to sulfur amino acid building blocks in proteins. The sulfur amino acids are *methionine*, *cysteine*, and *taurine*. Sulfur is present in all proteins. Numerous enzymes require intact sulfur groups and many are *inactivated* by mercury. Lead binds with the sulfur groups on proteins and inactivates them. Lead suppresses neuron clusters in the brain, hindering brain development in children by stunting the mapping of sensory nerves.

One of the primary ways the body gets rid of metal compounds is through a pathway that goes from the liver into the bile where it is then transported to the small intestine and excreted in the feces. Inorganic mercury is complexed with glutathione in the bile, suggesting that glutathione status is a major consideration in the biliary secretion of mercury. This same pathway is affected by a mercury induced reduction of available **taurine** needed to produce bile acid *(taurocholic acid)*.

When the microflora of the intestine have been reduced through stress, poor diet, use of antibiotics and other drugs, fecal content of mercury is greatly reduced. Instead of being excreted in the feces, the mercury gets recirculated back to the liver. The person who is under stress, eating a poor diet, and/or taking antibiotics will tend to maintain a higher body burden of mercury derived from dietary sources–especially if they are eating diets high in fish. The following is a list of nutrients that facilitate the removal of heavy metals.

Mega H$^-$ The negative hydride ions in *Mega H*$^-$ alter the water consumed with the food and supplements in our diet, to have a **lower surface tension** and an **increased conductivity**. A low surface tension in the extra cellular fluids is also important in the removal of toxins from the cells and into lymph and venous blood for removal from the body. Tap water has a surface tension of approximately 73 dynes/cm. The water around our cells has a surface tension of approximately 45 dynes/cm. The body must **reduce the surface tension of water** consumed for *nutrients* to pass through cell walls and for *toxins* to pass out of the cells.

Glutathione contains *cysteine, glycine* and *glutamic acid.* The liver manufactures glutathione whenever extra *cysteine* is available. Blood glutathione levels change in direct proportion to the amount of *cysteine* in the diet. One 50 milligram capsule or tablet, three times a day taken on an empty stomach is a good starting dosage. Individuals with insulin deficiency should not take glutathione.

Methionine levels are a major determinant in the liver's concentration of sulphur-containing compounds, such as *glutathione* and *cysteine.* As methionine is the **precursor for the manufacture of cysteine** in the body, extra supplementation of this critical amino acid should increase available cysteine. One 200-500 milligram tablet two-three times a day is indicated for glutathione. The desired intake is 1000 mg/day.

N-Acetyl-L-Cysteine (NAC) forms *L-cysteine, cystine, L-methionine, glutathione* (GSH), and mixed *di-sulfides*. Stimulates the body to produce large amounts of cysteine and glutathione, thus greatly augmenting plasma and red blood cell content of both cysteine and glutathione.

Methylsulfonylmethane (MSM), like fresh garlic, provides a bioavailable dietary source of sulfur. MSM exerts a direct beneficial effect in ameliorating a variety of allergic responses and pain associated with systemic inflammatory disorders.

Milk Thistle (silymarin) provides support and protection against liver toxins which can cause free-radical-mediated oxidative damage. Silymarin is many times more potent in antioxidant activity than vitamin E. In addition, it increases liver production of glutathione and protects red blood cell membranes from peroxidation and hemolysis.

Chlorella: Is a food-like all purpose mild chelator of heavy metals; it is a specially processed green-algae type of food that is taken with meals and is quite tolerable and pleasant for many. But since chlorella is so easily contaminated, the manufacturer's quality control is important. Nature's Balance is a source of high quality chlorella that can be taken as a part of a person'd detox program.

Cilantro stimulates the body's release of mercury and other heavy metals from the brain and CNS into other tissue. This facilitates the ability to remove heavy metal from the body using other dietary protocols, such as Chorella and other chlorophyll containing herbs such as Nettles and Alfalfa. These herbs aid in detoxifying by denaturing the toxins, protecting and restoring normal cellular functions while promoting elimination. The major constituents of the volatile oils are: myrcene (1.71%), d-linalool (52.26%), citronellol (4.64%), geraniol (9.29%), safrole (2.67%), aterpinyl **acetate (1.07%) and geraniol acetate.** A typical dose is orally 6-15 drops *1/2* hr. before or 1 hr. after meals 2x/day. For 5 days. 2 day rest and continue. Or Apply ¼ *to* ½ dropper on wrists, joints, or affected areas twice a day.

Vitamin B_6 is needed in the metabolic process that converts *methionine* to *cysteine* and then into *glutathione*. B_6 is capable of reducing and controlling the swelling and pain associated with the routine tissue and bone trauma resulting from normal dental operative procedures. You can also use *Pyridoxal-5-phosphate* (P5P), the active form made in the body.

Vitamin B_1 is capable of reducing pain that may be associated with routine dental operative procedures. B_1 is one of two B-vitamins containing sulfur, the other is *biotin*.

Magnesium availablility is essential for the proper functinoing of the immune system as well as hundreds of enzyme systems critical to human health. Organically amino acid-bound forms of magnesium are more easily absorbed and are less irritating to the gastrointestinal tract.

Activated Charcoal taken immediately with *chlorella*, 15 minutes before drilling/chunking out amalgam, will bind any swallowed mercury and also prevent recirculation in the liver. **Refrain from taking any supplements that contain iron and copper.** Mercury amalgam removal alone does not put an end to the mercury poisoning.

The mercury which leached from the fillings in the mouth is stored in cells throughout the body and continues to exert its damaging influence. It is not unusual to see patients who have had their amalgam fillings removed and replaced ten to fifteen years prior to testing still having elevated levels of mercury in the body. Once mercury toxicity has been demonstrated, by tests such as high electrogalvanism, high mercury vapor emissions, and/or high urine or stool mercury excretion after a challenge, mercury amalgam removal and replacement with alternate, non-toxic materials is the recommended step. Botanical substances to assist in removing the mercury include *cilantro* and *chlorella* which are particularly effective.

Clay

Clay has been used for thousands of years by the Egyptians, Mayans, and the Native American Indians, and yet no one has been able to pin down what makes it a healer. Various observers offer differing perspectives how clay works. Raymond Dextreit, the French naturopath who popularized the clay cure in his own country, believes clay's powers, particularly from *bentonite*, a particular kind of clay, transcend its purely three-dimensional physical properties. "From a *thermodynamic* point of view," he writes, "clay cannot be the sole source of energy of the phenomenon it produces. Clay is a dynamic presence–a *catalyst* rather than an *agent* itself. This is possible because clay is alive." Most of the poisons in the body Dextreit notes, are *positively* charged, whereas clay has a *negative* electrical attraction. Thus, he writes, "These toxins cannot resist being drawn toward the clay." Bentonite's minute particles create a **large surface area** in charged particles or toxins.

The crystalline lattice of clay gives it the ability to store energy and then re-emit it. Certain bentonite clays are a powerful agent of *stimulation, transformation* and *transmission* of energy. It has a natural magnetic action and transmits an extraordinary strength to the organism, and helps to rebuild vital potential through the liberation of latent energy. This natural Earth remedy is a quick and inexpensive way to pull those toxic substances out of the body. It is crucial to use 'clean clay.' One example of a clean clay is from *LL's Magnetic Clay Detox Baths* The industrial clays found in may health food stores, contain *aluminum*, and contain *chemical emulsifiers*, defeating the whole purpose of the treatment. The clays can be used for hydrotherapy immersions, or consumed orally to detox the system.

Sweating

The skin is the body's largest detoxiification organs and sweating can help draw mercury from the body. Saunas are a useful adjunct to safe mercury removal because they induce copious sweating. Initiate sweating and increased circulation by exercising 20 minutes three times a day on a rebounder (mini trampoline). Immediately following the exercise, sit in a sauna or under infrared lights (infrared sauna) for up to 30 minutes, then take a cool shower. The temperature from a "low heat" sauna should be between 140 to 180 degrees F. in contrast to the 200 to 210 degree F. for a non-therapeutic standard sauna.

The sauna may be followed by a plunge into a bath or under a shower whose temperature is 65 degrees F. Over a period of three to four days, increase your time in the sauna to a total of up to two hours, divided into 30-minute periods with a short cooling-off period in between. It's important to shower and towel dry because the removal of sweat prevents reabsorption of toxins. While doing the sauna program, consume adequate amounts of water to avoid dehydration. This is a minimum of two quarts before and after entering the sauna. Replace the electrolytes lost to perspiration with grape or prune juice, and drink vegetable juices to replace calcium and magnesium lost through the skin.

Heavy Metal Chelators

DMSA and DMPS are heavy metal chelators. They are both effective at that function, but **either one can be very dangerous.** *Dimercaptosuccinic acid* (DMSA) is a drug which is approved by the FDA for use in acute metal poisoning. Its trade name is *Chemet*. DMSA is considered to be much safer than DMPS. In research studies, DMPS proved to be **three times more toxic than DMSA**. DMSA is much less likely to bind to the beneficial minerals, as DMPS does. DMSA and DMPS actually bind to and mobilize mercury. It takes properly functioning excretory systems to then move the chelator-bound metal out of the body. So in order to get the heavy metals out of your body, you have to dislodge them from their present locations, and move them so that the liver and kidneys can excrete them.

Whenever heavy metals are moved, there is an increasing risk of damage done to the body. Anywhere along the way, the chelator can lose its grip and drop the metal. If the excretory systems are not functioning well, the metal the chelator has mobilized will be unable to be excreted, and the mobilization will just do more damage.

Two of the most important factors in determining chelation safety are *dosage* and *frequency*. Aspirin is generally considered to be a safe drug, but if a whole bottle of aspirin is taken all at once, it can kill a person. It is no different with chelators. Too *much* can be not only toxic, but lethal. Too *little* is ineffective. Very few doctors know how to use any of these chelators safely and effectively. DMSA and DMPS are available only by prescription. Respected toxicologists claim that these chelators should only be used in cases of acute metal poisoning, or as a last resort for intractable chronic poisoning.

DMPS

A protocol for diagnosing chronic mercury toxicity is the "DMPS challenge test". A patient is injected or infused with approximately 250 mg of DMPS. After this infusion, the patient provides a 24-hour urine sample to a testing laboratory. The results will always show high levels of mercury, even in patients with no discernible health problems. There's a simple reason for this. It's because the reference values, or *norms* to which they are comparing the patient's urine are for healthy populations who have *not* had an injection of a metal chelator like DMPS. It is a misleading, even fraudulent report. Some physicians are as fooled as the patients. They don't understand that the results are skewed.

Dimercapto-propane sulfonate (DMPS) is **not approved by the FDA**. FDA approval occurs when a new drug has gone through monitored clinical trials which assess the drug's metabolic effects on the various physiological systems. From such trials, protocols for safe and effective use are developed, and side effects and contraindications are made known. This has not been done for DMPS. The majority of patients who try DMPS will not have a serious adverse reaction. Most patients will have only mild side effects, but a minority of patients experience serious adverse reactions. Because neither physicians nor patients are reporting these adverse reactions, it is not known just how frequent they are.

DMPS frees up stored mercury, but is unable to maintain a secured bond to all that it has shaken loose. That permits the loosened mercury to enter the bloodstream and be redistributed to other places in the body, doing new damage. These chelators merely *mobilize* mercury. It takes properly functioning excretory systems to *remove* the DMPS-bound metals from the body. EDTA, DMPS or DMSA draws the metal toxins out of the cells and bones where the body *sequesters* (binds) them as conju gates with glutathione, metallothionine and phosphates, respectively, and then dumps them into the bloodstream where they can poison the immune and nervous systems, and vital organs. Consequently these poor individuals can remain extremely toxic and incapacitated for years.

The *informed consent form* lists the following adverse effects: *pancreatitis* (inflammation of the pancreas), *nausea, headache, muscle pain or weakness, gastrointestinal symptoms* (nausea, diarrhea, stomach pain), *rashes, sensomotor neuropathy, decreased urination, cardiac arrhythmias* and *allergic reactions*.

A scientific monograph on DMPS from Heyltex (*DMPS-Heyl* is the *parenteral* form, *Dimaval* is the *oral* form), revealed the following: "Contraindications: DMPS should not be used in the presence of hypersensitivity to DMPS or its salts. Special care is required on injection of DMPS-Heyl in patients with allergic asthma symptoms. Side effects: Occasionally shivering, fever or skin reactions, presumably of an allergic nature, such as itching and exanthema or rash may occur, which are generally reversible on withdrawing treatment. In isolated cases severe allergic skin reactions have been reported. Long-term use of DMPS can influence the mineral balance, especially for elements zinc and copper. Administration of DMPS causes mobilization of mercury taken up in the body. In isolated cases therefore, **Clinical symptoms of mercury poisoning may be produced.**

In individual cases there may be raised levels of certain enzymes (*transaminases*). After ingestion of *Dimaval* (DMPS) nausea may rarely occur. Cardiovascular reactions may occur, especially on too rapid injection of DMPS-Heyl and is apparent as a fall in blood pressure, nausea, dizziness and weakness generally a short time after injection." DMPS should not be given to any patient who has metal in his/her mouth. The drug can quickly enter the saliva, and begin to dissolve the metals in the mouth, pulling them into the body, and resulting in "acute poisoning of the mucosa of the gut."

More researchers are recommending that synthetic chelators be avoided for six-months to a year after amalgam replacement. A person is more likely to have an adverse reaction to DMPS if s/he is allergic to sulfa drugs, or sulfites. DMPS can also combine with copper to form more toxic complexes.

Oral Metal Chelation

Metal Free

Recent clinical experience with the use of a new heavy metal *clathrating* agent "Metal Free" suggests that it is more efficient and quicker acting than chlorella, cilantro, *DMPS*, garlic, lipoic acid and a niacin/sauna detox. It is classified as a 'dietary supplement,' is **non-toxic**, and is **not a drug**. It removes heavy metals from the tissue, brain and nervous system simultaneously. Patients who previously had little to no improvement with up to two years treatment with DMPS experienced total abatement of associated symptoms in a short time taking *Metal-Free*.
Ingredients include:

* Microactivated algae
* Peptidyl gluconase
* Hydrated colloidal silica
* Ionic minerals from sea water rich in calcium potassium and magnesium.
* Glutathione
* Vitamin C
* Hyaluronic Acid
* Fulvic, Ferulic and Lipoic acids
* Chlorella
* N-Acetyl-L-cysteine
* Proprietary ratio of 12 beneficial flora ferments including *lacto bacillus bulgaricus, acidophilus, salivarius, strep, hemophilus*, sub species and beneficial soil bacteria.

The peptide in *Metal-Free* binds to metals and other matter at *several* sites rather than at just *one*. This creates a *non-competitive* irreversible bond. On the other hand, with intravenous chelation of heavy metals, a *competitive* reversible bond is created, allowing the possibility of metal reattachment within the body. The peptide's affinity to metal is 10 orders of magnitude stronger than other chelators. This means that when a metal is picked up by *Metal-Free* it will not lose the particle on its way out of the body. Metals may be removed in the urine, sweat or fecal matter. Furthermore, the product is orally active as it is absorbed into the oral mucosa and crosses the *blood brain barrier*. **Actions**:

* Engulfs (clathrates) and removes heavy metals prioritized according to the descending order of their valence (heaviest first)

* Clathrates *lipopolysaccharides*, cell wall residue of microorganism, nucleic acid fractions from microorganisms, endotoxins
* Anti-microbial effects noticed in hepatitis A and C and renal failure
* Beneficial effects noticed in Hepatitis B and renal failure
* It is a cleanser and tonic for the liver
* Is completely non-toxic
* Does not pull beneficial minerals out of the body

A *peptide ligand* binds with greater affinity to cell receptor sites than heavy metals thereby releasing the heavy metals. A companion molecule straps onto (*clathrates*) the toxin keeping it soluble and flowing in the circulation for elimination. The cell receptor sites in the body have a lesser affinity to heavy metal as compared to *Metal-Free*. This means the locations in the body where metal is being stored will release this metal when the product pervades its area. When the metal is released from the receptor site, a molecule in the *Metal-Free* formula attaches itself onto the metal or toxin, which keeps it soluble and in circulation for removal. The formula attaches itself using all three methods of bonding (*ionic, covalent*, and *hydrogen* bonds) while DMPS uses only *ionic*. This prevents the metal from being carried away and reattaching itself into another area of the body. Delivery via:

1. Silica water
2. Borosilica water
3. Peptide water
4. Protein water–small spherical particles of the colloid, nanometers in diameter, provide water with the *hydrogen bond angle* increased to 180 degrees (linear water) thus lowering the surface tension and making the water 'wetter," therefore penetrating via the mucosa more efficiently.

Metals are clathrated in the following order: lead, thallium, cadmium, arsenic, aluminum, mercury. Because the mercury goes into a methyl form, it can hide in the fatty tissues and is thus more difficult to remove. If a person has more lead (or any other heavier metal) than mercury and you are only measuring mercury in the urine, you will not see the mercury go down until the lead (or other metals) has been clathrated. Any metal that belongs in the body has an enzyme system suited to it, as it is part of a living system, and is thus well protected and tightly bound.

Heavy metals do not belong in the body and do not have natural enzyme systems to protect them. *Metal-Free* goes after non-complexed, loosely bound metals. It does not interfere with Cu, Fe, or Se. If, however, there is an excess of a mineral, for example Ca in plaque, it will bind with it. *Metal-Free* penetrates inside the cell and reaches the *mitochondria* because it is recognized as a nutrient. Methods of analysis utilize *neutron activation analysis, atomic absorption spectrometry* and *atomic fluorescence spectrometry*.

Any other tests are not recognized as accurate by the analytical chemistry profession, including *flame ionization* coupled with *mass spectrometry* as utilized by many popular labs. Final analysis is performed using continuous flow vapor generation coupled to *Atomic Fluorescence Spectrometry*. One dose of *Metal-Free* lowers the measured ppm of heavy metal by 1 ppm. A 150 lb. person with 50 ppm mercury in the urine would require approximately 50 doses. A sense of improvement is usually noticed by patients when the challenge reveals they are down to about 17 ppm. When they get down to about 7 ppm, they report a tremendous improvement in mental function, clarity, memory, and vitality as well as abatement of a host of associated symptoms. This generally happens within weeks (as compared to years on DMPS), as their urine levels of mercury go down.

NDF (Nanocolloidal Detox Factors)

NDF is an example of an aggressive chelating agent that is not a drug. It is manufactured from chlorella, cilantro and other natural and food-like products that have been processed into a tiny particle size for enhanced absorption. NDF is a product that aims for heavy metal detox without a healing crisis. With NDF, your body may feel good while detoxifying. It doesn't strip enzyme bound beneficial minerals from your body.

Based on the results of comparative 24 hour urine samples analyzed by an independent clinic and lab, a person can safely excrete up to 920% (9.2 times) more heavy metals per month taking NDF daily as compared to doing one DMPS intravenous injection per month. This greatly shortens the time required to achieve detoxification, an average toxic adult person requiring a maximum dose of 2 mls. twice a day for a period of about two months. NDF also removes other toxins from the system. The predominant route of excretion is via the urine, thus accelerating the excretion rate of the mobilized metals as compared to the fecal route, decreasing the possibility of enzyme and leaky gut mediated resorption through the bowel, and decreasing the burden on the liver. The majority of the metals to be mobilized and eliminated per dose are quickly detectable in the first urination following the dose. Because the NDF does not use the sulfhydryl bonds it does not bind to the kidneys. Fecal element studies show an average of 38.4% reduction in fecal metals following 5 days at maximum dosage while urine levels remain elevated. Individual pathways of elimination have been noted.

Compared with DMPS, NDF eliminates nine times as much heavy metal toxin in the first month. And in contrast to DMPS, NDF is able to detoxify the brain; and tests on patients show NDF has a beneficial effect on the electrical activity of the brain. Independent real time digital EEG studies show a beneficial effect on the electrical activity of the brain, specifically raises the heavy metal suppressed beta waves to normal levels (from within 5 to 113 minutes post ingestion and lasting at least 4 hours) with a concurrent dramatic increase in the urinary excretion of heavy metals and patient reports of subjective improvement. This proves that no 'healing crisis' is required during heavy metal detox while using NDF.

Ingredients:

2 milliliters (2 droppers full or 52 drops) contain:

- 50 mgs.–Nanocolloidal cell wall decimated Chlorella Pyrenoidosa
- .12 mls.–Nanocolloidal Cilantro
- 10 mgs.–Nanocolloidal **PolyFlor*
- 75 mgs/liter nanocolloidal Silica
- Grain neutral spirits 18% as a preservative

**PolyFlor* microorganisms include: 12 strains of lactobacillus (including *casei, acidophilus, salivarius, bulgaricus, sporogones* and *plantarum*), 3 strains bifidobacterium including *longum* and *bifidum*, *streptococcus thermophilus*, and *b. laterosporus*.

Why "Nanonize" the Ingredients?

NDF is based on whole-food and bacterial components that have been "nanonized," (made very small to enhance absorption). Chlorella is known in mining to bind heavy metals to its cell wall. Yet many people have taken Chlorella with no benefit. The reasons are that all of the available chlorella is not really 'cell wall broken' and that most of it is already contaminated with heavy metals.

Most of the cell walls are in tact, but individual diatoms are tightly clustered in groups of about 500 units each. This is very difficult to digest and may explain why some people get gastro intestinal distress when taking normal chlorella but not with NDF. Nanocolloidal cell wall decimated chlorella has never been available so far! In addition to binding to heavy metals, Chlorella has other beneficial effects, augmented by putting it through this process, including: increased elimination of toxins, growth hormone regulation, a powerful nutritive impact and protection from radiation.

Why does it work?

The following is essential to the understanding of this supplement: The ingredients are in a nanocolloidal form. There is at least a 500-fold increase in available surface area and a dramatically reduced particle size, thus rendering each ingredient more bioavailable and effective. That means the effective bioavailable dose is roughly one five hundredth of the dose required compared to using a dose of the original ingredient. This is why 50 milligrams of nanonized chlorella achieves what 25 grams of normal chlorella cannot. Most toxin-burdened people have compromised assimilation and utilization and can't benefit from macromolecules. In the past, Chlorella was only known to mobilize a small amount of heavy metals via the bowel.

In NDF, because it is nanonized, 'molecular components digested off the nano particles can be absorbed across the GI wall into the bloodstream and have a possibility to enter the brain depending on the molecule' – a possible explanation of why it can facilitate elimination via the urine. *PolyFlor* contains fulvic acid. This could be the underlying reason why healthy bowel flora is so vital to good health. However, just taking a flora supplement will not provide heavy metal detox of the same magnitude as NDF (www.fulvic.com).

The major health benefits of both live and cell wall broken beneficial bacteria are described by recent clinical research in *The Handbook of Probiotics*. Lee, Nomoto, Salminen, and Gorbach. Pub. Wiley & Sons, Inc. '99. Unfortunately, once the amalgams are put into the teeth, or the toxic body burden becomes too great, or if a person only consumes processed and pesticide grown foods, these powerful allies no longer stand a chance of sharing their benefits.

Duration of Therapy

So far, only how much metal is being excreted can be measured, not the total body burden, so it is impossible to exactly predict the duration or cost of therapy. We do know that there is a linear relationship between the volume of the dose and the amount of excreted metals. Therefore, the more they can take, the quicker the detox will be. However, it is preferable to maintain the dose at the level that the patient continuously reports subjective improvement as a 'healing crisis' is not required to effectively remove the heavy metals with NDF.

Cost Effectiveness / Compared to DMPS

It was recently determined by an independent, comparative 24-hour urine tests conducted by Dr. J. Wright via Doctors Data that a single, 2-dropper dose of NDF pulled out 20% as much metals as an IV dose of DMPS on the same patient. Since NDF can be taken daily, and DMPS only once a month (per the protocol presented by Drs. Klinghart and Mercola), this means that up to **920% (9.2 times) more metal can be excreted per month** using 2 droppers of NDF twice a day (maximum dose) without the side effects and mineral deficiencies associated with DMPS. Since there is a linear relationship between amount of the dose and percentage increase in excreted metals, 6 drops twice a day would take out about 107%, or roughly the same amount of metals per month as DMPS, making NDF very cost effective, especially when you consider that very little additional supplementation is required while using NDF. Retail is $150 for a one-month supply, equal to the cost of one DMPS IV push.

Homocysteine Redux

Products such as MSM (*methylsulfonylmethane*) have surfaced on the market to provide an outside source of sulfur that in turn may hopefully be incorporated into the body and utilized for all the reactions and building blocks requiring sulfur. When the homocysteine pathway is functioning correctly, the end-product is natural sulfur, which is manufactured in the body and is already *endogenously* (inside) present for beneficial results. Additionally, MSM can create a molybdenum deficiency because *exogenous*, (outside) sources of sulfur will drain molybdenum resources because the molybdenum is essential for sulfur metabolism. On the contrary, *natural* provision of sulfur makes what the body needs, and does not create an excess pool which then must drain molybdenum to be metabolized.

Nutra-West company (nutriwestfl.com) formulated a product called *Homocysteine Redux*, to optimize the correct functioning of the homocysteine pathway it contains all of the necessary, synergistic nutrients (including molybdenum) to ensure that all the reactions that depend on the homocysteine pathway are optimized. These reactions include: 1) The synthesis of building blocks for cartilage/tissue repair that depends on the natural sulfur molecule; 2) The liver detox path that utilizes sulfur to detox insults to the system (especially metals such as lead, mercury, and cadmium); 3) The methyl donations from SAM (*S-adenosyl methionine*), which are used for the synthesis of neurotransmitters, and essential cell components such as *phosphatidylcholine* and *phosphatidylserine*.

SAM has also been used by itself as a nutritional supplement, but look at the pathway–unless you have all the necessary ingredients to optimize the efficiency of the whole pathway (nutrients that are in *Homocysteine Redux*), SAM can metabolize to the toxic homocysteine in just two more metabolic steps! There is another reason that addressing the correct functioning of the homocysteine pathway is important–if the necessary nutrients are not present, homocysteine can build up and become toxic. A synergistic balance of the nutrients can recycle homocysteine to methionine to avoid toxicity (vitamin B_{12}, folic acid, and methyl donors such as choline or betaine (*trimethylglycine*). Reducing homocysteine levels has been associated with reducing the risk for a whole host of conditions, from heart disease to osteoporosis, and MSM doesn't have that claim associated with it.

Rectal Chelation

New Delivery Method for Chelation Therapy

The newest, easiest, most convenient and efficacious technique for detoxifying heavy metals out of the body is by means of rectal chelation therapy. The method is to self-apply *Detoxamin*, a patented, trademarked and registered over-the-counter suppository. People exhibiting toxic metal burdens now are able to chelate themselves while sleeping by use of this non-prescription chelator. Merely insert the firm gelatin pill into the rectum, go to sleep, and awake in the morning partially detoxified. Repeat the procedure until testing show that there is no more metal poison remaining in the body. With this suppository method, the main obstacle to intravenous EDTA chelation therapy has been eliminated. **Rather than spending three or more hours per infusion session in a clinic, hooked to an IV, you may take less than a minute to insert the Detoxamin**

suppository at home before bedtime. Since many people cringe at the thought of getting stuck with a needle for twenty or more such IV treatments, use of a suppository eliminates this psychologically stressful and time-consuming obstacle. **Rectal administration is less invasive, in no way uncomfortable, and generally greatly preferred over IV treatments.**

Taking 3-5 suppositories over a 30-day period. This is medically equal to approximately 2-EDTA IV treatments. When on Detoxamin maintenance one box of Detoxamin lasts 6 to 10 months. Taken every night for 90 days or every other night for 180 days provides the medical equivalence of approximately 30 IV Chelation treatments.

Rectal chelation therapy does the job of detoxifying in a low-cost way to effuse EDTA through the bowel's walls and into your blood stream to clean toxic metals from all body cells. **Detoxamin has a time-release mechanism that allows the EDTA to absorb through the colon wall over an eighty-minute period while you sleep.** Almost all the blood from the rectum makes its way to the *superior hemorrhoidal veins*, a tributary of the portal system, so that absorption through the rectal wall carries the EDTA in Detoxamin to the portal vein.

The lower and middle hemorrhoidal veins bypass the liver-and do not undergo first pass metabolism. This means that **the EDTA in Detoxamin goes directly to the organs of your body without being filtered through the liver first.** Because of this, the EDTA contained in Detoxamin is very productive. Detoxamin also introduces EDTA directly into the systemic circulation, efficiently bypassing the portal circulation and the liver metabolism on the first pass. **Rectal absorption may also occur through the lymphatic system and, in some cases, largely through the blood via the vena cava.**

Detoxamin offers many advantages both over the expensive intravenous method of EDTA chelation. With the use of needles via the intravenous method, and risk of AIDS and other communicable blood-borne diseases, Detoxamin is becoming the logical choice over I.V. EDTA chelation and the poorly absorbed oral EDTA. **The rectum has a more neutral pH and is not as acidic as the stomach, which makes this area much better for EDTA absorption** because it is not buffered and has a neutral pH, unlike the stomach. It also has very little enzymatic activity, thus

enzymatic degradation does not occur. The rectal mucosa (rectum) is much more capable than the gastric mucosa (stomach) of tolerating various drug-related irritations. This is why patients who can't tolerate oral pain medication are given the same medication in suppository form. In fact, absorption with any oral EDTA tablet is so low that 135 (500mg) oral EDTA tablets are equal to just 5 Detoxamin suppositories.

Detoxamin removes most harmful toxins from the body, safely and effectively. Detoxamin is taken at night prior to bedtime, each Detoxamin suppository contains 750mg of *Calcium-disodium EDTA*, and is made in a cocoa-butter base (melts on body contact), which is very therapeutic for the rectal mucosa and the colon wall. The Ca-sodium form is able to bond (chelate) effectively because **it does not lower the blood pH to a level that would prohibit the bonding action.** The Ca added to the salt is important in this mode of administration as it buffers the acidic quality of the active ingredient keeping the suppository from being abrasive to the mucous membrane of the rectum area. Ca-disodium EDTA has both a *scientific justification* for therapeutic effectiveness as well as a *clinical history* of effectiveness.

The Calcium EDTA in Detoxamin has an extra chemical bond compared to the older Disodium EDTA. **This gives Detoxamin EDTA an affinity for Mercury.** Mercury is also excreted from the body through the feces and, because Detoxamin utilizes the colon wall for EDTA assimilation; it is a powerful Mercury chelator.

Metal Removing Nutrients

Calcium & Vitamin C: Just as lead will displace calcium, calcium is an excellent nutrient to utilize for displacing mercury and lead. A combination of minerals, such as magnesium and calcium, is even more effective in clearing metals from the body. Increasing vitamin C intake is a reasonable cost-effective way to control toxic metal levels in the population. Several studies implicate lead in causing cavities, and at least one study suggests that almost 3 million cavities in children result from lead. Vit. C and calcium supplementation are recommended for protection.

Chlorophyll: Chlorophyll binds to heavy metals very well. In fact, it is imperative to choose a reputable source (which screens for toxins and heavy metals) for your chlorophyll, or you may be getting more than you want. Juiced raw, organic greens. are a good source of chlorophyll.

Fiber: Fiber, such as oat bran and apple pectin, will bind to metals and help draw them out of the body. *Montmorillinite* clay also binds extremely well to toxins and metals for clearance. Fiber, such as red beet root, is high in *proanthocyanidins* and antioxidants and facilitates clearance of metals through the liver.

Lipoic Acid: Lipoic acid is a potent antioxidant and has a high affinity for binding to metals. This makes it an excellent choice as a supplement to bind and clear mercury and lead from the system. It is best utilized in combination with conjugating nutrients.

Minerals: A mineral-rich diet acts as a chelating agent. Many minerals will chelate metals, including calcium, magnesium, zinc and selenium. Mercury interferes with some functions of selenium, including its powerful antioxidant function and its ability to bind to metals. A good source of bioavailable minerals is raw sea vegetables and grass juices from wheat, barley, alfalfa, kamut, etc.

Milk Thistle (silybum marianum): Milk thistle is a renowned liver herb, and supports this major detoxification organ. Milk thistle contains *silymarin*, a bioflavonoid that is a very potent remedy for the liver. Silymarin inhibits free radical damage; free radicals have an adverse effect on the detoxification enzymes of the liver *cytochrome P450* system, while silymarin protects those enzymes. Glutathione is destroyed by lead. Silymarin not only prevents the depletion of GSH (glutathione), it even increases this liver-detoxifying enzyme. A sulfur pathway in the liver detoxes lead, and milk thistle helps to boost liver function.

Molybdenum: Large amounts of exogenous sulfur (from outside the body) will usurp the body's stores of molybdenum to metabolize it. An easier solution is to use the nutrients which will facilitate the homocysteine pathway. Homocysteine is a toxic substance; however, the pathway itself, when properly supported, is essential for a host of metabolic functions. When the pathway is facilitated, sulfur is generated as a natural by-product at the end (molybdenum changes the toxic *sulfite* molecule to the much-needed *sulfate).* Vitamins B_{12}, B_6 and folic acid, along with *trimethylglycine* and *dimethylglycine* recycle *homocysteine* to *methionine*, and allow for *Sam-e* to methylate *phosphatidylserine*, an important brain nutrient. Usually the people who are the most deficient in sulfur will be the most sensitive to metal toxicity and vice versa.

Parotid Glandular: Parotid glandular accelerates the clearance of chemicals/heavy metals from tissues. It is best utilized in combination with detoxification nutrients that will pull the metals out of the body by detox pathways such as the bowel, kidney, lymph, lungs, blood, skin, and liver.

Sulfur: Lead steals sulfur from important proteins, which could be enzymes, hormones, or cell receptors. Conversely, sulfur is needed in the liver detox pathway to hook onto lead and clear it from the body. So, lead depletes sulfur, the very nutrient needed to detox the lead overload. A depletion of sulfur will also adversely affect joint connective tissue growth, since sulfur is an essential precursor to the building blocks of cartilage, namely *glucosamine sulfate, chondroitin sulfate*, and *hyaluronic acid*. Good sources of sulfur are garlic, kelp, kale, turnip, raspberries, onions, cabbage, and mustard.

Zinc: Zinc and copper get displaced from *metallothionine*, the protein that binds and carries them. This destroys many of the zinc-dependent enzymes. Zinc is important for proper functioning in a host of major metabolic pathways; it is a component of over 90 *metalloenzymes* in the body. Lead has always been known as a neurotoxin, with the brain being particularly susceptible to attack. Lethargy is a common symptom of lead toxicity; lead inactivates the zinc-dependent enzymes of the Kreb's cycle, which produces our energy. Zinc is also a part of the antioxidant enzyme *Zn-SOD*, which fights *superoxide* radicals.

Symptoms of lead toxicity are similar to zinc deficiency symptoms because lead can bring on a zinc deficiency. Zinc deficiency has been implicated in a variety of neuropsychiatric disorders, including dyslexia, epilepsy, mental depression, and attention deficit disorder. The symptoms of *lead toxicity* are similar to *zinc deficiency* because lead destroys zinc-dependent enzymes.

The "Q" instrument: The Q2 Water Energy System uses a foot bath device to treat amalgam free persons. The energized hydrotherapy detoxifies the last vestiges of microbes and toxic metals, especially mercury, deeply lodged in the cells and tissues.

Fluoride

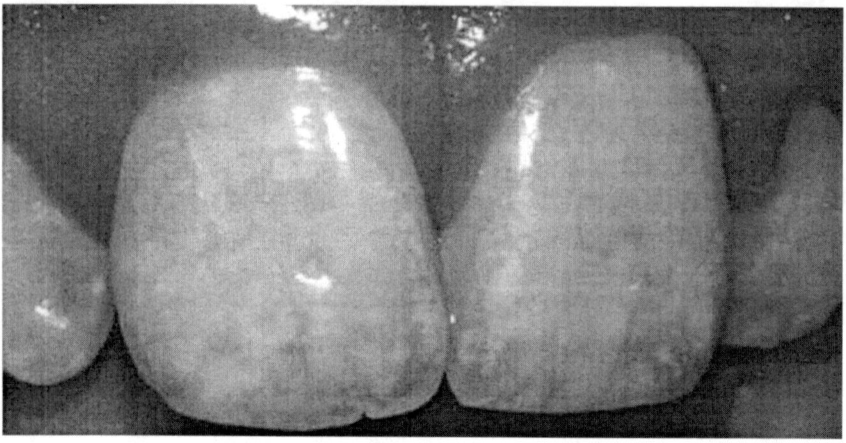

Fluorosis of Teeth

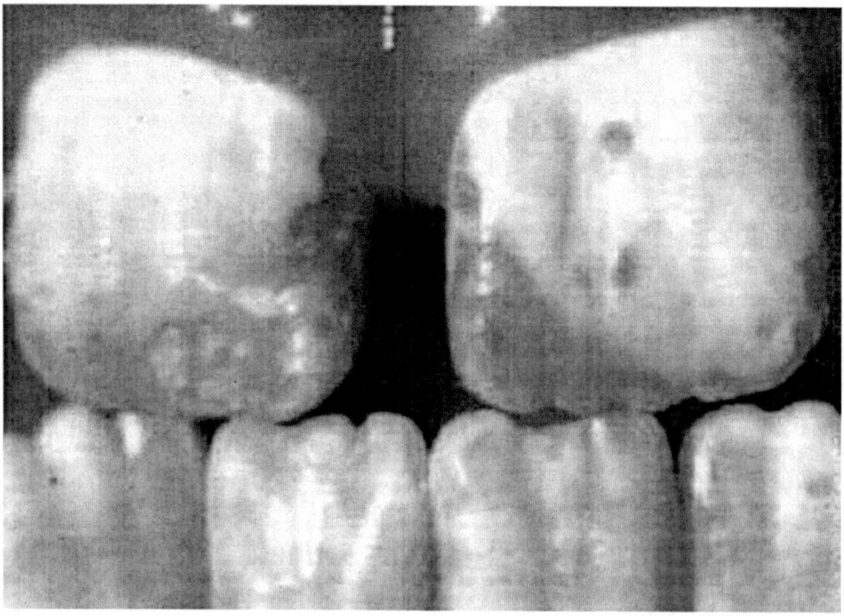

Fluoride

Controversial fluoride is one of the basic ingredients in both *Prozac* (*FLUoxetene Hydrochloride*) **and Sarin nerve gas** (*Isopropyl-Methyl-Phosphoryl FLUoride*). **Sodium fluoride, a hazardous-waste by-product from the manufacture of aluminum and phosphate fertilizer, is a common ingredient in rat and cockroach poisons, anesthetics, hypnotics, psychiatric drugs, and military nerve gas**

Historically it has been quite expensive to properly dispose of, until some aluminum industries with an overabundance of the stuff sold the public on the terrifically insane but highly profitable idea of buying it at a 20,000% markup, injecting it into our water supplies, and then drinking it. Yes, a 20,000% markup: Fluoride—intended only for human consumption by people under 14 years of age—is injected into our drinking water supply at approx. 1 part-per-million (ppm), but since we only drink 1/2 of one percent of the total water supply, the rest literally goes down the drain as **a free hazardous-waste disposal for the chemical industry, where we pay them so that we can flush their expensive hazardous waste down our toilets.**

Independent scientific evidence repeatedly showing up over the past 50 years reveals that **fluoride allegedly shortens our life span, promotes cancer and various mental disturbances, accelerates osteoporosis and broken hips in old folks, and makes us stupid, docile, and subservient, all in one package.** There are reports of aluminum in the brain possibly being a causative factor in Alzheimer's Disease, and evidence points towards fluoride's strong affinity for aluminum and also its ability to "trick" the blood-brain barrier by looking like the hydrogen ion, and thus allowing chemical access to brain tissue

There are reportedly more than 11 million Americans with diabetes. Since many diabetics drink more liquids than other people, then according to the *Physicians Desk Reference* these 11 million Americans probably shouldn't drink fluoridated water, because in doing so, they'll receive an excessive dose of fluoride. Kidney disease, by definition, lowers the efficiency of the kidneys, which is your main route of fluoride elimination. So those people with kidney disease also shouldn't drink fluoridated water. Cases are on record (Annapolis, Maryland, 1979) where kidney patients on dialysis machines died, due to a fluoride overdose in the city water supply.

***Sodium fluoride* is the most violent protoplasmic poison known to science.** The National Library of Medicine's computerized data service on toxic substances rates fluorides **4-5 (very toxic–extremely toxic)** on a scale of five. Scheele discovered *fluorine* in 1771, but Moissan did not produce it in gaseous elemental purity until 1886. Fluoride is added to the water supply of most American cities for the purpose of dental hygiene. The reader will be amazed to find out that such a result is not only unlikely but the reverse of the actual outcome. The U.S. has been fluoridating drinking water for so many decades people hardly think about it.

Very few articles appear about fluoridation in newspapers and magazines anymore. At least chlorine will evaporate from a glass of water if you let it sit for an hour or so. Not so with fluoride. Even cooking, food processing, filtration, or digestion will not remove fluoride. Fluoride goes right up the food chain. It accumulates in fat cells when ingested or absorbed through the skin or mucous membranes. Fluoride drops, tablets, and vitamins are more likely to *damage* children's teeth than to *prevent cavities*, according to mainstream dental groups such as the Canadian Dental Association and the Western Australia Health Department's Dental Service. Both organizations have *stopped* recommending regular fluoride supplementation.

In the past, the American Dental Association (ADA), the American Medical Association (AMA) and the World Health Organization (WHO) have all endorsed fluoridation, and many established scientific bodies have declared that its advantages are not debatable. But, recently, the tide has been changing, and what the fluoride promoters will not reveal to their targeted legislators, City Council members, County Commissioners, or even their unsuspecting well-intended supporters: The July 2000, peer-reviewed cover story of the *Journal of the American Dental Association* (JADA) clarifed for every dentist in America that **ingestion of fluoride does not provide any significant reduction in the incidence of tooth decay--any beneficial dental effect is a result of topical application.**

The American Dental Association and the American Academy of Pediatrics have revised their recommendations for controlled-dose fluoride which restricts a doctor from prescribing fluoride to a child of 6 months to 3 years of age to **0.25 milligrams per day, the amount found in one cup of fluoridated water, and none to an infant**–meaning that, as a public policy, fluoridation mass medicates at a higher expected dosage than a doctor in a non-fluoridated community can prescribe.

The August 17, 2001 *Morbidity and Mortality Weekly Report* (MMWR) from the Centers for Disease Control and Prevention (CDC) despite its touting of fluoridation, included: "The prevalence of dental caries in a population is not inversely related to the concentration fo fluoride in enamel, and a higher concentration of enamel fluoride is not necessarily more efficacious in preventing dental caries." In short, **dental cavities are not a result of a lack of fluoride exposure, and more fluoride is not better in the prevention of tooth decay.**

In a Congressional investigation by the House Committee on Science, the Environmental Protection Agency (EPA), the CDC, National Sanitation Foundation, and the Food and Drug Administration (FDA), all replied to inquiries that they **have no scientific studies on the actual fluorine-bearing substances used in 90% of the nation's fluoridaiton programs.** The FDA, in a December 2000 communication, stated that "Fluoride, when used for the diagnosis, cure, mitigation, treatment, or prevention of disease in man or animal is a drug that is subject to Food and Drug Administration regulation." and that **"No fluoride substance intended to be ingested for the purpose of reducing tooth decay has ever been approved for safety and effectiveness."**

On June 29, 2000, at the *U.S. Senate Congressional Hearing on Arsenic, Radon, and Fluoride,* held by the subcommittee on Fisheries, Wildlife, and Water, J. Willam Hirzy, Ph.D. testified on behalf of the union (that consists of and represents all of the toxicologists, biologists, chemists, physicians, statisticians, epidemiologists, attorneys, engineers, scientists, and other professionals at the U.S. Environmental Protection Agency, Washington, D.C.), **calling for a moratorium on all fluoridation.**

In his testimony to Congress, Hirzy cited scientific evidence that the union of scientists have in their possession, and court findings in three different states, whose conclusions have never been overturned on the merits, that found, with reasonable certainty (i.e. beyond speculation and guess), and by preponderance of the evidence, including the testimony of experts learned in the field, that **fluoride in public water supplies causes or contributes to the cause of cancer, genetic damage, intolerant reactions, chronic toxicity, dental fluorosis, bone pathology and neurological injury in humans, and that fluoride in public water supplies aggravates malnutrition, iodine deficiencies and other existing illnesses.**

Before fluoridation's implementation in 1945 and popular acceptance in 1950, *sodium fluoride*, **a by-product of aluminum manufacture**, was known as **an intractable industrial pollutant**. Waterworks engineers warned that **water containing 1 part-per-million (ppm) fluoride is contaminated**. The devilish plot to put fluoride in drinking water has been backed in Washington since **an ex-employee of the Aluminum Company of America was made Secretary of the Public Health Administration**. Fluoride is a very toxic substance, which is why **it is the active ingredient in a number of pesticides**.

Two grams of fluoride is enough to kill an adult, and 500 mg. is enough to kill a child. A tube of toothpaste can have as much as 1,500 mgs., and fluoride gel contains up to 6,000 mgs. In the U.S., people have died, and many have become sick, when faltering fluoridation equipment has pumped excess fluoride into the water. Poor nutrition exacerbates the toxic effects of fluoride exposure, which is one reason why it's wrong to target poor communities with fluoridation (poor nutrition is more prevalent in low income communities).

Subsets of the population may be unusually susceptible to the toxic effects of fluoride and its compounds. These populations include the elderly, people with deficiencies of calcium, magnesium and/or vitamin C, and people with cardiovascular and kidney problems. Ninety-eight percent of Western Europe has rejected water fluoridation. This includes Austria, Belgium, Denmark, Finland, France, Germany, Italy, Luxembourg, Netherlands, Norway, and Sweden. The predominant reason for Europe's rejection is the belief that public drinking water is *not* the appropriate vehicle with which to deliver medication to a population.

Fluoride is not an essential nutrient, which means that no human disease (including dental decay) has ever been linked to a fluoride deficiency. **Fluoridation adds between 0.1 and 1.6 parts per billion (ppb) arsenic to drinking water**, and therefore violates the EPA's *Maximum Contaminant Level Goal* for arsenic—which is 0 ppb. When water fluoridation began 50 years ago, it was believed that fluoride needed to be ingested in order to be effective. This is no longer the view of the dental establishment, which now generally concedes that fluoride's benefits are derived primarily from topical application.

No fluoride products designed for ingestion have ever been approved as safe or effective by the U.S. Food and Drug Administration (FDA). Fluoridated water can appropriately be classified as **an unapproved prescription drug.** Fluoride is ineffective at preventing the most common type of dental decay—*pits* and *fissures*. Pit & fissure decay—which is the decay found in the crevices of the chewing surfaces—accounts for upwards of 85% of dental decay now experienced in the U.S. Despite the fact that nearly all large U.S. cities have been fluoridated for decades, dental decay is currently rampant in virtually all poor urban areas.

Routinely prescribed to U.S. children who don't drink fluoridated water (starting with toothless six month olds), **fluoride supplements were never tested for safety and efficacy** by the F.D.A. These supplements comprise one category of many different medications the FDA officially "grandfathered" in, (they were sold before drug testing was required by law). Current research shows that many of the old fluoride studies were flawed. Fluoride's benefits are merely *topical*, not *systemic*, as was once thought.

Moreover, ingested fluoride can result in **unwanted side effects**, including *dental fluorosis* (spotted, stained, or pitted teeth). Brian A. Burt of the University of Michigan School of Public Health states that "fluoride supplements should no longer be used for young children in North America...**the risks of using supplements in infants and young children outweigh the benefits**." Euan Swan, author of the Canadian Dental Association's (CDA) new fluoride supplement guidelines, said, "The evidence supporting the effectiveness of dietary fluoride supplements is relatively weak. There's better evidence indicating that they contribute to dental fluorosis."

"The notion that systemic fluorides are needed in nonfluoridated areas is an outdated one that should be abandoned altogether," says Canada's leading fluoride authority, Hardy Limeback, head of the Department of Preventive Dentistry at the University of Toronto and past president of the Canadian Association for Dental research. He says, "We are now spending more money treating dental fluorosis than we would spend treating new decay if water fluoridation was halted."

Forms of Fluoride

There are five forms of fluoride that are often discussed and sometimes get confused. First, there is ***elemental fluorine***, which is a gas and the most reactive element in the periodic table. It reacts with every other element except three of the noble gases. It even reacts with asbestos. Free fluorine is not produced in nature. Fluorine is not put in our drinking water! Fluorine is found in the form of ***hydrogen fluoride,*** another gas. It etches glass. It dissolves in water to form a weak acid. It is a pollutant emitted by metal smelters, the oil industry, ceramic and brick industries, coal fired power stations, incinerators, and a number of other industries. It's been responsible for many deaths in air pollution incidents. Then there is the ***fluoride ion.*** The fluoride ion cannot be placed in a bottle by itself. It is a *negative ion*; it must be accompanied by *positive ions*.

Negative ions are formed when metals react with non-metals (fluorine is a non-metal). When this happens, the metal transfers one or more of its electrons (negative particles) to the non-metal. The result is a positively charged metal ion and a negatively charged ion. In the solid form, these positive ions and negative ions appear in a tidy three-dimensional arrangement. This internal arrangement gives rise to the crystalline shape of these substances. For example, table salt has crystals in the shape of a cube. When these substances (salts) are dissolved in water the positive ions and negative ions separate.

Sodium chloride is very soluble in water; calcium fluoride is far less soluble. Ten percent of the water fluoridated in the U.S. is fluoridated with sodium fluoride. Complex ions are positive metal ions that are surrounded by negative ions or neutral molecules that have a stronger bonding than simply electrostatic attraction. Thus they have different properties from the parent ions. Thus, (AlF_4^-) has different properties from the parent Al_3^+ ion and the F^- ions. It is this ability of the fluoride ion to form complexes with so many ions, including a lot of toxic ones, and others that are needed by the body, which might help to explain why this unreactive species (in the chemical sense) can be so biologically active and dangerous. Another form of fluoride that we meet is ***hexafluoro silicic acid*** (H_2SiF_6) and its sodium salt ***sodium fluorosilicate*** (Na_2SiF_6). **These substances are used to fluoridate 90% of the fluoridated water in the U.S.** They are waste products from the superphosphate industry.

Pro-fluoridation people claim that when these substances are diluted and dissolved in water, they completely dissolve into SiO_2 and fluoride ion. This is disputed, as there are still some silicon fluoride complexes left when the water reaches our taps. These complexes **facilitate the uptake of lead into the blood**. Over 50% of the communities in the United States use *fluorosilicic acid* or *sodium fluorosilicate* to fluoridate drinking water. Neither the EPA nor the Centers for Disease Control and Prevention can provide one safety study proving the product is safe for long-term, low-level consumption.

Not one clinical study with animal models has ever been done with the products. Interestingly, all the people who say this product is 'safe' have no concept of how it is produced. The last form of fluoride that we meet is the ***organofluoride*** group. These are compounds which have fluorine covalently bonded to carbon atoms. One of the organofluorines, which you have probably handled, is the plastic PTFE. This is *poly tetra fluoro ethyle*ne, used in non-stick frying pans. It consists of long chains of carbon attached to itself with two fluorines attached to each carbon. It is very stable and resistant to chemical attack.

Fluorine is frequently added to pharmaceuticals. These drugs, when they are metabolized, break down in the body and produce fluoride ion. The net result is that these drugs carry fluoride into very sensitive places, like the brain, where it can cause problems. Little investigation has been done on this aspect of organofluorines. There are other organofluorines that are very toxic in their own right– the toxicity has nothing to do with the fluoride ion itself; or the formation of the fluoride ion. Substances like *fluorocitrate* are very toxic because they bind to an enzyme involved in sugar metabolism, and they don't let go–they block it–they prevent it from handling the citrate, and it usually changes into something else.

This rather unreactive chemical species called *fluoride ions* can interfere with biological systems in three profound ways: a) by forming hydrogen bonds with key groups in proteins and nucleic acids, b) can complex with metal ions like aluminum, beryllium, lead and carbon) can interfere with enzymes that use magnesium ions as a co-factor. For many enzymes, magnesium helps to align the enzyme with the substrate it is working on, and fluoride can interfere with this alignment. We're swallowing more fluoride each day with every glass of water.

Since 1945, when fluoride was first put into the municipal water system in Newburgh, New York, 75% of the United States water supply has been fluoridated. Other countries are taking a suspicious look at fluoride. Sweden abandoned fluoridation on the recommendation of a special fluoride commission. Denmark, Holland, Finland, France, Germany and Japan have also rejected it, citing public health concerns. Plans to make fluoridation mandatory in Britain were suspended in 1998 after the British Home Secretary intervened and urged the Health Secretary to review the negative evidence. Disreputable and power-hungry persons in high places have been know to experiment with fluoride to see if it "could not be **used to subjugate the people of a whole community more quickly than fighting them into submission**," according to William Guy Carr, a retired commander from the Royal Canadian Navy.

Mass Medication

The first occurrence of fluoridated drinking water on Earth was found in Germany's Nazi prison camps. The Gestapo had little concern about fluoride's supposed effect on children's teeth; their alleged reason for mass-medicating water with sodium fluoride was to sterilize humans and force the people in their concentration camps into calm submission. (Ref. book: "The Crime and Punishment of I.G. Farben" by Joseph Borkin.)

The following letter was received by the Lee Foundation for Nutritional Research, Milwaukee Wisconsin, on 2 October 1954, from Mr. Charles Perkins, a chemist:

"I have your letter of September 29 asking for further documentation regarding a statement made in my book, The Truth About Water Fluoridation, to the effect that the idea of water fluoridation was brought to England from Russia by the Russian Communist Kreminoff. "In the 1930's, Hitler and the German Nazi's envisioned a world to be dominated and controlled by a Nazi philosophy of pan-Germanism. The German chemists worked out a very ingenious and far-reaching plan of mass-control which was submitted to and adopted by the German General Staff. This plan was to control the population in any given area through mass medication of drinking water supplies. By this method they could control the population in whole areas, reduce population by water medication that would produce sterility in women, and so on. In this scheme of mass-control, sodium fluoride occupied a prominent place...

"Repeated doses of infinitesimal amounts of fluoride will in time reduce an individual's power to resist domination, by slowly poisoning and narcotizing a certain area of the brain, thus making him submissive to the will of those who wish to govern him. [A convenient light lobotomy]

"The real reason behind water fluoridation is not to benefit children's teeth. If this were the real reason there are many ways in which it could be done that are much easier, cheaper, and far more effective. The real purpose behind water fluoridation is to reduce the resistance of the masses to domination and control and loss of liberty.

"When the Nazis under Hitler decided to go into Poland, both the German General Staff and the Russian General Staff exchanged scientific and military ideas, plans, and personnel, and the scheme of mass control through water medication was seized upon by the Russian Communists because it fitted ideally into their plan to communize the world. ...

"I was told of this entire scheme by a German chemist who was an official of the great IG Farben chemical industries and was also prominent in the Nazi movement at the time. I say this with all the earnestness and sincerity of a scientist who has spent nearly 20 years` research into the chemistry, biochemistry, physiology and pathology of fluorine—any person who drinks artificially fluorinated water for a period of one year or more will never again be the same person mentally or physically." CHARLES E. PERKINS, Chemist, 2 October 1954.

Quoting Einstein's nephew, Dr. E.H. Bronner (a chemist who had also been a prisoner of war during WWII) in a letter printed in *The Catholic Mirror*, Springfield, MA, January 1952: "It appears that the citizens of Massachusetts are among the `next` on the agenda of the water poisoners.

"There is a sinister network of subversive agents, Godless `intellectual` parasites, working in our country today whose ramifications grow more extensive, more successful and more alarming each new year and whose true objective is to demoralize, paralyze and destroy our great Republic—from within if they can, according to their plan—for their own possession.

"The tragic success they have already attained in their long siege to destroy the moral fiber of American life is now one of their most potent footholds towards their own ultimate victory over us.

"Fluoridation of our community water systems can well become their most subtle weapon for our sure physical and mental deterioration.

"As a research chemist of established standing, I built within the past 22 years, 3 American chemical plants and licensed 6 of my 53 patents. Based on my years of practical experience in the health-food and chemical field, let me warn: fluoridation of drinking water is criminal insanity, sure national suicide. Don't do it.

"Even in small quantities, sodium fluoride is a deadly poison to which no effective antidote has been found. Every exterminator knows that it is the most efficient rat-killer. ... Sodium fluoride is entirely different from organic calcium-fluoro-phosphate needed by our bodies and provided by nature, in God's great providence and love, to build and strengthen our bones and our teeth. This organic calcium-fluoro-phosphate, derived from proper foods, is an edible organic salt, insoluble in water and assimilable by the human body, whereas the non-organic sodium fluoride used in fluoridating water is instant poison to the body and fully water soluble.

The body refuses to assimilate it. "Careful, bonafide laboratory experimentation by conscientious, patriotic research chemists, and actual medical experience, have both revealed that instead of preserving or promoting `dental health,` fluoridated drinking water destroys teeth, before adulthood and after, by the destructive mottling and other pathological conditions it actually causes in them, and also creates many other very grave pathological conditions in the internal organisms of bodies consuming it. How can it be called a "health" plan? What's behind it?

"That any so-called "doctors" would persuade a civilized nation to add voluntarily a deadly poison to its drinking water systems is unbelievable. It is the height of criminal insanity. "No wonder Hitler and Stalin fully believed and agreed from 1939 to 1941 that, quoting from both Lenin's Last Will and Hitler's Mein Kampf: "America we shall demoralize, divide, and destroy from within."...

"Are our Civil Defense organizations and agencies awake to the perils of water poisoning by fluoridation? Its use has been recorded in other countries. Sodium fluoride water solutions are the cheapest and most effective rat killers known to chemists: colorless, odorless, tasteless; no antidote, no remedy, no hope: Instant and complete extermination of rats. ... "Fluoridation of water systems can be slow national suicide, or quick national liquidation. It is criminal insanity—treason!" Dr. E.H. Bronner, Mfg. Research Chemist, Los Angeles.

Earliest available Russian fluoride evidence: "I, Oliver Kenneth Goff, was a member of the Communist Party and the Young Communist League, from May 2, 1936, to October 9, 1939. During this period of time, I operated under the alias of John Keats with number 18-B-2. My testimony before the Government is in Volume 9 of the Un-American Activities Report for 1939.

"While a member of the Communist Party, I attended Communist training schools in New York and Wisconsin ... and we were trained in the revolutionary overthrow of the U.S. Government."... We discussed quite thoroughly the fluoridation of water supplies and how we were using it in Russia as a tranquilizer in the prison camps. The leaders of our school felt that if it could be induced into the American water supply, it would bring about a spirit of lethargy in the nation, where it could keep the general public docile during a steady encroachment of Communism.

We also discussed the fact that keeping a store of deadly fluoride near the water reservoir would be advantageous during the time of the revolution, as it would give us opportunity to dump this poison into the water supply and either kill off the populace or threaten them with liquidation, so that they would surrender to obtain fresh water.

Expert Does About-Face on Fluoride

Hardy Limeback, B.S., Ph.D. in biochemistry, D.D.S., and head of the Department of Preventive Dentistry at the University of Toronto and president of the Canadian Association for Dental Research, now opposes the use of fluoride in drinking water or toothpaste. Asked by *The Tribune* of Mesa, Ariz., why he had reversed a pro-fluoride position he had embraced for decades, Limeback responded: "It's been building up for a couple of years.

But certainly the crowning blow was the realization that we have been dumping contaminated fluoride into our water reservoirs for half a century. The vast majority of all fluoride additives come from Tampa Bay, FL., smokestack scrubbers. The additives are a toxic byproduct of the super-phosphate fertilizer industry. Tragically, that means we're not just dumping toxic fluoride into our drinking water. **We're also exposing innocent, unsuspecting people to deadly elements: lead, arsenic and radium, all of them carcinogenic. Because of the cumulative properties of toxins, the detrimental effects on human health are catastrophic."**

A new study at the University of Toronto supports Limeback's argument: "Residents of cities that fluoridate have doubled the fluoride in their hip bones vis-à-vis the balance of the population. Worse, we discovered that it is actually altering the architecture of human bones." Skeletal fluorosis is a debilitating condition that occurs when fluoride accumulates in the bones, making them extremely weak and brittle.

"Mottled and brittle teeth" are the earliest symptoms, Limeback said. "In Canada we are now spending more money treating dental fluorosis than we do treating cavities. That includes my own practice." "Here in Toronto we have been fluoridating for 36 years," Limeback said. "Yet Vancouver, which has never fluoridated, has a cavity rate lower than Toronto's." Cavity rates are low, he said, across the industrialized world, including Europe, which is 98 percent fluoride-free.

*The Tribun*e pointed out that the Centers for Disease Control ran a puff piece all across America saying the stuff was better than sliced bread. "Unfortunately," Limeback replied, "the CDC is basing its position on data that is 50 years old and questionable at best. Absolutely no one has done research on fluorosilicates, which is the junk they're dumping into the drinking water. On the other hand, the evidence against systemic fluoride intake continues to pour in."

Limeback recently apologized to faculty and students at the University Of Toronto Department Of Dentistry. "I told them I had unintentionally misled my colleagues and my students. For the past 15 years, I had refused to study the toxicology information that is readily available to anyone. Poisoning our children was the furthest thing from my mind."

Fluoride In Toothpaste

Contrary to its public image as a benign substance used solely to reduce tooth decay, fluoride is **extremely corrosive**, more toxic than lead and just slightly less toxic than arsenic. *Sodium fluoride*, the active ingredient in most brands of toothpaste, was originally sold as a **rat poison**. If a three-year-old ate **half a tube of the toothpaste, it could kill him**. "Fluoridated toothpaste contains 1,000-2,000 mgs. of fluoride. Fluoridated drinking water contains one to four parts per million. **Fluoride is absorbed through mucous membranes in the mouth.** A child may not consume the whole tube, but smaller amounts daily are certainly a hazard to anyone. It is estimated that **children swallow or absorb approximately 1 mg. of fluoride at each brushing** with such toothpaste.

In 1987 the *Journal of Pediatrics* issued a warning that children should use **no more than "one-third of one pea-sized dollop of toothpaste**" when brushing their teeth. Allowing for the 4 ppm standard to which the EPA has raised fluoride, and based upon accurate water consumption figures, approximately **50% of children under five are receiving a daily dose of fluoride known to cause skeletal fluorosis.** Is the possible saving of 0.8% of one tooth surface over a seventeen-year period worth the risk of skeletal fluorisis, cancer or AIDS? Implementation of sound nutritional principles, removal of pollutants that reduce natural immunity and appropriate health education proves more effective in resolving the problems of tooth decay along with many other modern degenerative diseases. Just as you lock your doors against unwanted intrusion, you must take the necessary steps to protect yourselves from this daily poisoning. It will have to be done by you. **No one else will do it for you.**

Terry Leader, a dental hygienist from Long Island, witnessed, in 1969, **a child given topical fluoride, who then went into convulsions and died in the dentist's chair**. She pleads: "I just wish parents would read before they subject their children to something so dangerous. It's not going to save them money. **Good oral hygiene prevents tooth decay; fluoride doesn't.** The mystique behind many 'miracle' drugs is the belief that, like heat-seeking missiles, they will zoom right to the enemy symptom and zap it neatly out of existence. So with fluoride, our bodies should deliver all the fluoride directly to our teeth where it will supposedly harden the enamel and form an indestructible barrier to tooth decay. Such magical thinking bears little relationship to biochemical reality.

Fluoride In Water

Corporations have a lot invested in fluoridation, which allows them to dispose of industrial pollution via dilution. Today, the most common product used for fluoridation is *hydrofluosilicic acid*, which is not a natural substance but a waste product coming straight from the scrubbers of the phosphate fertilizer industry. When phosphate is mined, they have to get rid of the attached fluorine or it would kill the plants. So they put the phosphate through a sulfuric acid wash to separate the fluorine out into what is called *hazardous waste liquor*. The fluorine is captured by a scrubber system since they can't let it go out into the air because it would kill all the plants and animals around.

If they had to dispose of this liquor as hazardous industrial waste, it would cost them $1.40 a gallon or more neutralize it—depending on how much cadmium, lead, uranium, and arsenic are also present. They don't want to pay that, so instead they call it a product and we pay them approximately 3 cents a gallon to dump in our water. Data collected in the largest survey to date—of over 39,000 American schoolchildren ages 5 to 17 in 84 communities, showed that children living in fluoridated areas had tooth decay rates nearly identical with those in non-fluoridated areas.

The cells that produce the collagen matrix that forms enamel are poisoned to the point that they can no longer produce opalescent pearl-like enamel. Fluorotic enamel is irregular in texture, porous, chalky white to brown in color and brittle. In severe cases, the enamel forms incompletely and corners easily break off the teeth. Even proponents of fluoridation acknowledge that fluorosis increases with the level of fluoride in the water.

Currently, an estimated 22% of American children exhibit the symptoms of fluorosis. This is not just a cosmetic flaw; it's proof of the fact that the body has been overdosed with fluoride and has not been able to handle it. Bottle-fed babies (whose formula is made with fluoridated water) are most likely to develop dental fluorosis. Mother's milk has virtually no fluoride present. Those children who are deficient in protein, calcium, magnesium, phosphorous, and vitamin C are especially vulnerable to fluoride poisoning. The accumulation of fluoride is greatly increased if the person has impaired kidney function. In short, the weakest members of our society, the undernourished and the underfed, are the very children that fluoridation was to allegedly benefit.

In some poorer communities, as much as 80% of the children have fluorosis. But don't assume that if your child is healthy and well nourished, he or she runs no risk. Look at the toothpaste, and read the directions—Children 2 to 6 years: To minimize swallowing, use a pea-sized amount, and supervise brushing and rinsing until good habits are established." Tempted by bubble-gum flavors and artificial sweeteners, a child can easily ingest more than the recommended amount. Studies show that children under four inadvertently swallow 50% to 100% of the toothpaste they put in their mouths, simply because they lack a fully developed gag reflex. **The American Dental Association will not give toothpaste its seal of approval unless it includes fluoride.**

Dental fluorosis is just the first, visible evidence of much more serious changes in the body. When fluoride accumulates at high concentrations in the bones, they become weak and brittle. Victims of this debilitating condition, called *skeletal fluorosis* can only hobble forward, stiff and hunched. The osteoarthritis that afflicts many people in this country may actually be a misdiagnosed stage of skeletal fluorosis. Recent studies have linked fluoride to an increased incidence of **hip fractures, damage to the central nervous system**, and **cancer**.

In China, researchers correlated dental fluorosis with a **10 point reduction in I.Q.** Low levels of fluoride in the drinking water of test animals produced pathological changes in the brain similar to those in humans with Alzheimer's disease. Another study demonstrated how fluoride interferes with the brain's pineal gland and inhibits its production of melatonin. What will happen when the first generation of fluoride-fed children turns 70, after accumulating this poison over a lifetime in their bones?

Cavities are not life-threatening, but fluoridation comes with real risks and negligible benefits. Even if you believe in the value of fluoride, no one should be allowed to use our drinking water as a delivery system. A lot of people consider Vitamin C beneficial, but so far it doesn't flow out of the tap. Water is our most precious resource, and we have no business adding anything to it, other than what's necessary to make it safe to drink. It is our responsibility to maintain this gift, as pure and pristine as possible, for each and every person to enjoy. In 1990, Dr. William Marcus, chief toxicologist for the EPA's Office of Drinking Water, was disturbed to find data from a study reporting specific fluoride-related cancers **altered or omitted** in the final National Toxicology Program report.

When he demanded an independent review of the raw data, **he was fired.** Later, an investigation by the Senate Environment and Public Works Committee corroborated his charges and produced evidence that government scientists had been pressured to portray fluoride more positively. Because fluorine is the most negatively charged and interactive element of all, it bonds with practically everything and does not exist separately in nature, despite its rank as the 13th most abundant element in the earth's crust. But most of it stays buried, unless it is mined and brought to the surface or created as a by-product of various manufacturing processes.

Fluorine is kind of a bully; it aggressively seeks out other electrons and is prized for its ability to disrupt and reconfigure other molecular bonds. One reason people have been reluctant to expose the problems of fluoride is that it cuts across so many industries. In its various forms, fluoride is used to etch glass, ceramics and computer chips; refine petroleum products; separate out heavy metal and power rockets. Our air is contaminated by fluoride emissions from the production of iron, steel, copper, aluminum and plastics. **Fluoride is one of the world's most widely used pesticides.** If you walk past a house tented for termites, they're probably spraying *sulfuryl fluoride* (*Vikane*) to kill the bugs.

Fluorinated Drugs

Many psychoactive drugs are fluorinated. The fluorine atom is attached to the active ingredients in many drugs in order to allow them to penetrate into the brain or other targeted organs more easily. Because the fluoride enhances the penetrating power of the active ingredient, less of the active ingredient needs to be made, and the manufacturer can save money. But the side effects of all the fluoride-containing medications is scarcely ever discussed as a general health issue.

The primary ingredients of most psychoactive drugs suppress enzyme production, and the **fluorine ion is also an enzyme inhibitor**. The one particular side effect common to almost all fluorinated drugs, which is mentioned in the Physician's Desk Reference, is **memory loss**. These drugs, including *Prozac* (*fluoxetene*)—and *Paxil*–antidepression drugs, contain **three Fluorine atoms in each molecule** that **quickly kill the brain-issued enzymes** that normally maintain mood stability. *Prozac* and *Paxil* contain the fluoride containing *Fluorophenyl* compounds and are also known to cause liver disease.

Organic fluoride compounds undergo extensive transformation in the liver, and in many instances the resulting metabolites may have higher activity and/or greater toxicity than the original compound. Prozac has caused hepatitis and has also been shown to promote tumors in the liver. *Rophypnol* (*flunitrazepam*, or "Roofies,")—the date rape drug—is **fluorinated *Valium***, which is about **20-30 times more potent than *Valium* alone.** *Phen-Fen* (*Fenfluramine)* a weight-loss drug, fluorinated corticosteroids and fluorinated psychoactive drugs all contain fluoride. In 2000, a U.S. district judge approved a $3.75 billion national settlement of health claims stemming from *Fen-Phen*. More than 9,000 lawsuits have been filed against American Home Products, maker of *Fenfluramine*. People taking such drugs might exceed 5 mgs. in just one prescribed application.

We are essentially putting psychoactive drugs into the water supply. If you go in for surgery, you'll usually be given a fluoride-based anesthetic because fluoride is virulent enough to throw you into an immediate coma. *Sevoflurane,* one of many fluorinated agents used in anesthesia, such as florinated *Halothane*, is thought to be responsible for **renal failure**. *Hydrogen fluoride* is the **only** toxic element in the nerve gas *Sarin* (**1500 times more poisonous than cyanide**) used in the Japanese subway attack.

On August 8th, 2001, *Baycol*–a cholesterol-lowering drug taken by 700,000 Americans–was pulled off the market. It had been linked to 31 U.S. deaths. Bayer AG, the maker of the drug, would not disclose the total number of deaths worldwide. Scientists have found that **all fluoride compounds interfere with thyroid hormones**. Numerous **congenital abnormalities** have been reported due to first trimester exposure to *Fluconsazole*, a systemic anti-fungal agent. There have been numerous fluorinated drugs removed from the market recently. Most have been shown to cause serious **adverse cardiac effects**, probably due to fluoride's adverse effects on thyroid hormone activity.

Fluoride in the Food Chain

So now we have fluoride in our water, which means we're mass-medicating the population, although we can't control the dose because everyone drinks varying amounts. Back when safety levels in the water were set at 1 ppm, there was basically no other source.

Since then, fluoride has been added to toothpaste, mouth rinses and dental floss. Dentists treat the teeth topically with fluoride, and doctors prescribe fluoride supplements. And, of course, if fluoride is in the water, it's in the food chain.

Food is irrigated, washed, and processed with fluoridated water; we're consuming much more fluoride than we think. Independent lab reports show high levels in common products: .98 to 1.2 ppm in *Coca-Cola*, 1 ppm in *Minute Maid* orange juice, 2.1 ppm in *Fruit Loops*, 10 ppm in *Wheaties*, 6.8 ppm in *Gerber's* white grape juice which is often used as a sweetener in baby foods. Grapes are commonly sprayed with an insecticide that contains fluoride.

A 1996 study published in the *Journal of the American Dental Association* warned parents to limit their children's intake of juices due to excessive fluoride content. In fact, according to a 1993 government survey, children in non-fluoridated communities are already receiving at least 3 times the amount of fluoride recommended for total consumption, while children in fluoridated communities are receiving 4.6 to 7 times the recommended amount. The National Research Council of Canada has done extensive research on the many environmental sources of fluorides and the multiple avenues by which they enter the human food chain.

Most packaged foods are processed with fluoridated water, and many fruits and vegetables contain fluorides in pesticide and fertilizer residues. When fluoridation first began, exposure to fluoride from sources other than fluoridated water was minimal, but today that is not the case. **People now receive fluoride from a whole host of sources**, including pesticide residues, fluoridated dental products, mechanically de-boned meat, fluoride air pollution, and processed foods & beverages prepared with fluoridated water (soda, juice, beer, cereal, etc).

It has now reached the point where most people receive the "optimal" 1 mg./day of fluoride without ever drinking a glass of fluoridated water. **Foods such as sardines, tea, lettuce, spinach,** and others have particularly high fluoride contents. **If fluoride is ingested**, even though a person is eating a nutritious diet and taking the best supplements in the world, **all the good nutrition is rendered almost completely ineffective, and development or advancement of degenerative disease will ensue**.

The harmful effects of fluoride have been known for over one hundred years. How much more evidence is needed before we, the victims, stop this behavior modification program, being literally forced down out throats? **Some beer-drinking men consume over six liters of fluoridated water a day from beer alone**.

Fluoride in Nature

In any case, fluoride is unavoidable in the diet, since it is the **thirteenth most abundant element** and is **extremely reactive**, forming many compounds available to the human body. Fluorine occurs in nature as *calcium fluoride*. **Sodium fluoride is an industrial waste product** from the aluminum and phosphate fertilizer industries. **Since the 1920s and 1930s, it has been sold as a potent roach and rat killer**. Sodium fluoride (NaF), is **over five hundred times more soluble than calcium fluoride** (CaF_2). It requires eighty times more CaF_2 to kill a rat than NaF. Fluoridation critics never accepted the transformation of sodium fluoride from *dangerous chemical* to *benign cavity fighter*.

Fluoride in Industry

The first fluoride compound purposely put in the public water was sodium fluoride, a toxic by-product of the aluminum industry. During World War II, as Alcoa accelerated production to meet the need for more warplanes, they produced more of this pollutant and faced mounting damage claims. Eager to put a positive spin on fluoride, the U.S. Public Health Service–then under the command of Treasury Secretary Andrew Mellon, a founder and major stockholder of Alcoa–sent a company employed dentist to investigate certain towns where fluoride occurs naturally in water

This dentist observed that the inhabitants had fewer cavities than average, although they also had stained and eroded teeth. In 1939, a scientist funded by Alcoa solved the disposal problem when he proposed adding fluoride to drinking water to reduce tooth decay. Then in the 1940s the unimpeded production of fluoride became a matter of national security–**fluoride was the key substance used to separate the uranium isotope to build the atomic bomb**. Millions of tons of fluoride were required. In 1944, according to declassified documents, an accident at a DuPont plant in New Jersey producing fluoride for the Manhattan Project released large quantities into the atmosphere. Crops were poisoned, animals were crippled, and people were sickened.

The fluoride even etched windows in the local school. Scientists scrambled to gloss over the adverse effects in the interests of the war effort. Defense contractors and the government needed to create public support for fluoride and protect themselves from liability as well.

Fluoride's Effects on Physiology

The average consumer of fluoridated water is usually not aware that **sodium fluoride**, or *hydrofluosilicic acid*, is rated as **more toxic than lead** in chemistry indices and only **slightly less toxic than arsenic**. **Fluoride is not an essential nutrient** and, according to the National Academy of Sciences, has never been shown to be necessary for human life. Drs. Roger Berry and Wilfred Trillwood at Oxford United Hospitals, concluded that **sodium fluoride kills human cells at 1/20 the strength of fluoridated drinking water**. Biochemical research has established that chemical poisons like fluoride **form hydrogen bonds with protein *amide* groups** together

Thus, since DNA strands are connected by hydrogen bonds, **fluoride will damage chromosomes**. *General Chemistry*, McQuarrie and Rock, Univ. Cal., 1984, discusses fluorine: **"Because its electro-negativity is higher than that of any other element, fluorine occurs with a positive oxidation state in any compound."** Thus, **fluorine is the most reactive element known to chemists,** and **its greatest affinity is for calcium.**

Dr. Sam Epstein, Professor Emeritus of Environmental and Occupational Medicine at the University of Illinois, Chairman of the Cancer Prevention Coalition and author of *The Politics of Cancer*, wrote on May 29 in support of British MP John Butterfill's motion (EDM 1258) opposing water fluoridation: "Fluoridation of water reflects high receptivity to the fluoride industry, and indifference with significant public health penalties to the UK population. I should further note that some 100 leading national and international cancer prevention scientists and representatives of consumer and environmental organizations have endorsed the Cancer Prevention Coalition's opposition to fluoride in its *Stop Cancer Before It Starts* campaign report. "Fluoride used for this purpose comes from highly contaminated industrial-grade fluorosilicic wastes; contaminants include heavy metals. Furthermore, there is significant experimental evidence that fluoride induces a dose-related incidence of bone cancer in rats.

This is further supported by epidemiological studies incriminating fluoride and bone cancer in young men. It should further be noted that fluoride is currently added to the water supply of about 60% of the U.S. population. This is in sharp contrast to only 2% of the European population, which has much lower rates of dental caries."

An article in *Nature, The International Journal of Science*, Jan. 15, 1987, let the cat out of the bag, further exposing the fluoridation fiasco. It published university studies showing that **water boiled in an aluminum utensil for 10 minutes acquired 0.2-ppm of aluminum**, which is a cause of **Alzheimer's disease. If water is fluoridated at 1ppm, in ten minutes, 200 ppm of Aluminum are released–1,000 times more aluminum! Fluorine causes irreversible loss of potassium from human red cells. Fluorine increases excretion of iron–leading to anemia.**

Even at 10 mg. per liter, fluorine causes *anemia*, *lymphocytosis* and *leukopenia*. Blood levels of vitamin B_{12} are lowered. Damaging effects of fluorine are found in the stomach, duodenum, small intestines, liver, spleen, lungs, brain, pancreas, adrenals and thyroid. Fluorine causes liver and muscle glycogen depletion as well as lactic acid accumulation, with increased blood sugar.

Especially serious damage occurs in the spinal cord, with neurological symptoms following. **The pituitary gland takes up several times as much fluorine as any other soft tissue**, which is especially dangerous because **the pituitary is the master gland of the endocrine system. Fluorine may cause anoxia in newborns and shorten their survival. Fluoride inhibits neuromuscular activity.** *Human Biochemistry*, Orten and Neuhause, 9th Ed., tells us, "**Calcium is needed by all cells**. It is required for physiologic balance."

A particular and important effect of the calcium ion is on nervous tissue. **If the ionic calcium of the blood falls, the nervous system becomes hyperirritable**. "**Calcium is the main structural mineral in the body**. *Osteoporosis* is a result of calcium loss in the skeleton. During the last trimester of pregnancy, between 200 and 300 mg. of calcium are deposited every day in the skeleton of the fetus. **Pregnant women are given synthetic prenatal vitamins with added fluoride.** Anyone with a calcium deficiency can experience **muscle spasms and convulsions.**

Also, the tissue levels of two poisonous metals, *lead* and *cadmium,* increase, and **blood clotting is adversely affected** causing *thrombosis* and *embolism*. **Oxygen deprivation in heart muscle** is increased, with calcium deficiency causing *arhythmias*.

Fluoride is a mutagen. Rats dosed with fluoride had a statistically significant increase in bone tumors. Fluoride-dosed rats had tumors of the thyroid, oral cavity and rare tumors of the liver. **Female infertility** is associated with elevated levels of fluoride (>3 ppm). One ppm. of fluoride in water facilitates the uptake of aluminum into the brain of rats, producing the type of brain tangles (amyloid deposits) that are associated with Alzheimers disease and other types of dementia. Fluoridated water was associated with elevated levels of lead in children's blood. Lead is associated with a variety of neurological problems, including reduced intelligence, aggression and hyperactivity.

Recently released reports by the New York State Department of Public Health and an expert panel appointed by the U.S. Surgeon General dispute the American Dental Association's blanket claim that there are no adverse health effects from fluoridation. Fluoridation's effectiveness may be less than earlier studies had indicated, according to a new study by the National Institute for Dental Research. The largest study in the fifty years since fluoridation of U.S. water supplies began covers almost 40,000 children, aged 5 to 17, in 84 areas across the country. The *Journal of the American Dental Association*, Vol. 23, 1936, pp. 569-570, states. "There is an increasing amount of evidence of the injurious effects of fluorine, especially the **chronic intoxication** resulting from the ingestion of **minute amounts of fluorine over long periods of time**." It adds: "Toxicity data suggests that **fluorine, lead and arsenic belong to the same group**, as far as the ability to cause some symptoms of toxicity in minute dosage is concerned." Small daily doses of lead or arsenic are believed to be harmful. Fluoride is in the same category.

The U.S. Department of Agriculture in 1939 surveyed and reported on the effects of fluoride. Fluorine was shown to be the cause of a disfiguring dental disease known as *mottled enamel* or *fluorosis*.
Fluorine interferes with the normal process of calcification of teeth during the process of their formation, so that affected teeth, in addition to being unusually discolored and ugly in appearance, are **structurally weak** and **deteriorate early in life**.

For this reason, it is especially important that fluorine be **avoided** during the period of tooth formation, **from birth to the age of 12 years**. Pediatricians report that **over 30% of U.S. children have some degree of dental fluorosis, or mottling of the teeth from exposure to excessively high levels of fluoride**.

There is an almost infinite array of fluoride-based toothpastes, mouthwashes, dentifrices, tablets and vitamins on pharmacy shelves, many of which warn (in very tiny print) that ***they should not be used if the fluoride concentration in drinking water exceeds*** **0.7-ppm.** The sources of fluorine intoxication are...(among others)...**drinking water containing 1 ppm or more of fluorine**." It is estimated that approximately 40 million Americans suffer from arthritis, the most common type being osteoarthritis. Fluoride stimulates abnormal bone development. High dose fluoride treatment increases bone mass, but the **newly formed bone is structurally unsound**. Thus, instead of reducing hip fracture, **high doses of fluoride increase hip fracture**.

Kyphosis (skeletal fluorosis spinal curvature) was very prevalent among a community whose drinking water contained 7.4 ppm fluoride. It's alarming to learn of these adverse effects of fluoride at 1.1 parts per million when the Environmental Protection Agency raised the safe level for fluoride up to 4.0 parts per million. Who is being protected, the people or the firms that sell fluoride and the manufacturers who produce fluoride as a by-product they can't get rid of? Yes, **the fluoride producers cannot dispose of this waste product unless all of us drink a little bit each day**.

Thyroid Dysfunction

Up until the 1950s, European doctors used fluoride to reduce the activity of the thyroid gland for people suffering from overactive thyroid (hyperthyroidism). The daily dose of fluoride which people are now receiving in fluoridated communities (1.6 to 6.6 mg/day) actually exceeds the dose of fluoride found to depress the thyroid gland (2.3 to 4.5 mg/day). Hypothyroidism is currently one of the most common medical problems in the U.S. ***Synthroid***, the drug doctors prescribe to treat hypothyroidism, **was the fourth most prescribed drug in the U.S. in 2000**. Symptoms of hypothyroidism include *depression, fatigue, weight gain, muscle and joint pains, increased cholesterol levels* and *heart disease*.

From a recent University of York report, considered the "final word on fluoridation," it was shown that **symptoms** described in the literature on fluoride's adverse health effects **are identical to those observed in thyroid dysfunction**, and the condition known as *dental fluorosis* is a direct result of *fluoride-induced iodine deficiency* during the time of enamel formation. It showed an increase in thyroid cancers in the fluoridated areas when compared to non-fluoridated areas.

In China, where entire villages are being relocated due to fluoride contamination, fluoride is being openly acknowledged as the **cause of** *thyroid cancer, Kaschin-Beck disease,* and *iodine deficiency.* It has been established since the 1930s that the **thyroid hormones control tooth eruption**. Fluoridation delays the eruption of teeth because of its hypothyroid effect. ***Dental fluorosis* is a sign of thyroid dysfunction.** Any anti-thyroid substance administered during the time of enamel formation will produce the effects seen in *dental fluorosis*. **Fluorides actually cause cavities.**

There are countless papers—some of them found in the *York Report*—clearly state that the dental defects seen in fluorosis **predispose the teeth to caries**. *Hyperthyroidism*, caused after iodine was added to public water supplies in the early 1920s, led to the use of fluorides as **anti-thyroid medication**. Fluorides are the worst **endocrine disruptor** imaginable. What was once known as *fluoride-iodine antagonism* can now be explained in detail by thousands of papers showing the fluoride power on *G-protein activation*. The biochemical activity of fluoride mimics TSH (thyroid-stimulating-hormone) on G-protein activation—molecular on/off switches by which all thyroid hormone activity is regulated.

Three-quarters of the world's population is suffering from **iodine deficiency** in areas which are identical to endemic fluorosis areas. Tooth decay is an epidemic in certain U.S. populations, whether or not they live in fluoridated cities. Eighty percent of decay occurs in 25% of the population, most of them poor and minorities. Well-meaning, but misguided dentists and hygienists are still pushing to get more of the U.S. fluoridated by the year 2010, primarily because they believe it will help poor children who suffer every year from needless dental pain that interferes with their eating, learning, and sleeping.

One problem is that dentists want more money to actually treat poor children. **Well-nourished children who practice good dental hygiene usually have less decay.**

Politics and Suppression of Truth

When the fluoridation campaign began, it was determined that the optimal dose was 1 milligram per day, which translates to 1 part per million (ppm) in the water supply (assuming an individual drinks 1 liter of water a day). Officials concurred that concentrations of 2 ppm would not be acceptable because that would produce too many cases of dental fluorosis. But over the decades the maximum allowable contaminant level (fluoride is classified as a contaminant by the EPA), inched up to 2.4 ppm. Then in 1985 when the EPA increased the allowance to 4 ppm, something unprecedented occurred.

The union representing employees at EPA headquarters in Washington D.C.–some 1500 scientists, engineers and other professionals–revolted against their own management and filed an *amicus curiae* brief in court to support a lawsuit brought by the National Resources Defense Council against the EPA. As the brief stated, in their professional opinion, allowable fluoride levels should have been *reduced* rather than *raised*. They alleged that evidence of adverse effects was manipulated or ignored in order to arrive at a preordained political conclusion. Why was this allowed when the *Federal Register* of November 14, 1985, stated that the Office of Drinking Water received 11 out of 12 studies confirming the ***carcinogenicity*** (cancer-causing potential) of fluoride during a comment period on the safe allowable levels of fluoride in drinking water?

An article titled "*Chronic Fluorine Intoxication*" in a 1943 issue of the *Journal of the American Medical Association* (JAMA) declared, "**Fluorides are general protoplasmic poisons**, probably because of their capacity to modify the metabolism of cells by **changing the permeability of the cell membrane** and by **inhibiting certain enzyme systems**."

Slander and smear campaigns have been commonplace in the frenzy of the fluoridation wars. The late Dr. John A. Yiamouyiannis, a biochemist and former biochemical editor of the prestigious *Journal of the Chemical Abstracts Service*, the world's largest chemical information center, was **removed from his post in 1969 when he began to publish articles critical of fluoridation**.

Since thousands of articles routinely passed through his hands, many of which showed the **negative effects of even miniscule amounts of fluoride on enzyme function and the immune system**, he began to question its use for human consumption. He says he was told by his editor-in-chief at the time, Dr. Russell Rowlett, that the Chemical Abstracts Service's federal funding ($1.1 million) was in jeopardy and that **if Yiamouyiannis did not "cease and desist" in his attack of fluoridation, he would be fired**. When Yiamouyiannis did not comply, he was put on probation and ultimately forced to resign.

He continued to be an outspoken critic of fluoridation until the time of his death, and wrote a paper saying the NIDR data show **no difference in decay rates between areas with fluoridated and unfluoridated water supplies.** Research scientists have produced a report saying the same data, showing **18% less decay** in the fluoridated areas, a difference they call significant, but which is far below the **40 to 60% reduction** claimed by the ADA.

In the summer of 1988, an article in the 100,000-member American Chemical Society's trade journal *Chemical and Engineering News*, examined the evidence on safety and effectiveness of fluoride and found many unresolved questions: "If the lifeblood of science is open debate of evidence, scientific journals are the veins and arteries of the body scientific. Yet **journal editors often have refused, for political reasons, to publish information that raises questions about fluoridation**." Submissions critical of fluoridation are returned as "inappropriate for publication." **The bulk of the social science literature on fluoridation is scientifically proven and indeed scientifically unquestionable. The many studies that fall into this category make no examination of the scientific evidence, but rely entirely on the endorsements of dental and medical authorities.**

Those promoting fluoridation have had almost exclusive access to the resources of authority, even while claiming that scientific truth was their strongest plank and that opponents to fluoridation are spurred by personal or political motivation. Therefore, **opposition to fluoridation has always been treated as an anomaly, to be explained away as the activity of fringe groups and "quacks**." The problem began in 1950 when key public health and professional bodies such as the United States Public Health Service and the ADA came out supporting fluoridation.

Almost overnight, the scientific issues were treated as closed. Fluoridation was considered scientifically proven and, furthermore, criticisms of fluoridation were treated as political rather than scientific. **Opponents were classified as cranks rather than as rational critics**. The climate is the same today. The combination of direct attacks on public opponents of fluoridation, fears about loss of grants, and the general labeling of them as ignorant and misguided, combine to discourage scientists from doing research or speaking out on the issues.

The relative lack of open opposition, in turn, encourages a perception of the fringe nature of critics. The pro-fluoridationists, through their control over dental and medical associations, their control over health authorities, and their influence over editorial policy of journals and publishers, have **exerted power to stop expression of anti-fluoridation views by professionals**. Nevertheless, not all critics of fluoridation have been effectively silenced.

Brian Dementi, toxicologist at the Virginia State Department of Health, discussed in his 1981 report, *Fluoride in Drinking Water*, the many scientific papers **showing fluoride to be both *mutagenic* and *carcinogenic***. Dementi contends that **there has not been nearly enough research done to warrant the claim that fluoridation is absolutely safe**. He concludes, "The weight of the evidence from studies on mutagenic effects of fluoride indicates that the substance is **mutagenic** (causes mutations) **at low concentrations**.

He adds that "there appears to be virtually **no margin of safety for fluoride** of the nature generally sought after or required for exposures to toxic substances." Dementi's report includes a 1969 study that shows an average 48% reduction in the activity of the enzyme *succinic dehydrogenase* in the kidneys of golden hamsters that drank water containing 1-ppm sodium fluoride. He discusses a study done in 1975, in which monkeys exposed to fluoride at the 1-ppm level for 18 months **exhibited *cytochemical* changes in their kidneys**.

A 1979 report stated, "The available evidence suggests that **some patients with long-term renal failure are being affected by drinking water with as little as 2-ppm fluoride**." In Dementi's report, which was deleted from Virginia Health Department files because it was "too old," Dementi chronicles the research on *fluoride mutagenesis*.

He writes that in 1977 researchers observed *leucocytes* in cows suffering from *fluorosis* (a systemic poisoning caused by excessive fluoride which can lead to severe crippling). The *chromosomal aberration rate* was over twice that of controls. The authors concluded, "These data suggest that **inorganic fluor compounds represent a potential genetic hazard to mammals**."

Similarly, another 1977 study by a team who added sodium fluoride to drinking water at various concentrations and noticed the effects on mouse cells (bone marrow and *spermatocytes*), showed "**statistically significant increases in chromosomal aberrations in both types of cells** even at drinking water levels as low as 1-ppm sodium fluoride." Dementi states, "Any perturbation of this complex system must be viewed, a priori, as cause for concern."

The largest epidemiological study ever done on fluoridated water and *carcinogenicity* was conducted in 1977 by Yiamouyiannis and Dr. Dean Burk, retired head of *cytochemistry* at the National Cancer Institute, in which they monitored cancer rates over a twenty-year period in ten fluoridated American cities and ten non-fluoridated ones. After controlling for population differences in age, race and sex, the researchers found **an increased cancer mortality rate in persons over age forty-five in fluoridated cities**. The study was validated in three courts of law in the U.S.

Further studies on DNA and DNA-repair systems have shown that **fluoride inhibits or interferes with the ability of DNA to repair itself**, thus providing a clue as to how fluoride might exert a carcinogenic impact on human cells. The New Jersey Department of Health had conducted a study and found the incidence of *osteosarcoma* to be significantly higher in fluoridated communities versus non-fluoridated ones. The New Jersey findings supported similar ones by larger national studies and by the National Toxicology Program.

In a 1989 *Medical Tribune*, a weekly publication for health professionals revealed that a panel appointed to study the issue in 1983 by C. Everett Koop, then surgeon general, also raised questions about health effects. **All mention of those issues was edited out of the panel's final report.** The omission of health concerns from the panel's final report is "shocking," charged Robert Carton, an EPA scientist and president of the union that represents the agency's scientific staff.

The immune system, the body's National Guard, so to speak, using white blood cells, **is disrupted and rendered much less effective from the effects of fluoride**. These **white blood cells are calcium dependent**. One consequence is hypersensitivity or "allergy" which will bring increased, more severe or longer-lasting colds, flus and other ills. Since studies have revealed that **fluoride, taken over a long period of time, breaks down the immune system**, some researchers feel that it is therefore **conducive to AIDS**.

The *Cape Cod News*, August 20, 1986, observed that **the three longest fluoridated areas in the U.S.**–New York, Washington D.C. and San Francisco–**are the most prolific with AIDS**. Los Angeles and San Antonio, on the other hand, have never been fluoridated, and this plague has been miniscule in these cities." **Though these two cities have large homosexual communities, AIDS isn't as prevalent.**

Dean Burk, Chief Chemist Emeritus at U.S. Cancer Institute, states, "In point of fact, **fluoride causes more cancer death, and causes it faster than any other chemical**." (*Fluoride and Cancer*," Congressional Record H7176-6, July 21, 1975, by Dean Burk and J.A. Yiamouyiannis).

Several studies, including one carried on over a period of years at the University of Wisconsin and published in 1963, show that **fluoridated areas have an exceptional number of stillbirths**. Scientists know that **fluoride passes through the placenta**. Dr. Ionel Rapaport, University of Wisconsin, "carried out two studies showing that ***mongolism***, a birth defect characterized by mental and physical retardation, **occurs more often in areas where there is a relatively high fluoride content in the water**."

According to the *Grand Rapids Press*, July 28, 1955, following widely publicized fluoridation experiments in Grand Rapids, Michigan: "**Deaths rose sharply after four years of fluoridation** which began in 1945. **Deaths from cancer, heart disease, intracranial** (brain) **disease, diabetes and hardening of the arteries increased 25 to 50 percent** over those in Michigan as a whole."

The *J.A.M.A.* for Feb. 10, 1961 states, "**Fluorine also tends to accumulate in the bones, leading to hyper-calcification and brittleness. Ligaments and tendons also become calcified**.

Serious symptoms may ensue, such as **loss of mobility of joints, easy fracture** and **pressure on the spinal cord**. Other defects include **baldness** in young men, **anemia** and **decreased blood clotting** power. In women, **painful menstruation, lowered birth rate, high incidence of fracture, thyroid alterations** and **liver damage**."

When one drinks *sodium fluoride* (NaF) in water, they excrete *calcium fluoride* (CaF2) in their urine. **This calcium was stolen from the body**. In 1936, fifty percent of Americans were calcium deficient. The AMA journal of the same year reported that out of 4,000 persons checked in at a New York hospital, only two were not suffering from calcium deficiency. The situation is worse today. **Fluoride in drinking or cooking water can disrupt the enzymatic activity of proteins.** Dr. John Yiamouyiannis *(Fluoride The Aging Factor*, Health Action Press, 1983) observed, "If the shape (or conformation) of the protein is greatly distorted by fluoride, the body's immune system will no longer be able to recognize the protein and will attempt to destroy it."

The summer 1959 issue of *Clinical Physiology* reported on page 96, a study done by experimental embryologist James D. Eberrt and published in *Scientific American* March 1959. It relates: "...he found that **sodium fluoride** in low concentrations **blocked,** almost completely, **the regions destined to form heart muscle** but left the developing brain and spinal cord intact." He correlated this with the **high incidence of *ventricular septal defect*,** which was **relatively uncommon before the 1950s, and fluoridation**. Most of the advanced Western European countries have banned fluoridation or given it up. **The United States is the most fluoridated country, and it has the highest tooth decay rate in the world**! So is fluoridation the "biggest hoax ever inflicted on humanity" or a modern miracle opposed by a small, ignorant minority?

Non-fluoridated toothpaste is available at your local health food store or co-op. Children and parents who are truly concerned about their children can refuse fluoride "swish" programs in public schools. The Union of Scientists and professionals at EPA headquarters has voted to **oppose** fluoridation and has called upon Congress to issue a "national moratorium" on the sixty year old policy. The toxicity of fluoride is so great and the purported benefits associated with it are so small—if there is any at all—that requiring every man, woman and child in America to ingest it criminal behavior on the part of the government.

Antibiotics

Antibiotics

Antibiotics in our bodies cannot tell the cops from the robbers. With no discretion, they kill *friendly* as well as *harmful* bacteria. It is usually not recognized that for every *injurious* or *parasitic* microbe, there are dozens of *beneficial* ones. The majority of bacteria are helpful, actually working for us, and are a source of nutrition, like the *microflora* in our intestines. **Antibiotics kill the friendly bacteria** that manufacture vitamin B_{12} in the gut. Where's the logic in depressing our immune system to fight an infection artificially? Humans and other animals don't produce antibiotics, nor do they need to, if their endocrine, immune, and nervous systems have the mineral, vitamin, protein, and enzyme substances found in foods grown on mineral-rich soil. Armed with these tools, the Earth's highest forms of life–*humans and animals* are well equipped to fight the Earth's lowest forms of life–*bacteria and fungi*. This has kept human beings surviving for aat least 100,000 generations. **Nature's track record for being right should inspire our trust.** Dr. Richard Novick, Public Health Research Institute, New York City, on the subject of antibiotics, says, **"Doctors use them as a crutch for an easy way to take care of patients, and drug companies have a financial stake in selling them as fast as they can."**

Today, about 15 million lbs. a year, **nearly half of U.S. production of antibiotics, is fed to farm animals**, primarily cattle, poultry and pigs–$270.9 million worth in 1983. It has been shown how antibiotic-resistant bacterium, in addition to residual antibiotics, can make their way from the barnyard to the dinner table and into the humans who eat it. **Antibiotics have not made any significant changes in the plague of human diseases**. Pathologist Widmann of Duke University stated, "Wonder drugs have not eradicated infectious disease; they have merely changed the conditions and natural history of many infections. They have, however, contributed to *immunosuppression*, perhaps **setting the stage for AIDS**. Antibiotics, instead of assisting the inflammatory repair process, **inhibit both *chemotaxis* and *phagocytosis***, which are essential to the healing of damaged tissue. **Antibiotics have been implicated in causing as many as 300,000 disease reactions per year with up to 90,000 deaths per year resulting therefrom.** Antibiotics have caused immunologic reactions such as: (a). *anaphylaxis*, (b.) *urticaria*, (c.) *Coomb's-positive hemolytic anemia*, (d.) *serum sickness* and (e.) *morbilliform eruptions,* resembling measles.

Antibiotics cause gastrointestinal reactions by direct irritation of the mucous membrane, destruction of normal, natural bacterial flora or by creating bacterial overgrowth of abnormal forms. Antibiotics eliminate organisms from the normal flora of the skin, oral and genito-urinary mucosa and promote growth of drug-resistant organisms. **Oral or vaginal candidiasis** (thrush) **often follows the use of broad-spectrum antibiotics**. Now, if the Ehrlich/Metchnikoff germ theory was still a contender in the ring of disease causation, which it's not, the antibiotic approach to disease treatment might have some credibility. It is worth noting that the term *antibiotic* is from root words that mean **"against life"** and is defined by the medical dictionaries as: (1) **destructive of life**, (2) a chemical substance produced by a microorganism, which are able to kill other microorganisms.

The layman's dictionary simply tells us that antibiotics are substances having the power to arrest or kill microorganisms called germs. **The incidence of infections in wounds caused by injury or operations has not decreased despite the use of antibiotics for more than twenty-five years**, declared bacteriologist and surgeon Dr. William Altemeier to a meeting of the American College of Surgeons. His study revealed that antibiotics may actually have increased the number and complexity of problems related to infections.

In 1972, the U.S. Senate Small Business Monopoly Subcommittee held hearings about drug abuse, and Dr. Henry E. Simmons made known some very important facts about antibiotics. At that time, Dr. Simmons was director of the Bureau of Drugs in the FDA and blamed doctors who prescribed antibiotics routinely for creating additional problems. Simmons explained that **"the inappropriate use of an antibiotic can result in the appearance of resistant strains of bacteria with an increased number of superinfections."** He explained to the subcommittee that one of the major problems in medicine today was the sharp rise in hospital-treatment-caused superinfections he called blood poisoning.

Simmons and other doctor-witnesses testified to the facts that: (1) "Antibiotics possibly cause 100,000 to 300,000 *iatrogenic* cases each year of which 30% to 50% are fatal." (2) "60% of hospital patients who receive antibiotics don't need them." (3) "Production of antibiotics has increased 300 percent in 10 years–in 1972 reaching 2.4 million kilograms."

This would mean, that in 1972, enough antibiotics were produced to give every man, woman and child in the U.S. 50 doses, a drop in the bucket compared to production in 1982. (4) In a letter by FDA to national medical groups, pertinent excerpts pointed out that: (a) **antibiotics are being massively introduced when not indicated and are often misused.** (b) **Indiscriminate or inappropriate use of antibiotics is detrimental.**

Robbins and Cotran's *Pathologic Basis Of Disease*, 1979, tells us that over 90% of hospital isolates of *staphylococci* from patients with serious infectious diseases are penicillin-resistant and that *gonococci* have become resistant to the *tetracyclines*, *streptomycin* and *sulfonamides*. "Drug resistance has been documented for many microbes, and so it has become a race between the ingenuity of man in developing new drugs and the ingenuity of the microbes in achieving methods of survival." Or, could it be that an intelligent Creator designed the microbe to adapt to chemical insult, in order to continue its scavenger function of dissolving dead cells so that man can keep living in spite of his **evolutionary ignorance**? In 1972, Harry Dowling, a former chairman of the Council on Drugs of the AMA, testified before the Senate Monopoly Subcommittee and cited FDA data that doctors prescribe 10 to 20 times as many antibiotics as are medically justified. Dowling said, **"It is doubtful that the average person has an illness that requires treatment with an antibiotic more often than once every five or ten years."**

The late Dr. Robert Mendelsohn, M.D., in his book, *Confessions of a Medical Heretic*, had a few remarks about antibiotic misuse and told us: (1) "...these 'miracle' drugs that were once extremely valuable are now extremely dangerous. (2) "Penicillin and other antibiotics do not shorten the course of the disease, do not prevent complications, and do not reduce the number of pathogenic organisms in the nose and throat. They do no good at all. (3) "...Chloromycetin (*chloramphenicol*) has the common, fatal side effect of **interfering with the bone marrow's production of blood**. About *Chloromycetin*, Mendelsohn says that if a person's life is at stake, using this drug could be an acceptable risk to take. But if a child suffers nothing more than a sore throat, "is the non-relief *chloromycetin* might bring worth risking depression of the child's bone marrow, requiring multiple transfusions and other therapies, none of which will guarantee complete recovery?" (4) *Tetracycline* became so popular it became known as the "house call" antibiotic.

He relates that the FDA finally required a warning on all packages informing that in late pregnancy, infancy, and to the age of 8–it can cause permanent yellow-gray-brown discoloration of teeth including malformed tooth enamel. Mendelsohn, who was an Associate Professor of Medicine, warns that 8 to 10 million Americans go to the doctor, each year, for a cold. **Ninety-five percent get a prescription and at least 50% are for antibiotics, which are not even indicated for a cold.** He says, "Not only are these people duped into paying for something which has **no effectiveness against their problem**, but **they are set up for the hazards of side effects and the risks of deadlier infections**."

Daniel L. Azarnoff, M.D., University of Kansas Medical Center, writing in the book *Controversies in Therapeutics*, 1980, comments, "A study of 50 randomly selected charts from one week in June 1973, at a well known medical center showed that 56 courses of antibiotics were given. Of all the prescriptions for antibiotics, 63% were considered not indicated, inappropriately selected or given in wrong doses." Dr. Azarnoff, in his study entitled *Monitoring and Control of Physician Prescribing Are Needed* tells us a few things that are hard to believe: **The average doctor writes approximately 8,000 prescriptions per year.** In one study involving 1,608 patients receiving antibiotics, **62% had no evidence of infection**, which would not indicate a need for antibiotics. Of 254 patients receiving the drug *spironalactone* in a university hospital, 104 were also receiving potassium chloride, which in combination, frequently has deleterious effects on humans. He warns: "If misuse of drugs occurs at teaching institutions that have strong peer review and supervision, what's happening in less-well-supervised situations? In one recent year, nearly 7 million ounces of antibiotic *Tetracycline* syrup was prescribed.

Ninety-nine percent went to children under 8 years of age. This particular drug produces symptoms similar to **brain tumors** and can cause **mouth and kidney infections, rectal disease, kidney failure, permanent tooth damage** and **inhibition of bone growth**. This information comes from Dr. Summer Yaffe, chairman of the Committee of Drugs for the American Academy of Pediatrics in Philadelphia. Dr. Yaffee warns, **"You don't need tetracycline. It's not effective,** and **it's toxic.** In small children, **it can cause the skull to bulge."** The condition mimics a brain tumor so closely that in some cases **babies had to undergo surgery**. The anguish and expense parents go through makes it clear that more stringent controls should be put on this drug.

Friendly Bacteria

Antibiotics (prescription or residues in meat & poultry) **cause improper or insufficient bacteria in the bowel**. The ability of intestinal flora to metabolize nutrients, hormones, bile acids, cholesterol and carcinogens is well established. **Over 400 species of microorganism inhabit the healthy human gut and contribute four pounds to overall body weight.** The ecology of these microorganisms is very important to the health of the human body. The balance of this ecology can significantly affect **lactose tolerance, serum cholesterol levels, tumor growth or suppression, serum steroid hormone levels, immune function, the proliferation of pathogenic organisms in the gut, bowel transit time and other aspects of metabolism**. Relatively few bacteria, between 10 and 100 organisms per ml. of stomach contents, are commonly found in the healthy human stomach. Concentrations of one trillion organisms per ml. of content are common in the colon.

Immune Suppression

Scientific American Medicine, 12/80, 7:-1, states, "In the past decade, there have been major advances in the use of immunosuppressive drugs in organ transplantation. An important side effect, however, has been the creation of a group of patients with major defects in host defense against infection. Therapeutic programs that may have an adverse effect on a patient's ability to withstand infection include *antibiotics, radiation therapy, corticosteroids* (cortisone-prednisone), and *cytotoxic agents*. Thus, antibiotic therapy should be as specific as possible and should not be used needlessly." One type of adverse reaction from antibiotics is called *cytotoxic* and an antibody theoretically mediates it. By whatever mechanism, the drug serves as a *haptene* and results in an *immugenic* action. Some of the adverse consequences of the "cytotoxic response" include *hemolytic anemia, agranulocytosis* and *thrombocytopenia* associated, supposedly, with the autoimmune mechanism. This ignores the true cause–**drugs**–and sets up a make-believe situation that blames the consequent pathology on patients' natural ability to cope with any physiological insult, as well as the drug insult.

Penicillin and *streptomycin* are more often associated with *hemolytic anemia*; a break down of the red blood cell wall, while *streptomycin, chloramphenicol*, antihistamines and sulfonamides, like HEAVY METALS, **interfere with the body's ability to produce neutrophils,** which is called *neutropenia*.

The periodical *Current Therapy*, 1983 revealed a few side effects from Penicillin. They are:

1. **Skin reactions**–a. *exfoliative dermatitis*; b. *maculopapular eruptions*; c. *necrotizing dermatitis*; d. *purpura* (hemorrhagic disease).

2. **Kidney reactions**–a. *angiitis* (renal artery inflammation); b. *glomerulonephritis*; c. *acute nephritis*.

3. **Other reactions and symptoms**–a. *eosinophilic pneumonia*; b. *photoallergic sensitivity*; c. *drug fever*; d. symptoms such as *dyspnea, fever, bleeding, nerve damage* and *painful muscles*.

4. ***Systemic Lupus Erythematosus*** has been induced by *Procainamide, Isoniazid, Quinidine*, and *Griseofulvin,* as well as by *penicillin*.

Not only are antibiotics not needed nor even indicated, they are classified as *immunosupressive* drugs, which impair the human immune system. How many fatal cases of AIDS are, in truth, the after-effect of irrationally prescribed antibiotics? Many antibiotics have a *nephro* (kidney) *toxicity* factor of 20% and several antibiotics have *hepa* (liver) toxicity factor more than 20%. Since most antibiotics inhibit chemotaxis and phagocytosis, **they definitely impair the immune system**, and, in turn, can and will contribute to AIDS. In the *Journal, Diseases of the Chest*, (39, 630-642: 1961), two chest specialists, Sidransky and Pearl, blatantly cautioned, "*Invasive pulmonary aspergillosis* almost always follows antibiotic or steroid (cortisone/prednisone) therapy and is increasing in incidence."

In other words, the administration of antibiotics or steroids **destroys the normal, needed bacteria in the respiratory tract**, which digest and destroy yeast cells. Devoid of proper bacterial flora, the stage is set for the invasion of yeast organisms such as *aspergillosis* and *histoplasmosis* spores. Both conditions can lead to pneumonia and influenza-type illness. *Fatal Aplastic Anemia* after *Chloromycetin* and *Tagamet* has been reported in the *Physicians Drug Alert*–April 1982. On day 32, the marrow was aplastic, on day 34, the patient died. **Both *Chloromycetin* and *Tagamet* can cause bone-marrow suppression.**

Chloromycetin causes reversible and irreversible ***pancytopenia.*** Most cases of *Chlormycetin*-induced *aplastic anemia* occur 2 weeks to 12 months after oral administration. Three cases of *Tagamet*-associated *pancytopenia* have been reported with marked marrow *hypoplasia* in one patient. How many unreported cases? Pancytopenia (PCP) exists when platelets, white cells and red cells are all diminished; an indication of **bone marrow depression**. When due to drugs, it is also called *secondary aplastic* (hypoplastic) *anemia.* Most cases of *Leukopenia*, which means a white blood cell count under 4,800, are usually due to **a decrease in neutrophils**-called *polys* or *polymorphonuclear leukocytes.* Neutrophils, as already mentioned, constitute the body's first line of defense when tissues are damaged. By chemotaxis, neutrophils promptly migrate to areas of inflammation and *phagocytize* (engulf) foreign matter and other necrotic debris.

Dr. W. Eugene Sanders, associate Professor of Medicine and Microbiology, University of Florida College of Medicine, was quoted in the *Health Bulletin*, Vol.9 No.3, that, "there was a time when there was so much penicillin used on hospital wards that one could detect minute organisms of penicillin in the air." He cautioned that **doctors prescribe antibiotics too frequently, in too high doses** or when they are not needed and this is upsetting the ecology of the human body and making it more difficult for the natural defense system to do its job. He goes on to state, **"This is not just a problem confined to physicians...It is prevalent in the best teaching institutions of this country."** Killing the myth is much more difficult than killing bacteria. The mystery of the effectiveness of antibiotics is decided in the *petri dish* or culture plate. Antibiotics *in vitro* (test tube or petri dish) kill microorganisms by weakening the cell walls.

But...in the body–*in vivo*–the real effect is the **enzymatic blockade of reactions** of cellular biochemistry needed for repair or replacement. A problem in this area was made manifest by F.K. Widmann, M.D., assistant Professor of Pathology at Duke University School of Medicine. Dr. Widmann stated that **culture contamination is by no means uncommon** and that detergents, alcohol sponges or other skin cleaners are not adequate when doing venipunctures to obtain blood for culturing. With millions of bacteria inhabiting a single breath of air and thousands of bacteria being pushed under the skin and into the bloodstream with each hypodermic needle insertion–it becomes evident that sterility of specimen and non-contamination of Petri cultures is a **sheer impossibility**.

Gram-positive or *gram-negative* bodies resembling yeasts may be seen in spinal fluids shortly after myelograms...obviously an artifact introduced into the spinal fluid by the hypodermic needle. In the case of tetracyclines, they enter the *mitochondrion* (power plant of the cell) and induce defective *oxidative phosphorylation*, which brings inflammatory repair to a halt. Steroids such as *Cortisone* and *Prednisone* are pharmacologically designated as anti-inflammation agents and do just that...**stop inflammation**. All authorities on chemotherapy of microbial diseases relate that in the selection of antimicrobial drugs and treatment guidelines, identification of the causative organism is essential to the appropriate antimicrobial drug selection and successful treatment of infections. If microorganisms cause disease, it would, naturally, be of scientific benefit to identify the culprit and then administer an effective chemotherapeutic agent with *selective toxicity*. Selective toxicity means the ability to kill (*bactericidal*) or inhibit (*bacteriostatic*) microorganisms without harming or killing the host (patient). Bactericidal type chemotherapeutic agents called *antimicrobials* include: 1. *Penicillins*; 2. *Cephalosporins*; 3. *Aminoglycosides* such as *Streptomycin*, *Neomycin*, *Kanamycin*, *Gentamycin*, *Tobramycin* and *Amikacin*; 4. *Vancomycin*; 5. *Polymixin*, *Polymixin B* and *Colistin*.

Bacteriostatic agents include the following: 1. *Sulphonamides* (SO_2NH_2), sulfa-like compounds; 2. *Trimethoprim*; 3. *Tetracyclines*; 4. *Chloramphenicol*; 5. *Erythromycin*; 6. *Lincomycin* or *Clindamycin*. This specificity factor has been determined in a petri dish by *disk diffusion*. The problem, or example, is seen in the fact that almost 100% of salmonella bacteria are susceptible, in vitro, to *Gentamycin* or *Colistin*, but in vivo (in the body) are diagnosed as systemic *salmonellosis*, **there's no therapeutic benefit derived from this antibiotic**. Also, *subacute bacterial endocarditis* is supposedly caused by the bacteria *viridans streptococci*. **In the dish, *chloramphenicol* destroys the microorganism almost 100% whereas in the blood, the antibiotic has no clinical benefit at all.** If you stop the first phase of the biochemistry of inflammation by administering an antihistamine, which neutralizes the histamine and relieves brawny induration or swelling...**relief of symptoms occurs, but there is no repair**. If you give an *antipyretic* and stop the *hyperemia* with its accompanying heat or fever, you have symptomatic relief, but **there is no repair**. You can administer an antibiotic or steroid hormone with abatement of symptoms, but **there is no repair**.

Cipro

Cipro is *ciprofloxacin*, a *fluorinated quinolone*, belonging to a class of **fluorinated antibiotics,** which also include *enoxacin, temafloxacin, grepafloxacin, norfloxacin, sparfloxacin, tosufloxacin, fleroxacin, lomefloxacin, ofloxacin*, etc. Ciprofloxacin has been in use since 1987 for a variety of indications and is the most widely used *fluoroquinolone* in humans and animals worldwide. In 2000, the FDA approved its use in treatment of inhalation anthrax under their "accelerated approval" regulations. They had actually taken the unusual step of urging *Bayer*—the sole manufacturer—to file for such approval, supposedly in order to protect the public from future terrorist attacks. The U.S. Department of Defense had already ordered reserves of *Cipro* during the 1991 Gulf War.

Adverse Effects

Along with Baycol (*cerivastatin*), other fluorinated drugs like *temafloxacin* and *grepafloxacin* (fluoroquinolones) have been withdrawn from the market because they had caused **severe liver and renal damage**—and **death**. Fatal liver failure associated with ciprofloxacin was reported in the *Lancet* in 1994. Ciprofloxacin has been implicated in several cases of acute renal failure and is the most established fluoroquinolone to cause such renal dysfunction. The most common side-effects reported due to Cipro are gastrointestinal in nature and similar to those reported when children accidentally ingest "too much" fluoride from their toothpaste—nausea, diarrhea, vomiting, and abdominal pain. Ciprofloxacin administration results in elevated serum fluoride levels. In a series of tests evaluating the safety of ciprofloxacin in children, serum fluoride levels increased after 12 hours in 79% of the children; on day 7, the 24-hour urinary fluoride excretion was higher in 88.9% of children observed. Just as other fluorinated drugs, Cipro can cause **musculo-skeletal disorders** such as *rhabdomyolysis*.

Since the introduction of fluoroquinolones on the market in 1987, more than 200 cases of rhabdomyolysis, tendonitis, tendon rupture, etc., have been reported in the literature. In October 1994, the Japan Pharmaceutical Affairs Bureau was first to amend the product information for fluoroquinolones to state that rhabdomyolysis may occur. In 1996, the FDA also issued directives to manufacturers to include warning statements on all fluoroquinolone product inserts, to alert patients and caregivers to the potential for *tendonitis* and *tendon rupture*.

Also in 1996, the Sri Lanka Drug Evaluation Sub-Committee decided that the product information of fluoroquinolone antibiotics should include a warning stating "The onset of tendon pain calls for immediate withdrawal of fluoroquinolone antibiotics." **Achilles tendon rupture** was shown to occur even after withdrawal of the drug. Pathologically, there was ultrastructure alteration in *tendinocytes*. Just as in other cases of fluoride poisoning, studies in animals show that magnesium deficiency aggravates the induced *tendinopathy*.

Drug Interactions/Death

Drug interactions with ciprofloxacin have resulted in fatal outcomes due to ***potentiation*** of the effects of another drug, such as *theophylline*, *methadone*, or *warfarin*. As in other fluorinated drugs, ciprofloxacin is a **potent inhibitor** of the thyroid hormone-regulated *P450* enzyme detoxification system in the liver. Of all fluoroquinolones, *ciprofloxacin* and *enoxacin* have shown the **greatest inhibitory capacity**. P450 IA2 prevents the metabolism/inactivation of *methylxanthines*, thereby causing increased serum concentrations of drugs like theophylline and caffeine, which, in turn, causes excess CNS and cardiac stimulation. Cipro also elevates serum fluoride levels. The liver has been identified as a target organ of fluoroquinolone toxicity in animal studies. Already in the 1930s, the same was shown by Bayer's scientists, who found that all organic fluoride compounds tested interfered with thyroid hormone activity in liver and muscle tissue. Meanwhile, they showed "anti-bacterial" activity. This led to the development of many fluorinated medications, including the numerous compounds then used very successfully in the treatment of hyperthyroidism.

One scientist developed many fluorinated "medications." When it was discovered that some of these organic compounds had the same detrimental effects on teeth and bone as inorganic fluoride—although much less actual fluorine was involved—he even filed patents, using these compounds in dental preparations. Pregnant women should never take ciprofloxacin. **Cipro transfers through the placenta.** It inhibits P450 IA2, which has been shown to be critical for neonatal survival, by influencing the physiology of respiration in neonates. Mice lacking this cytochrome died shortly after birth and showed symptoms of **severe respiratory distress**. Respiratory distress is a side-effect of ciprofloxacin in adults also. Cipro also **transfers through breastmilk**.

Resistance to Bacteria

Taking ciprofloxin can spur germs to mutate so that future bacterial infections become untreatable. During the last decades a dramatic increase in bacterial strains multiresistant to antibiotics, particularly Cipro, has been reported. *Clostridium difficile* has become one of the most common acquired organisms in hospitals and long-term care institutions. The organism typically infects patients whose normal intestinal flora has been disturbed by the administration of a broad-spectrum antibiotic such as Cipro. The diarrhea and inflammatory colitis associated with infection represent a serious medical and surgical complication leading to increased morbidity and mortality, and prolonging hospital stays by an average of nearly three weeks. This is especially true for the elderly and for patients with serious underlying diseases who are the most likely to develop the infection.

C difficile associated diarrhea represents a major economic burden to the healthcare system, conservatively estimated at **$3-6 billion per year in excess hospital costs** in the U.S. alone. The emergence of this "antibiotic resistance" is a result of the overwhelming use of antibiotics in human and veterinary medicine. High rates of fluroquinolone resistance have been reported in many countries. In Asia, Cipro no longer can be used to treat gonorrhea because the disease has become resistant to the drug. While the FDA in August 2000 approved *Cipro* as the first line treatment against anthrax, a few months later (October 2000) it asked Bayer to remove *Baytril*, its equivalent for animals. The FDA proposed banning the fluoroquinolones, which chicken and turkey farmers had given to birds in their water since 1995, to help shield animals from infection.

The agency acted after linking the drugs to a jump in *Campylobacter* bacteria immune to the medications. Nearly 18% of one common strain that infects humans are now *immune* to the very same drugs which were considered the *last line of defense* against the infection. *Campylobacter* is the **leading bacterial cause of food poisoning** in the U.S. Typically contracted through **raw or undercooked meat**, the germs afflict more than 2 million people and kill some 500 each year in the U.S., according to the CDC. While Abbot voluntarily *withdrew* its version of the antibiotic (*SaraFlox*), Bayer decided to *challenge* the FDA. The company had the option to comply with the proposed ban or seek a hearing to determine whether such a move was justified. Bayer refused to comply with the ban, a move that kicked off a lengthy process that **could take years**.

Meanwhile Bayer gets to ***poison*** the world and make huge ***profits*** from it. The AMA has advised its members to prescribe Cipro very *cautiously*, saying **the worldwide problem of antibiotic resistance poses future dangers, worse than the anthrax attacks of today**.

Photosensitivity

Photosensitization can result when *light* interacts with *chemical agents* in the skin and eyes. This process can produce undesirable clinical consequences, such as *phototoxicity* (exaggerated sunburn), *photoallergy*, or *photocarcinogenicity*. People receiving Cipro or any other fluoroquinolone are warned on the product inserts **not to expose themselves to direct sunlight**. Rashs develop on the areas exposed. Upon UVA-radiation, the "fluorine" of numerous fluoroquinolones such as *lomefloxacin* and *fleroxacin*, are "lost" as fluoride. Anions can activate visual photoreceptors in the dark. One *anionic activator* is the commonly used dental agent **fluoride**. These anions modulate photoreceptor *biochemistry* and may effect photoreceptor *sensitivity*.

Other Cipro Side Effects

Abnormal dread or fear, achiness, bleeding in the stomach and/or intestines, blood clots in the lungs, blurred vision, changes in color perception, chills, confusion, constipation, convulsions, coughing up blood, decreased vision, depression, difficulty in swallowing, dizziness, double vision, drowsiness, eye pain, fainting, fever, flushing, gas, gout flare up, hallucinations, hearing loss, heart attack, hiccups, high blood pressure, hives, inability to fall or stay asleep, inability to urinate, indigestion, intestinal inflammation, involuntary eye movement, irregular heartbeat, irritability, itching, joint or back pain, joint stiffness, kidney failure, labored breathing lack of muscle coordination, lack or loss of appetite, large volumes of urine, light-headedness, loss of sense of identity, loss of sense of smell, mouth sores, neck pain, nightmares, nosebleed, pounding heartbeat, ringing in the ears, seizures, sensitivity to light, severe allergic reactions, skin peeling, redness, speech difficulties, sluggishness, swelling of the face, neck, lips, eyes, or hands, swelling of the throat, tender red bumps on skin, tingling sensation, tremors, unpleasant taste, unusual darkening of the skin, vaginal inflammation, vague feeling of illness, weakness, yellowed eyes and skin.

Cipro causes fluoride poisoning. The ADA has **shielded** all from proper knowledge of fluoride toxicity.

According to *ABC News* (Thur. Sept. 27, 2001), sales of *Bayer*'s antibiotic *Cipro* have skyrocketed 1,000 percent since September 11. Peter Jennings reported anxious consumers are spending $700 per person for a two-month supply of the drug. Alternative antibiotics effective against anthrax are readily available for as little as $20. Nowhere in the *Physician's Desk Reference* (2000) is it claimed that *Cipro* is especially indicated for anthrax. In fact, *Bacillus anthracis* is **not even mentioned**. What *is* mentioned is that, "although effective in clinical trials, *ciprofloxacin* is not a drug of first choice in the treatment of presumed or confirmed pneumonia secondary to *Streptococcus pneumoniae*.

This organism, like anthrax, is an *aerobic gram-positive* microbe. (Likewise, *Bacillus anthracis* causes pneumonia in the form of commonly terminal *hemorrhagic bronchopneumonia*.) Furthermore the PDR states: "WARNINGS-THE SAFETY AND EFFECTIVENESS OF CIPROFLOXACIN IN PEDIATRIC PATIENTS AND ADOLESCENTS (LESS THAN 18 YEARS OF AGE), PREGNANT WOMEN, AND LACTATING WOMEN HAVE NOT BEEN ESTABLISHED."

Alternatively, numerous bioweapons experts have consistently recommended far less costly and time-tested antibiotics to fight anthrax, including the natural and synthetic *penicillins, erythromycin, cephalosporins*, and the *tetracyclines*. In an open letter to FBI officials and members of congress, Dr. Leonard Horowitz, a consumer health advocate, and Harvard School of Public Health graduate, is urging an investigation. At issue is the unprecedented July 29, 2000 single drug endorsement by the FDA for *Cipro*. A conspiracy to commit fraud is indicated.

Black's Law Dictionary defines fraud as "a concealment of a material fact to induce another to act to his or her injury." "In this context," Dr. Horowitz wrote, "ABC's special segment on anthrax and *Cipro* sales may be seen as a form of 'white collar bioterrorism.' Through this savvy and fraudulent form of drug promotion, consumers are being disadvantaged, over-charged, and placed at risk of injury from the potentially dangerous side effects of an antibiotic that offers no significant advantage over less costly alternatives for anthrax." A list of alternative antibiotics recommended for anthrax is provided on the doctor's website at http://www.tetrahedron.org.

The Bayer Corporation maintains several serious skeletons in its corporate closet. The CIA (currently overseeing public health and infectious disease departments for national security reasons) took over the I.G. Farben/Bayer building at the close of WWII, as they helped many Nazi scientists and wealthy German industrialists escape to America and elsewhere during *Project Paperclip*. Hermann Schmitz, Bayer's president at the time, and overseer of Farben–controlled labor camps, was sentenced to only four years of imprisonment at his Nuremberg trial. The company emerged from the holocaust virtually unscathed. Bayer maintained intimate ties to the German chemical/pharmaceutical cartel known as *I.G. Farben*. This consortium produced the earliest pesticides, drugs, and war gasses, including *Zyclone B* **used in concentration camp gas chambers**

According to the first CIA director Allen W. Dulles, as reported by CBS News war correspondent Paul Manning, the Farben cartel **provided the chief economic and industrial engines behind the rise of the Third Reich and Hitler**. The Bayer Company evaded U.S. government controls during and following the holocaust, in which millions of Jewish people were used as experimental subjects in medical atrocities overseen by I.G. Farben's president Hermann Schmitz, who directed the German-multinational Bayer A.G.

Colloidal Silver

Colloidal silver is the product of an electromagnetic process that pulls microscopic particles from a larger piece of silver into a liquid, such as water. These microscopic particles can more easily penetrate and travel throughout the body. Colloidal silver is pure silver divided so finely that **fewer than 15 atoms** of it cluster together in a particle. The FDA considers it a dietary supplement and does not restrict its sale in any way as long as it is properly manufactured. Colloidal silver works as a catalyst, disabling the enzyme that all one-celled bacteria, fungi and other microorganisms use for their oxygen metabolism. In short, the bad guys suffocate. Colloidal silver is nontoxic, making it safe for children and adults, as well as pets. Anything bigger than one cell seems to like it. Ayurvedic, Chinese and homeopathic practitioners use silver regularly. In ancient Greece and Rome, people used silver containers to keep liquids fresh. Throughout history, royal families have eaten from silver plates and cups, with silver utensils, and they've stored food in silver containers.

In 1919, Alfred Searle, founder of the pharmaceutical conglomerate wrote that "applying colloidal silver to human subjects has been done in a large number of cases with astonishingly successful results. For internal administration, orally or hypodermically, it has the advantage of being rapidly fatal to parasites without toxic action on its host. It is quite stable. It protects rabbits from10 times the lethal dose of tetanus or diphtheria toxin." Mainstream physicians used colloidal silver extensively as an antibiotic treatment up to 1939. But back then it cost a lot to produce highly effective colloidal silver. The pharmaceutical industry wanted drugs that were cheaper and patentable. As a result, colloidal silver fell out of favor. But in the 1970s, doctors at Washington University in St. Louis, searching for effective treatments for burn victims, stumbled upon colloidal silver after trying many other medicines, and it became valued once again. In 1988, a bio-medical research team at UCLA's School of Medicine showed that destructive bacteria, virus and fungus organisms died within minutes of contact with silver.

The EPA approves colloidal silver water filters. NASA uses a silver water purification system for the space shuttle, as do the Soviets. Japanese firms remove cyanide and nitric oxide from the air with silver. Because it doesn't sting the eyes, it often replaces chlorine in swimming pools. British Airways, Swissair, Scandinavian Airlines, Lufthansa, Olympic, Air France, Canadian Pacific Airlines, AlItalia, KLM, Japan Airlines and Pan Am use silver water filters to curtail waterborne diseases. Because no known pathogenic organism can live in the presence of even minute traces of the chemical element metallic silver, colloidal silver is effective against **more than 650 different pathogens**, whereas a broad-spectrum antibiotic kills, at best, six different disease organisms.

It does this by attaching itself to the cell membranc of a bacterium, which disables its oxygen-metabolism enzyme, its chemical lung. Because it can no longer breathe, within a few minutes the pathogen suffocates and dies and is cleared out of the body by the immune, lymphatic and elimination systems. Many strains of pathogenic microbes, viruses, fungi, bacteria or any other single-celled pathogens resistant to other antibiotics are **killed on contact** by colloidal silver and are unable to mutate. However, silver is virtually non-toxic and does not harm tissue-cell enzymes and friendly bacteria. Unlike antibiotics, colloidal silver doesn't weaken the body's immune system. In fact, it gives the body a **second immune system**, creating a shield against disease of all kinds.

Physicians use silver compounds in seventy percent of all the burn centers in the United States. All pathogenic organisms that have been tested were sensitive to the electrically generated silver ion, including some that were **resistant to all known antibiotics**. In no case have any undesirable side effects of the silver treatment been apparent. Silver doesn't interact with any other medications. It doesn't upset the stomach, and, in fact, is a digestion aid. It does not sting in the eyes. Medical journal reports and documented studies spanning the past 100 years indicate **no known side effects** from oral or I.V. administration of colloidal silver in animal or human testing. Silver **stimulates bone-forming cells** into growing new bone where it had not healed for long periods of time. Silver profoundly **stimulates healing of skin and other soft tissues** in a way unlike any known natural process. An average adult dose might be anywhere from a tablespoon per day to a sixteen-ounce glass, or more, since **no toxic dose is known**.

When you apply current to silver in solution, metallic silver will always break off no larger than 1.26 angstroms or about 1/10,000 of a micron (0.0001 microns). This is misleading, however, because no colloid consists of individual silver ions or atoms of silver. Single atoms would, by definition, be dissolved. After the silver breaks off at 1.26 angstroms, atoms of silver aggregate into clusters that form new particles. The smallest aggregate of clusters creates a silver particle approximately 0.001 microns, or ten times larger than the smallest atom. These particles create colloidal silver that appears clear. Over time, as more electric current is applied, silver particles will aggregate into larger and larger particles much as they do in a silver plating process. For systems with particle diameters less than one-twentieth the wavelength of light, the light scattered from a polychromatic beam is predominantly blue in color and is polarized to a degree that depends on the angle between the observer and the incident beam. The blue color of tobacco smoke is an example of *Tyndall blue*.

As particles are increased in size, the blue color of scattered light disappears, and the scattered radiation appears white. The end result is that each particle size will interact with light at a specific wavelength, creating a variety of colored colloidal solutions. The *Tyndall Effect* is the visible scattering of light along the path of a beam of light as it passes through a system containing discontinuities. The luminous path of a beam of light is called a *Tyndall Cone*.

Any true colloid of silver, or any other metal, will produce a Tyndall Cone once a narrow beam of light pierces the medium. A laser pointer works best. As the light passes through the colloid, each particle of silver refracts the light across other silver particles. The colloid becomes a sea of submicroscopic mirror balls, creating a glowing tunnel of light much wider than the original beam. Therefore, even clear colloidal silver can be given a visual test that will prove the presence of incredibly tiny particles. Because clear colloids contain the smallest silver particles, the Tyndall cone will be faint but still visible to the unaided eye.

The Colors of Colloidal Silver

When examining the variety of bottled colloidal silver at a health food store, it becomes evident that most manufacturers favor yellow-colored silver. The very idea of silver being "yellow" is confusing for many people. Some individuals have speculated that the yellow color is the result of sulfur or iron contamination. Others say the yellow color is the result of stabilizers containing a yellow dye. The continuous change in color from yellow to blue corresponds to a change in the absorption maximum of the shorter to longer wave-lengths, with a decreasing degree of dispersion. This is a general phenomenon in colloid chemistry illustrating the relation between color and degree of dispersion. It turns out that all metals have a yellow phase when they are broken down into submicroscopic particles in water. This is because color is the result of a specific particle size—rather than the metallic content of that particle—and the spacing between the particles.

Therefore, colloidal silver can produce a yellow appearance when the particles fall somewhere between .01 to .001 microns (10-100 angstroms) and are evenly dispersed. This is the result of the absorption of *indigo* light by the colloid, which leaves its inverse color, *yellow*, to be refracted. In short, color equals particle size plus dispersion. This is why yellow colloidal silver appears clear for the first few hours after its manufacture. It takes several hours for the particles to evenly disperse through the water, creating a gradual deepening of color. The density of the colloid produces the intensity of the color. From 1 to 20 ppm, the color will range from very light yellow to yellow to amber. A shift in color indicates a new silver particle agglomeration size plus dispersion. From small to large, the spectrum reads as follows: clear, yellow, red, green and blue.

While trace elements can affect conductivity and, therefore, influence agglomeration rates, color is not always a function of trace elements per se. Of all the various colloids of the spectrum, clear colloidal silver is the highest quality simply because it consists of the smallest particle size. The yellow colloidal silver may be *less* effective than the clear colloid because of the slightly *larger* silver particles. Colloids are by nature the smallest particles into which matter can be divided, while still retaining individual characteristics of that matter. Reducing a piece of metallic silver to a cloud of submicroscopic particles greatly extends its total surface area, and its healing properties, while deepening its penetration into the body. The minute particles also afford ease of elimination and therefore the absence of toxicity. Upon ingesting the silver colloid, the silver particles quickly pass through the stomach lining and into the bloodstream, where they circulate for about a week before elimination. There is evidence that the majority of silver particles are eliminated within twenty-four hours, though this can vary with particle size and individual body chemistry.

Making Clear Colloidal Silver

Colloidal silver generators are available for home use. For a 12-ounce glass of distilled water at 72° F, (room temperature), approximately 30 minutes of applied current at 27 volts DC will produce 5 ppm. For a 16-ounce glass of distilled water at 72° F, approximately 45 minutes will be needed to achieve the same concentration of 5 ppm. Larger electrodes are helpful for working with larger volumes of water and for making higher concentrations. Do not add saline drops for making clear colloidal silver.

Coconut Oil

Coconuts are a source of important physiologically functional components, found in the fat part of whole coconut, in the fat part of desiccated coconut and in the extracted coconut oil. *Lauric acid*, the major fatty acid from the fat of the coconut, has long been recognized for the unique properties that it lends to nonfood uses in the soaps and cosmetics industry. More recently, lauric acid has been recognized for its unique properties in food use, which are related to its antiviral, antibacterial and antiprotozoal functions. These fatty acids are found in the largest amounts only in traditional lauric fats, especially from coconut. Natural coconut fat in the diet leads to a normalization of body lipids, protects against alcohol damage to the liver and improves the immune system's anti-in flammatory response. Certain fatty acids and their derivatives can have adverse effects on various microorganisms. Those microorganisms that are inactivated include bacteria, yeast, fungi and enveloped viruses.

Lauric acid is a medium-chain fatty acid which has the additional beneficial function of being formed into *monolaurin* in the human or animal body. Monolaurin is the **antiviral, antibacterial and antiprotozoal** monoglyceride used by the human and animal to destroy lipid-coated viruses such as *HIV, herpes*, *cytomegalovirus, influenza*, various pathogenic bacteria including *hemophilus influenzae*, *staphylococcus epidermidis* and group B gram-positive *streptococcus*, *listeria monocytogenes streptococcus agalactiae*, *helicobacter pylori,* groups A, F and G *streptococci*, gram-positive organisms, and some gram-negative organisms if pretreated with a chelator; also, a number of fungi, yeast and protozoa such as *giardia lamblia* have been found to be inactivated or killed by lauric acid or monolaurin. The fungi include several species of ringworm. The yeast reported is *candida albicans*. *Chlamydia trachomatis* is inactivated by lauric acid, capric acid and monocaprin. Some studies have also shown some antimicrobial effects of the free lauric acid.

Also, approximately 6-7% of the fatty acids in coconut fat are *capric acid*. Capric acid is another medium-chain fatty acid which has a similar beneficial function when it is formed into *monocaprin* in the human or animal body. Monocaprin has also been shown to have antiviral effects against HIV and is being tested for antiviral effects against *herpes simplex* and for antibacterial effects against *Chlamydia* and other sexually transmitted bacteria. The properties that determine the anti-infective action of lipids are related to their structure. The *monoglycerides* are active; *diglycerides* and *triglycerides* are inactive. Of the saturated fatty acids, *lauric acid* has greater antiviral activity than *caprylic acid*, *capric acid*, or *myristic acid*. The fatty acids and monoglycerides produce their killing/inactivating effect by *lysing* the plasma membrane lipid bilayer. The antiviral action attributed to monolaurin is that of solubilizing the lipids and phospholipids in the envelope of the virus, causing the disintegration of the virus envelope. One antimicrobial effect in bacteria is related to monolaurin's interference with signal transduction, and another antimicrobial effect in viruses is due to lauric acid's interference with virus assembly and viral maturation.

Research has shown that enveloped viruses are inactivated in both human and bovine milk by added fatty acids and monoglycerides and also by endogenous fatty acids and monoglycerides of the appropriate length. Lauric acid is one of the best inactivating fatty acids, and its monoglyceride is even more effective than the fatty acid alone. Monolaurin does not appear to have an adverse effect on desirable gut bacteria but, rather, only on potentially pathogenic micro-organisms.

X-rays

X-Rays

Wilhelm Roentgen discovered X-rays in 1895. Within the year, physicians were using X-rays for diagnosis and as a new way of gathering evidence to protect themselves against malpractice suits. Almost immediately—during 1895-96—it also became clear that X-rays could cause serious medical problems. Some physicians received burns that wouldn't heal, requiring amputation of their fingers. Others developed fatal cancers. Radiation treatment for benign (non-cancerous) diseases became a medical craze that lasted for over 40 years. Large groups of people were needlessly irradiated for such minor problems as ringworm and acne. Many women had their ovaries irradiated as a treatment for depression. Such uses of X-rays would today be viewed as quackery, but many of them were accepted medical practice into the 1950s.

Physicians weren't the only ones enthusiastic about X-ray therapies. If you get a large enough dose of X-rays, your hair falls out—so, beauty shops installed X-ray equipment to remove their customers' unwanted facial and body hair. Roentgen's discovery of X-rays in 1895 led directly to Henri Becquerel's discovery of the radioactivity of uranium in 1896, and then to the discovery of radium by Marie Curie and her husband Pierre in 1898—for which Becquerel and the Curies were jointly awarded the Nobel Prize in 1903 (twenty years later, Madame Curie died of acute *lymphoblastic leukemia*). Soon, along with X-rays, physicians were prescribing radioactive radium. Radium treatments were prescribed for heart trouble, impotence, ulcers, depression, arthritis, cancer, high blood pressure, blindness, tuberculosis, and other ailments. Soon radioactive toothpaste, then radioactive skin cream, was being marketed.

In Germany, chocolate bars containing radium were sold as a "rejuvenator." In the U.S.A., hundreds of thousands of people began drinking bottled water laced with radium as a general elixir known popularly as "liquid sunshine." As recently as 1952, *Life* magazine wrote about the beneficial effects of inhaling radioactive radon gas in deep mines. Numerous studies now indicate that the only demonstrable health effect of radon gas is lung cancer. Thus, the medical world and popular culture together embraced X-rays (and other radioactive emanations) as miraculous remedies, gifts to humanity from the foremost geniuses of an inventive age.

Non-Cautious Use of Medical Radiation

The *Law of Unintended Consequences* refers to the observation that human activities, in addition to their *intended* results, almost always have *unanticipated* consequences–ranging from unpleasant to tragic. One unintended consequence of the cold War has been a half-century of *non-cautious* use of medical x-rays, resulting in **premature death** for millions of Americans from cancer and coronary heart disease. "Non-cautious use of medical x-rays," means the use of x-rays for medical imaging at much higher radiation doses than the doses required to obtain good images. During the Cold War (1945-1991), both the *free world* and the *communist world* relied upon nuclear deterrence to protect their homelands from the presumed aggressive intent of the other.

The governments of both sides felt obliged to let "nothing, but nothing" interfere with the production and test-explosions of their nuclear weapons. The free world anticipated an inherent and serious disadvantage in this competition. The communist world permitted neither *free speech* nor a *free press*. And it did not tolerate citizens who tried to receive information across the Iron Curtain. By contrast, the free world has a free press, which meant that only in the free world would there be any public information about the peacetime health consequences from making and test-exploding nuclear bombs.

In the early 1950s, open-air explosions of nuclear bombs began at the Nevada test site. Radioactive fallout was landing virtually all over the country. When radioactive atoms decay, they emit ionizing radiaiton–which is the type of radiation emitted also by x-ray machines. Radioactive atoms are part of military and civilian nuclear enterprises at every step of the way–from *uranium mining*, to *plutonium production* in nuclear reactors, to the *fission products* created by operating nuclear reactors, to the fision products created by exploding nuclear bombs. **A civilian 1,000-megawatt electrical nuclear reactor produces as many long-lived radioactive atoms during each year of its operation, as does the explosion of about 1,000 Hiroshima-sized bombs**. As radioactive fallout from the bomb tests drifted down from the skies, vigorous protests erupted, with Dr. Linus Pauling in a leading role. Such protests were regarded by the U.S. government as a serious threat to national security during the Cold War. "Nothing but nothing" must weaken public support for nuclear deterrence. What if fear of fallout should evolve into the sentiment, "better Red than Dead?"

The government felt it had to quell public fear of *radiation*...which meant *ionizing radiation*. Back then, the public did not fear other kinds of radiation–microwaves, radio waves, infrared waves, ultrasound waves, visible and invisible light waves, etc. Prior to World War II, ionizing radiation was a known cause of human cancer (especially leukemia, and lung cancer), bone disintegration (from ingestion of radium), unhealable skin ulcers and skin disintegration (from excessive exposure to x-rays, gamma rays, alpha particles), and inheritable mutations (in animals). Peacetime nuclear activities (military and civilian) expose the general public to *low doses* of ionizing radiation. The government's solution to quell public fear of "radiation" was to have its agents assert–for decades after it was no longer true–that evidence of harm from ionizing radiation comes exclusively from exposure to *high doses*, and that evidence of human harm from low doses does not exist. The intended consequence was to convince fearful people that they were wimps with irrational fears of a danger which was too trivial to detect and "just hypothetical."

What the government and its agents failed to point out in the 1950s and early 1960s was that **no studies capable of producing evidence about low doses had ever been completed**. In the absence of evidence that low doses cause harm, the prudent position is that low doses *do* cause harm. And that is why the protestors against open-air nuclear-bomb testing finally prevailed. In 1963, the U.S.A., U.K., and the U.S.S.R. agreed to move such bomb-testing undeground. The U.S. government's position became–and remains–that it will behave as if there is no safe dose of ionizing radiation, to which it almost always adds that danger at low doses remains "just hypothetical" and "could be zero."

In recent years, Karl Morgan has described and criticized the work of the International Committee for Radiation Protection. Morgan says the ICRP has suffered from two major blind spots: the Committee has **never focused on harm to the public from excessive exposure to medical X-rays**, and by the mid-1960s, the ICRP began setting standards for radioactivity that **protected the nuclear industry rather than the public**. According to Morgan, **the ICRP began ignoring serious radiation hazards in the early 1960s**. He said the period of atmospheric testing of nuclear weapons by the United States, the United Kingdom, France and the U.S.S.R. is a sad page in the history of civilized man. Without question, **it was the cause of hundreds of thousands of cancer deaths**. Yet, **there was complete silence** on the part of the ICRP.

During the years 1960-1965, **most members of the ICRP either worked directly with the nuclear weapons industry or indirectly received most of their funding for their research from this industry**. They were reluctant to bite the hand that feeds them. In the 1970s, the situation grew worse after a series of studies revealed that radiation was **even more dangerous than previously believed**. In 1974, Baruch Modan showed that a woman's chances of breast cancer were increased by X-ray doses **as low as 1.6 rem**. In 1977, Thomas Mancuso and others reported that workers at the Hanford plutonium facility were dying of cancers from radiation doses as low as 3 rem, accumulated over many years. (The worker safety standard at the time was 5 rem per-year). Karl Morgan says **these studies threw the nuclear industry into a panic**.

"Concerned that its very existence was threatened if the public believed that there was an increased risk of cancer at these low levels of exposure, the nuclear-industrial-complex determined that it would respond vigorously to all challengers," Morgan reports in his autobiography. "As a result, health physics in recent decades has sacrificed its integrity," Morgan said in 1999. The ICRP turned a blind eye to other problems affecting public health: **excessive exposures from medical and dental X-rays**. Early in the 1950s, a series of studies had shown that X-rays were more dangerous than previously known. In 1950, H.C. March showed that **radiologists were nine times as likely as other physicians to die of leukemia**. In 1956, Alice Stewart showed that **a single X-ray of a fetus in the womb would double the likelihood of childhood leukemia**. The subject of excessive medical exposure was a no-no with ICRP because ICRP was founded under the auspices of the *International Congress of Radiology* (ICR), and **radiologists did not want any restraints or interference in their use of diagnostic X-rays**. There was a **serious conflict of interest** with ICR sponsorship of ICRP.

In the mid-1960s, Morgan's division of the Oakridge Laboratory studied the X-ray doses to which U.S. children were exposed from a mass chest x-ray program. Starting in the 1950s, portable X-ray machines in special trucks were brought to schools, and hundreds of thousands of US children were given chest X-rays. The Oak Ridge study found that each of these children was receiving an X-ray dose of 2 to 3 rem; Morgan knew that **children were getting a dose of X-rays 130 to 200 times as high as the dose needed to produce an adequate X-ray film**—not to mention that most of the children did not need a chest X-ray at all.

In the 1940s and 1950s, many shoe stores installed fluoroscopic (X-ray) shoe-fitting machines. By 1949, a study had shown that **shoe-fitting machines were giving children high doses of radiation**. Again, **the ICRP showed no interest in the subject**. Morgan and his colleagues calculated that **medical X-rays accounted for 90% of all radiation from human-created sources**. Morgan showed in 1963 that the average U.S. citizen was exposed each year to as much radiation from medical X-rays as from natural background sources. In other words **the use of medical X-rays was doubling the average person's exposure to radiation in the U.S**. Morgan's point was that **the same benefits could be achieved at much lower doses** by using up-to-date equipment and techniques. The medical community turned a deaf ear.

For many years, Morgan and others wrote about the hazards of excessive and unnecessary radiation exposures from medicine and dentistry—an effort he describes as "twenty years of frustrating failures." In his autobiography, Morgan says it was "a highlight of my life's work" when President Lyndon Johnson signed Public Law 90-602, the *Radiation Control for Health and Safety Act* of 1968, which set minimum federal standards for X-ray equipment. However, the law does nothing to curb unnecessary and excessive X-ray exposures, which still occur routinely.

With the Cold War now over, what explains the government's resistance to endorsing and disseminating the overwhelming evidence that danger from ionizing radiation is proportional to dose, right down to zero dose? Attachment to the "just hypothetical" line may arise from the estimated **half-trillion dollars** it will cost to *recapture* the radioactive poisons released from dozens of bomb-making facilities, and to *pay injury claims* from workers, soldiers, and other citizens. Fifty years of ridiculing the fear of low-dose ionizing radiation has had a tragic unintended consequence.

Two or three generations of practicing physicians and their professors at medical schools have mistakenly believed that danger from x-ray imaging procedures was either absent or trivial. The result is that x-ray practitioners have not made maximum efforts to reduce x-ray doses during imaging. They would not even know if their doses were falling or rising, because very few practitioners bother to measure the skin-doses they give to patients, although it is easy and inexpensive to do.

There is powerful evidence that **x-ray doses could at least be cut in half on the average and still produce good images**. About 250,000 persons each year in the U.S.A. are dying prematurely from cancer and coronary heart disease due to unnecessary x-ray doses they accumulated earlier in life during x-ray imaging procedures. This has been going on for 50 years and continues. Indeed, per capita dose from x-ray imaging is probably *rising* today, not *falling*, because of the increasing use (without dose measurement) of CT scans, and of fluoroscopic imaging during surgery and cardiac catheterization. Carcinogenic and atherogenic *x-ray-induced mutations* co-act with other agents to cause cancer and coronary heart disease. **The medical use of higher x-ray doses than necessary has killed millions of Americans already**. Each preventable death is a tragedy. The combined tragedies have occurred as an unintended consequence of the Cold War, because the Cold War inspired the fervent but mistaken assertion that danger from low-dose ionizing radiation was "just hypothetical" or trivial. Moreover, concerns about national security probably soothed the consequences of those who insulted and defunded the dissenters.

X-rays, Cancer and Heart Disease

For the past 20 years, another prominent scientist concerned about excessive exposure to X-rays has been Dr. John Gofman. In his autobiography, Morgan describes Gofman this way: "…John Gofman, a scientist, holds degrees in both chemistry and medicine. Along with Glenn Seaborg, Gofman co-discovered uranium-233, and he also was the first one to isolate plutonium. In spite of these achievements, Gofman has yet to receive the recognition due him; in my opinion, he is one of the leading scientists of the twentieth century." For 20 years or more, Gofman has been publishing studies about the hazards of low-level radiation. His latest book fills 700 pages addressing this hypothesis: "Medical radiation is a highly important cause (probably the principal cause) of cancer mortality in the United States during the twentieth century." Gofman believes that **medical X-rays are the major cause of cancer** and **heart disease in the U.S**. Gofman's work is careful, thorough and clearly written, so most of the health physicists of this world probably cannot be expected to take it lying down. John Gofman is a medical doctor with a Ph.D. in nuclear and physical chemistry. He is Professor Emeritus of molecular and cell biology at the University of California, Berkeley, and a member of the faculty at the University of California Medical School at San Francisco.

During his long career, he has pursued two separate fields of research: **heart disease**, and **the health effects of low-level radiation**. He has won several awards for original research into the causes of atherosclerosis, which is the growth of fatty "plaque" inside the blood vessels, often causing fatal heart attacks. In 1974, the American College of Cardiology selected him as **one of the 25 leading researchers in cardiology of the past quarter-century**. In the early 1960s, the U.S. atomic Energy Commission (AEC) asked Gofman to develop a Biomedical Research Division at the AEC's Livermore National Laboratory (LNL), to evaluate the health effects of all types of nuclear activities.

In 1970, **he became convinced that radiation is more dangerous than previously believed**, and he spoke out against Project Plowshare. He also called for a five-year moratorium on the AEC's plan to develop 1,000 commercial nuclear power plants. By 1974, Gofman's government funding was cut. He then began a series of books on the dangers of radiation. Gofman is a superb teacher. In his books, he interprets the raw data, where it came from, its shortcomings, how it might be improved (or why we're stuck with what we have). Nothing of importance is omitted. As a result, Gofman's books are lengthy—typically 500 to 900 pages filled with tables of data, accompanied by detailed explanations. His work has already changed the way the world views the dangers of radiation, and eventually, after a long fight—revolutionized the way the world looks at medical radiation. His work will save, cumulatively, tens of millions of lives.

In his latest (1999) book, Gofman presents strong evidence that **medical radiation is a major cause of cancer and of atherosclerosis** (coronary heart disease). By *medical radiation*, Dr. Gofman is referring mainly to **X-rays**, including **fluoroscopy** and **C.T.** (CAT) **scans**. The mechanism is simple: **Radiation causes genetic mutations that eventually give rise to disease**. Gofman is not saying that medical radiation is necessarily the only cause of cancer and coronary heart disease. He does not mean that cancer is not caused by smoking, poor diet, genetic inheritance, pesticides, diesel exhaust, dioxin and toxic chemicals encountered on the job. Cancer and heart disease both have multiple causes. For cancer (or an atherosclerotic plaque) to develop, **a cell must undergo several separate gene mutations**. Most occur from exposure to **gene-damaging substances in the environment**.

It is important to point out that Gofman is not opposed to medical X-rays. Rather, he is opposed to **unnecessary exposure** from X-rays. He and others have shown over the years that medical X-ray exposures in the U.S. could be cut by at least 50% with no loss of medical information. The careful use of modern X-ray equipment and techniques can reduce X-ray exposure by half (or more) without sacrificing any medical benefits. Thus, **at least half the cancers caused by medical X-rays are completely unnecessary**. Gofman calculates that **in 1993, 50% of all cancers in women and 74% of all cancers in men were attributable to X-rays**. About 500,000 people die of cancer each year in the U.S.

If 60% of these deaths are attributable to X-rays and half are unnecessary, we are talking about 150,000 unnecessary cancer deaths each year in the U.S. Gofman calculates that the proportion of coronary heart disease (CHD) attributable to X-rays is slightly higher than the proportion of cancers. Among men in 1993, 63% of CHD deaths were attributable to X-rays, and 78% among women. So, in rough numbers, 70% of CHD deaths are attributable to X-rays, Gofman believes. Since CHD caused roughly 460,000 deaths in the U.S. in 1993, then, if Gofman is right, 70% (or 322,000) of these deaths are attributable to X-rays, and half of these (or 161,000) are unnecessary. He found disease statistics for the entire U.S. population, broken down into nine census districts (1940 to 1990 for cancer, and 1950 to 1990 for coronary heart disease). Then he correlated these statistics, year by year, to the number of physicians per 100,000 population in each of the nine census districts. The density of physicians per 100,000 population provides a relative measure of the medical radiation per 100,000 population in the nine districts by year.

Gofman has shown that cancer death rates rise in lock-step with increasing density of physicians in a census district, while non-cancer deaths decline in lock-step with increasing density of physicians per 100,000 population, except in the case of coronary heart disease, which follows the rising pattern of cancer. Thus, Gofman's hypothesis, that **CHD is linked to medical radiation**, "fell out of the data." Because he had decades of experience researching the causes of CHD (he has written three books on heart disease), and because he knows the radiation literature so well, Gofman was able to put two and two together: **Radiation induces mutations in the coronary arteries, giving rise to** what he calls ***dysfunctional clones*** (mini-tumors) **in the smooth muscle lining the arteries**.

Using his "physician density" method, Gofman estimates that medical radiation caused 83% of female breast cancer in the U.S. in 1993. Using a completely different method, Gofman estimated in 1995 that medical radiation was responsible for 75% of U.S. breast cancer. The two estimates, by completely different methods, are remarkably similar.

What To Do?

It will not be easy to convince dentists and physicians to take special care to minimize radiation administered to their patients. Familiarity breeds contempt, and **many physicians and dentists treat X-rays as if they are entirely harmless**. Physicians and dentists want to document damage and injury for insurance purposes. But, a patient can scribble a note such as, "I broke my tooth (or any other condition), and I don't want an X-ray." Just sign it, and the insurance company is required to accept it.

Dental X-rays Go Digital

A 1997, Silicon Valley breakthrough in X-ray technology was destined to revolutionize medical care. This breakthrough is the digital X-ray, a development which means no more waiting for film to be developed. A radiologist will be able to look at an image as it's being taken and make an immediate diagnosis. The new device features a silicon-coated glass panel the size of a pizza box. The resolution is as good as film, and they reveal **greater detail than conventional X-rays**. Patients will still have to "open wide" and "bite down," but in place of dental film, they'll close their mouths around electronic sensors.

With the new technology, instead of the trip to the developing tank, dentist and patient will watch images come up on a computer screen seconds after the device is inserted into the patient's mouth. The images will be higher resolution than film images and will be stored in computer memory from which they can be easily retrieved, combined, and manipulated to supply more information. The chemical waste associated with film processing will be eliminated. Most significantly, patients will be exposed to **one tenth the x-ray dosage typically delivered today**. The conventional way to x-ray teeth is with a piece of thick film that is moderately sensitive to x rays. To increase its efficiency and lower the required dosage of X-rays, the film can be sandwiched between sheets of plastic called intensifying screens. The disadvantage of using the screens is that they scatter radiation, resulting in decreased spatial resolution and accuracy.

The ultimate aim is to avoid the use of film for medical x-ray imaging. They're starting small, making devices for dental radiography, because the electronics are easier to make. Eventually standard 11x14-inch radiology film and developing tanks will be replaced by electronic detectors, high definition display screens, and computer-stored data. These technologies will simplify procedures in a clinic or hospital's radiology department, and patients will be exposed to much lower doses of radiation.

Compatible Materials

Compatible Materials

In their 2001 readers' survey, the *Clinical Research Associates Newsletter* asked an interesting question: "What is your most deciding factor in choosing a Class 2 restorative material?" The answers were not unexpected: durability, 47%; patients' preference, 22%; esthetics, 12%; ease of use, 10%; biocompatibility, 4%.

Why is biocompatibility such a low priority? **Dentists are most concerned that their work is comfortable, good looking and long lasting.** The majority of dentists appear to believe that the biocompatibility of dental materials and procedures is a settled issue. It turns out, though, that their materials and procedures range from very benign to frankly toxic. Some of their all-time favorites, **mercury and fluoride, have a therapeutic ratio of one to one, meaning that their toxic effects emerge at the same concentration to which the patients are exposed for their intended effects.** By making distinctions–some obvious, and some subtle–among the available materials and procedures, dentists can reduce the impact on their patients' biological responses. A dentist's sense of duty to the well being of a patient should position biocompatibility as a high value. There are now so many ways to make the dentistry work, giving them the opportunity to do so.

It is important to determine a material's biological compatibility (biocompatibility). There are three different levels of biocompatibility to consider: *general, immunological*, and *bio-energetic*.

1. **General biocompatibility**–On this most basic level, we have to look at how the material reacts generally with human tissue. In other words, how toxic the material is at a cellular level. Does it poison cells? This toxicity tends to be an inherent property of the material, and all people will react to it in a similar manner. Using a toxic material such as mercury or nickel would always be a mistake.

2. **Immunological biocompatibility**–This level looks at materials from a standpoint of how an individual reacts to the material. The problem is analogous to what happens when someone with an allergy to mushrooms consumes an edible mushroom. The adverse reaction is due to an immunological and/or allergic type response based on teh patient's biochemical makeup.

A test like the *Clifford Materials Reactivity Test* (www.ccrlab.com) measures how antibodies in the blood react with the material (or, more accurately, its corrosion by-products). This blood test indicates if the material is suitable form an indiviedual reactivity point of view. When evaluating a Cliffor test, a material that tests ***NS*** (not suitable) should not be used. On the other hand, materials that test ***S*** (suitable) should, ideally, be further tested. Kinesiologic testing for biocompatibility can also be performed to determine the body's immunological response to substances.

3. **Bio-energetic biocompatibility**–For thousands of years Eastern medicine has studied the flow of energy through the human body and applied this to such healing arts as acupuncture. In more recent times, Dr. Reinhard Voll spent 40 years studying and documenting the relationship between teeth and organ systems. Using Electrodermal screening (EDS) and Applied Kinesiology (AK or Muscle Testing), it can be determined how a material reacts with the body on an energitic level. If energetically incompatible materials are used, interferences are created on the meridians associated with the teeth being restored. according to Eastern medicine, each tooth correlates with and potentially influences different organ systems.

To select a restorative material of the highest levels of compatiblility, start with materials that exhibit low toxicity to cells, then eliminate the ones that elicit an immunological response, and then, to further narrow down the choice, select from the remaining materials using either *EDS* or AK. Using such a multi-step approach should give you the highest probability of selecting a non-reactive, compatible material. Of course, many patients will skip the testing and simply ask to have a material used that has been found to generally biocompatible. However, in cases where patients are experiencing *multiple chemical sensitivity* (MCS), various illnesses, or are highly concerened about achieving the highest level of biocompatibility, specific testing as described above is indicated.

Once the final restorative material has been selected, it is important ot understand that other materials are used in order to get a finished product. In the case of a metal restoration, this usually involves only the dental cement used to adhere the crown to the tooth (unless the tooth is so broken down that it requires a build-up, in which case all of the following steps also apply). If the restoration is a ceramic or composite, a number of steps are required to complete the bonding process.

Biocompatibility Testing

The medical device industry has come a very long way in testing for biocompatibility, beyond the traditional cytotoxicity, carcinogenicity and sensitization tests. The current guide for safety assessment is the *International Organization for Standardization* (ISO) *10993 standard*, and its American version, the FDA's "Blue Book Memorandum G95-1." The ISO standard is a seventeen part guide for thorough, customized evaluation, including tests for systemic toxicity, chronic and sub-chronic toxicity, characterization and toxicity of breakdown products and leachables.

However, both the ISO and the FDA processes have a Grandfather Clause. **According to the FDA's section 510(k), a manufacturer need only demonstrate that a new device or material is "substantially equivalent" to one that was legally in interstate commerce prior to May 28, 1976.** Everything used in dentistry today, from amalgam to endosseous implants and sixth generation bonding agents, has been passed through to market under that rule. **Few dental materials have been subjected to anything like the kind of scrutiny mandated by the new standards.**

There are, to be sure, more specific guidelines and safety checks, but **the Grandfather Clause lets the big fish–dental amalgam–get away.** It's a biocompatibility nightmare. The scientific evidence has established beyond any doubt two propositions: that amalgam releases mercury in significant quantities, creating measurable exposures in people with fillings, and that chronic exposure to mercury, in the quantity released by amalgam, causes physiological harm. Dentists and dental staff members themselves have been shown to be affected adversely by their occupational mercury exposure. Toxicologists have not detected a minimum level of exposure at which there is no adverse physiological effect. From a practical standpoint, amalgam is totally unnecessary anymore. From the biocompatibility standpoint, it is totally insupportable. Yet the leaders of the dental profession persist in maintaining the old party line.

It's all in the scientific literature, although this information is typically mentioned in dental journals only in the form of editorial rebuttals. The evidence is instead published in many of the world's leading medical journals, where it has remained hidden from the independent dentist and the public alike

Materials Reactivity Testing

Because each of us possesses a unique biochemistry, substances we come in contact with daily effect each of us differently and in varying degrees. For some, the effects of certain substances (and their corrosion byproducts) can be toxic and hazardous, and may result in serious health problems. A substance which causes little or no reaction in one individual can prove harmful to another.

Since these effects may vary in each of us, it is vital that these factors be considered when choosing dental and other materials for use in the body, especially in patients with special or unique health concerns. The *Clifford materials reactivity testing* (www.ccrlab.com) provides dentists and other professional health care providers with extensive information about their patient's individual sensitivities so that least offensive materials can be chosen and used in their treatments.

When we come in contact with harmful substances, the body's natural defense system produces antibodies to counter these agents. Among other things, these *IgG, IgM* and *IgA* antibodies provide an immunological record of chemical families which have proven offensive. The Clifford materials reactivity test, developed by Walter J. Clifford, screens patient blood samples for these antibodies. Antibodies which have been specifically formed against harmful agents are detected and analyzed. The agents against which these antibodies were formed are then cross referenced against a list of over 2600 dental and medical trade-named products and narrows it down to a list of "suited: materials for personal suitability.

The Clifford materials reactivity test results allow a dentist or physician to quickly determine from an extensive list of materials that can be used with the least degree of risk in meeting needs. The report also lists trade-named products with simple *suited/not suited* indicators for rapid spot checks of products in question. It does not address issues of mechanical performance nor electro-activity between materials.

Composite Fillings

These materials consist of tiny glass particles suspended in a resin (plastic) matrix. The size and amount of the glass particles give the composite filling materials different characteristics, such as strength and polishability. Composites are used in areas where the fillings are relatively small and there is plenty of tooth structure for support.

Composite fillings are less durable than amalgam if the filling is large, but comparable in durability if the filling is small to average size. Composite fillings in back teeth are significantly more difficult and time-consuming to place than amalgam fillings, therefore more expensive. Composite materials are most commonly placed directly into the tooth (like amalgam fillings), but can also be prefabricated and bonded into place indirectly (like a crown). However, they are more natural-looking, require less tooth reduction to place, and are bonded in place for a better seal.

Composites are not totally compatible either. Most are made of the petrochemical *bis-phenol*, which some research indicates leaches out estrogen-like substances. Some composites are less biocompatible than others because of the amount of iron oxide, aluminum oxide, barium, and other materials in them. *Direct* composites can cause hairline cracks in the tooth from the hardening process, whereas *indirect* composites do not because they are hardened in the lab. Porcelain is more natural-looking than composites, but because it is harder and more brittle, it causes a wearing away of everything it contacts with and can crack instead of flex from stress.

All porcelains contain aluminum oxide. The one exception is **unshaded** *Dicor*, which is weaker and not very natural-looking (over a period of 3-4 months, unshaded dicor will pick up the shade of the tooth under it). If metal is not used in a crown or bridge, it is significantly weaker and has an increased risk of breakage during normal function. Gold fillings, porcelain fillings, indirect composite fillings, and crowns require more tooth structure to be trimmed away than for amalgam and direct composites, and take two appointments rather than one. Most "gold" crowns placed today contain from 1% - 40% gold and have nickel in them, which is inappropriate for those with a compromised immune system. Special order higher content gold will obviously cost more due to the cost of gold.

Studies of gallium alloys have reported problems with corrosion, durability, tooth fracture, and tooth sensitivity. More research and development is needed, but for now, it is recommended for use in baby teeth only. Some experts consider all metals, even non-allergenic or non-toxic metals, to be disruptive and therefore believe they should never be used in the body. Since nearly all composites and porcelains contain iron and aluminum oxides, some experts limit their choices to only a few.

Still others think the use of high quality metals like high content gold or titanium is acceptable, **but only if** one brand and formulation is used for the entire mouth. One must weigh *biocompatibility* against *function* and *durability*. Because of contractual language and statistics, use of titanium, high content gold, and composite for crowns, bridges, or fillings will probably result in **lessened insurance benefits**, even though the time, cost, and effort in doing them is the same or more as for standard gold alloy and porcelain materials. Cadmium is used for color stabilization, so cadmium-free materials may lose some color over time.

Filling Materials

Amalgam

Amalgam is the most commonly used material for back teeth. It contains approximately 50% mercury and varying amounts of silver (30%), tin, zinc, and copper. It is the least costly and least time-consuming to place. It does not hold its shape over time, corrodes easily, and is expected to last 5-10 years. The controversy is that it contains mercury, a known neurotoxin (poison to the nervous system).

Galloy

Galloy is a brand new material containing silver, tin, copper, indium, and gallium. It is meant to be mercury-free alternative to amalgam. Why is the American Dental Association developing & patenting this substitute for mercury amalgam if mercury amalgam is safe?

Direct Composite

A direct composite is a special plastic material that bonds to tooth structure, is tooth colored, is more easily repairable, and requires less tooth structure to be trimmed away than any other material. It is expected to last 5-7 years, although small to moderate size fillings may last longer. Research has shown that it reinforces the tooth and makes it stronger. Cost and time to perform is about 50-75% more than amalgam. Composites are a petrochemical derivative and, as such, are a possible problem for the environmentally sensitive.

Indirect Composite Inlay/Onlay

This type of restoration is used when ideal fit and durability is desired, which is seldom achieved with a direct composite filling. Cost is approximately 2-3 times that of an amalgam filling and takes two visits.

Porcelain Inlay/Onlay

Dental ceramics (sometimes referred to as dental *porcelains*) have come a long way! Until a few years ago, these materials were relatively weak (that's why they required support from a metal substructure) and abrasive (causing wear on the opposing teeth). Today there are many different types of ceramic systems: *Feldspathic, Leucite-reinforced, Polymer-reinforced, Zirconium-based*–each with unique properties. From rebuilding broken teeth to replacing missing teeth (even in the back of the mouth), there is a ceramic to do the job. However, they are more difficult to use than conventionally cemented (non-bonded) crowns.

Picking the right ceramic for the job, proper tooth preparation, quality laboratory work, and meticulous cementation technique are all needed for a successful tooth restoration. It costs about the same as an indirect composite inlay/onlay and takes two visits. Most ceramic and resin-based materials contain metals in the form of oxides (such as aluminum) or even heavy metals (such as cobalt, barium or cadmium). These are usually added to give the amterials strength and improve their appearance. Sometimes they are added to make the restoration show up on x-rays. The number of materials that do not contain any of these products is very limited. However, the advantage of being oxide-free is lost when these are bonded to the tooth using an oxide-containing luting agent.

Gold Inlay/Onlay

Because of gold's long history, it is the standard against which other materials are judged. This type of restoration is used when maximum strength is desired and appearance is not a factor. Gold is almost never used in its pure form; rather gold is used as an alloy with other metal elements. It costs approximately three to four times more than an amalgam and takes 2 visits.

There are many formulations of gold, varying from 1% to 99%. The other metals are added in order to give the gold strength and the ability to bond to porcelain (in the case of porcelain veneer fused to cover a gold crown). The most commonly added metals are palladium, silver, copper, and platinum. The composition and amount of each metal in the alloy determines whether it is classified as a "high noble," "noble," or "base" metal. "Noble" metals are defined as gold, platinum and palladium. The most expensive gold alloys are "high noble" and they are defined as hving at least 60% noble metals and at least 40% gold.

An alloy can still be called "noble" if it has at least 25% noble metal content. The cheapest materials fail even that test and are called "base" alloys–they have less than 25% noble metals. It is especially important for patients with metal sensitivities to avoid the base alloys since these usually contain toxic metals such as nickel and chromium;. But even the high noble materials can be incompatible for patients and even toxic; palladium, for example, is toxic.

Titanium Inlay/Onlay

Titanium is used when a gold alloy is not biocompatible; otherwise, the benefits, cost, and time to perform are the same as for a gold alloy, even though it is not a precious metal. It takes two visits.

Dental Material Philosophies

Conventional

Except in rare situations, currently used dental materials are safe in the mouth. The important criteria are how durable, natural looking, inexpensive, and practical they are for the dentist and dental laboratory to use. Concerns therefore are economics and aesthetics. Because some people have a sensitivity to certain substances, the choice of dental materials may have to be limited. A special blood test may be used to determine sensitivity to corrosion by-products of components.

Toxicity

Some dental materials contain toxic substances that, depending on exposure and other factors, may impact total toxic body load. Non-toxic alternatives should be used to decrease exposure to and accumulation of scientifically confirmed environmental toxins. Some dental treatment and materials can be disruptive to the normal flow of energy through the acupuncture meridians. Eastern philosophy believes chronic disruption of energy flow causes dysfunction and resultant health problems on the associated meridian; therefore, the choice of dental materials and treatments is limited.

Electrogalvanism

Dissimilar metals in the mouth, including different formulations of the "same" metal, create microamps of current which could cause oral pain, corrosion of the metal (black mercury amalgam fillings), dry mouth, metallic taste, erythema (red & swollen gums), and possible dysfunction of other organ systems, endocrine glands, etc. on that meridian.

Crown and Bridge Materials

Gold Alloy

A gold alloy is used when maximum strength is desired and appearance is not a factor. There are many formulations, varying from 1% to 99%.

Titanium

Titanium is used when maximum strength is desired, appearance is not a factor, and a gold alloy is not biocompatible. There are different purities of titanium, with grade-1 being the purest. This is used in joint replacement, dental implants, and bone pins. Cost is the same as for gold alloy.

Non-Precious Alloy

Non-precious alloys are used when maximum strength is desired, appearance is not a factor, but cost is most important. Since it does not contain any gold, cost is less. There are two basic formulations, one that contains nickel and one that is nickel-free. The controversial issue is that nickel, beryllium, cobalt, chromium, and palladium may cause immune problems and/or toxicity.

Porcelain

Porcelain is used when appearance and wear resistance is the most important factor. It is much more fragile than metal and may break easily. Porcelain alone is not normally recommended for bridges.

Indirect Composite

Indirect composites are used when appearance is an important factor but when the risk of porcelain fractures and wearing down the other teeth is to be avoided. These are not quite as wear-resistant or esthetic as porcelain but very acceptable for normal situations.

Zirconium Oxide

One of the most difficult areas in dentistry today is the restoration of dental structures with biocompatible materials that are strong enough to withstand the forces of chewing (500-1000lbs pressure on molar teeth). Recent technology from Germany now offers a material that has overcome most of the pitfalls of present day products. Patients now have a choice of a material that is esthetic, strong, pure, biocompatible and capable of being used for single and long span dental bridgework. That material is called Zirconium oxide.

Zirconium oxide has the following superior characteristics that make it the most ideal material available:

* Excellent biological compatibility: absolutely bio-inert.
* Outstanding physical and mechanical qualities:
* Hardness (Vickers) 1200 HV
* Compressive Strength 2000 MPa
* Bending Strength 1000 MPa
* Modulus of Elasticity 210 GPa
* Tensile Strength 7 Mpavm
* Wear characteristics (Ring on disc) <0.002 mm 3/h
* Absolute corrosion resistance: Ringer's solution 370C <0.01mg/ m2x24h
* Very small particle size: <0.6ym
* No glass phase for particle binding
* Extremely high density
* Porosity: 0%
* Purity (Zr/Hf/Y): 99.9%
* Translucence of the framework material makes excellent cosmetic results possible
* Equivalent fit to precision gold castings: edge opening 20-50 ym. Precludes the need to use adhesive cements.
* Zirconium oxide is manufactured and optimized industrially so that the material qualities remain unchanged through the complete pro duction chain.
* Optimal material for crowns: tasteless, radiopaque, no pulp irrita tion because there is no need to use adhesive cements and minimal invasive preparation by dentist.

Zirconium oxide forms the core of each crown and provides the cross-link that bridges the gap of missing teeth. The precision fit of the Zirconium core is derived from computer guided Swiss lathes that cut the form out of a solid Zirconium oxide block. The cutting instructions are obtained from a laser beam that reads 120 points per millimeter from the anatomy of a model of the prepared teeth. Once formed, new synthetic porcelain (99.9% pure) is baked on to the Zirconium core and then shaped like a tooth. Because of the extreme accuracy of the crown fit, the crowns can be cemented with biocompatible dental luting material. This avoids the use of an invasive procedure of etching the tooth with acid and injuring the pulp or nerve of the tooth. This latter procedure often times results in the pulp dying and necessitating root canal therapy.

Advantages of ET zirconium high performance ceramic

Zirconium oxide ceramic primarily stands out due to its high crack resistance. Crack resistance is the resistance with which the material counteracts the spreading of cracks. If a material is stressed, it usually comes to excessively high tension within a defect area (pores, surface deficiencies, cavities) or it cracks. While with metals under high tension in the area of cracks, plastic deformation appears and the top of the tension can be reduced by rounding the cracks; in ceramics due to missing plastic deformation possibility the cracks continue to grow.

The unusual feature of zirconium oxide, compared with other ceramics is that at the appearance of a high-tension area, a transformation of the crystal structure can take place. This process is also accompanied by a volume expansion, which builds wedges in the crack and therefore it reduces the continuation of the crack. While the critical tensile strength (KIC) e.g. of *Dicor, Vita Mark II* and *Empress* is in the area of 1-2.5 Mpam-1/2, zirconium oxide shows values in the range of 10 Mpam-1/2. Even *In-Ceram* (glass infiltrated Al203 ceramic) and *Procera aluminum oxide* (pure Al203 ceramic) show values less then 5 Mpam-1/2.

In connection with the tensile strength there also stands the characteristic of bending strengths. While conventional glass ceramics show results of 100-200 Mpa and aluminum oxide ceramics lie in the area of 400-600 Mpa, zirconium oxide reaches a bending strength of over 1000 Mpa. Because of the high tensile strengths exhibited in test results, it is now possible to fabricate posterior bridges with zirconium oxide. Further decisive advantages of zirconium oxide are its high resistance to corrosion; stability to hydrolysis and its high biocompatibility in comparison with other ceramics makes this material ideal for restorative dentistry. In medicine, zirconium oxide is being used more and more as the material of choice especially for hip prosthesis. For years there has existed substantial clinical tests and examinations which confirm the high quality of zirconium oxide.

Denture Materials

Dentures are usually made from acrylic, stainless steel, and chromium-cobalt, but can be made of nylon, a gold alloy, or titanium. **Most pink-colored acrylics and vinyls contain cadmium**, which is considered toxic and/or immune reactive. The alternative is to use cadmium-free pink or clear materials.

Metals are used to increase rigidity and increase retention of the prosthesis in the mouth during function. If metals are not used, the opposite is true, which is not desirable from a functional perspective.

Bonding

Since all direct fillings (composites) and most indirect restorations (inlays, onlays, and crowns) being placed today use a process called bonding, it's good to have a basic knowledge of how this process works. While there are a myriad of variations in this process, here are the basic steps:

Step 1–Prepare the tooth surface using a mild acid solution. This creates a "honeycomb" in the top layer of tooth.

Step 2–Paint a liquid resin-bonding agent on the tooth. It flows and "locks" into the honeycomb created in Step 1 (technically forming a hybrid layer that is part-tooth and part dental-resin). This layer is "cured" (hardened using a photo-chemical reaction) with a visible light source.

Step 3–Place luting cement if an indirect restoration (e.g., crown) is being used. Essentially, this material is a more liquid form of white filling material. It bonds to both the tooth and the pre-fabricated ceramic restoration and fills the gaps between them. The surface of the first layer of cured bonding agent is highly reactive and is easily bonded to with today's composite filling materials.

Advantages of Bonding

There are a number of advantages to using bonding. Besides allowing the placement of non-metal restorations, less removal of healthy tooth structure is required. The dentist needs to remove only the unhealthy tooth structure and a precisely fitted piece can be bonded into place to replace it. In the case of fillings, bonded restorations have other physical advantages over amalgam.

Even the ADA, in its *Journal of the American Dental Association (JADA)*, recently acknowledged, **"Resin-based composites eventually will replace amalgam as a direct restorative material because they possess many characteristics not inherent in amalgam. Some of the more important of these properties are esthetics, micro-mechanical bonding to tooth structure, smaller cavity preparations and better sealing potential."** (*JADA*, Vol. 132, August 2001, p. 1100).

New Advances

Breakthroughs in the development of dental materials and techniques are occurring on a regular basis. We have yet to find one single material that is compatible for everyone. Debate continues about how to best restore a patient's mouth to optimal health and no perfect solution has yet presented itself. The best we can do is to to keep an open mind and keep searching for answers. Only by thorough testing can it be determined which is most compatible for any one person.

I.A.O.M.T.

The *International Academy of Oral Medicine and Toxicology* (IAOMT) is an organization for that group of dentists, physicians, and allied researchers who consider biocompatibility to be their first concern, and who demand scientific evidence as their key criterion. Members of this group have, since 1984, examined, chronicled and supported research into the distinctions that can make dental practice more biologically acceptable.

A general principle of biocompatible dentistry would state that everything a dentist implants, or leaves, in and around a tooth represents a systemic exposure, whose impact must be accounted for. As dentists pursue the main agenda of dentistry, restoring function and eliminating disease, they have two very broad challenges. The first is choosing among the synthetic materials for restorative and esthetic functions, and the second is reducing the presence of pathogens.

Kinesiology

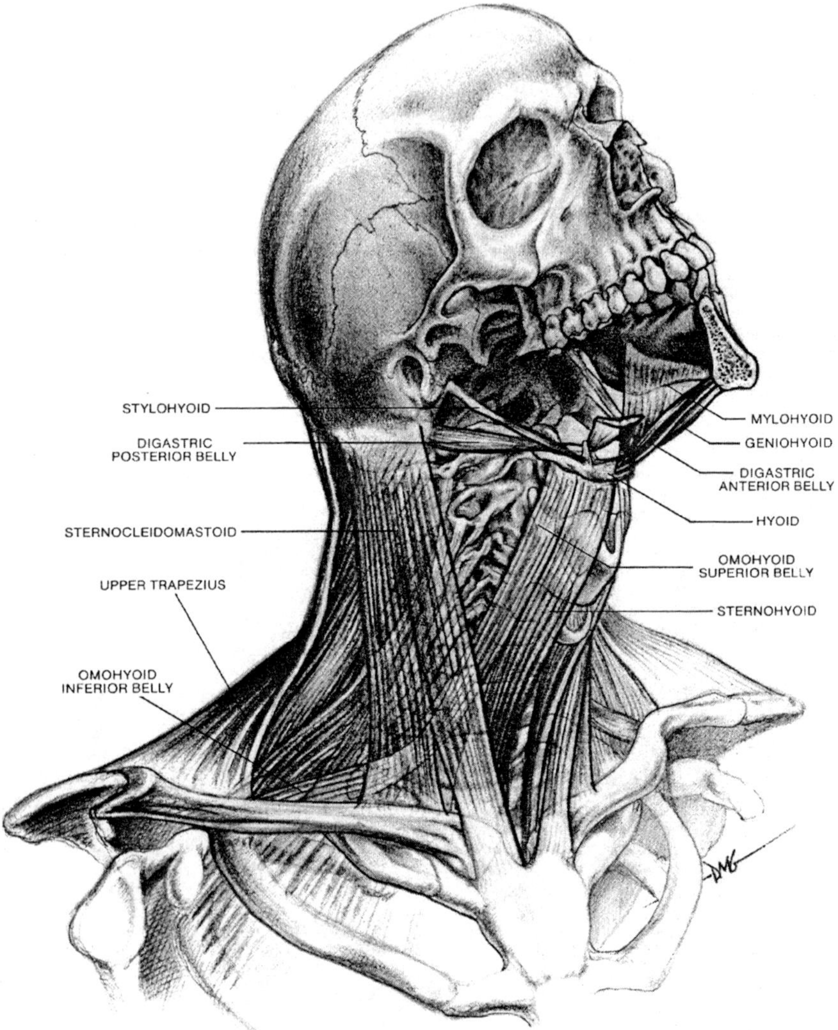

The Closed Kinematic Chain
of the Stomatognathic System

Kinesiology

The body heals itself by primary intent. It heals itself in a sure, sensible, practical, reasonable, and observable manner. The healer within can be approached from without. Man possesses a potential for recovery through the physiological homeostatic ***innate intelligence*** *of the human structure. This recovery potential, with which he has been naturally endowed, and which is his natural birthright, merely waits for the trained hand, the knowing mind, and the caring heart of the trained individual to bring it to physical manifestation, allowing health to come forth; this is man's natural heritage. It allows the same force which created the body to heal the body and allow it to operate unimpeded. This benefits man, both individually and collectively, and also the physician or therapist who has rendered the service.* —George Goodhart, Jr. DC, FICC Diplomate, ICAK, and founder of *Applied Kinesiology.*

Kinesiology: n. The study of muscles and their movements, esp. as applied to physical conditioning. [Gk. *kinesis*, movement (*kinein*, to move) + -logy.] *Kinesiologists*–those who discourse on movement–combining *anatomy*, the science of structure of the body, with *physiology*, the science of function of the body, to produce *kinesiology*, the science of movement of the body. The human brain is a wondrous computer, linked with a universal energy field, that knows far more than it knows it knows. Kinesiology is a well-established science of communicating with another person's nervous system or "database of consciousness," by testing an all-or-none muscle response to stimuli.

The kinesiologist uses muscle tests to find imbalances, tensions and blockages in the body, then makes corrections and rebalances the nervous system, and finally tests the muscles again to verify changes. Kinesiology is showing enormous success in dentistry, chiropractic, and allopathic medicine as well, and can be used to understand the tooth-body connection. This kinesiologic response reflects a capacity of the human central nervous system to differentiate between life-*supportive* and life-*destructive* patterns, to distinguish *positive* from *negative* stimuli, *anabolic* (life-enhancing) from *catabolic* (life-consuming) and, most dramatically, *truth* from *falsity*. It is also possible to test a person's intolerance and stress to things in the environment, i.e. over-sensitivity reactions (physical and mental). All attitudes, thoughts and beliefs are connected with various acupuncture energy meridians, to all of the body's organs, including the teeth.

Specific acupuncture points are linked with meridians, which serve, in turn, as energy channels to specific muscles and body organs. Kinesiology can tap into the inner wisdom that can discriminate *healthy* from *unhealthy*. Ideological validity can be appraised as an innate quality in any subject.

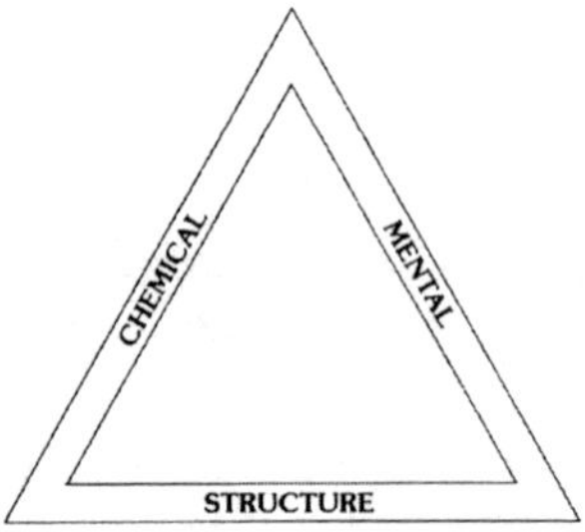

The Triad Of Health

The triad of health displays the three basic causes of health problems. They are *structural, chemical*, and *mental*, with structural as the base of the triad. Literally, all health problems, whether functional or pathological, are involved with one part or all of the triad. The physician who is aware of the triad of health, and evaluates every patient for all three sides, increases his/her ability to find the basic underlying cause of a patient's health problem. Unfortunately, most professionals in the health care system do not thoroughly evaluate for influences of the different aspects of the triad on the patient's chief complaint. Rather, they tend to stay on the side of the triad associated with their specialty.

Each side of the triad is represented by one or more specialties in both natural health care and allopathic medicine. Often, individuals in a specialty attempt to influence the other two sides of the triad by treatment in their area of expertise, creating a lopsided triangle. The efforts may be symptomatically effective, but they often do not give attention to the basic underlying cause of the patient's chief complaint.

Interplay Between Sides

Throughout applied kinesiology, the triad of health is an important principle evaluated in all types of conditions. It is of paramount importance because nearly all conditions, especially chronic ones, involve all three sides of the triad. The physician must consider all possibilities so that s/he is not treating secondary effects rather than primary causes. Almost always, the more chronic a condition, the more involved it is with the three sides of the triad. Even a simple acute condition, such as a sprained ankle–which is obviously structural only–can ultimately affect other structures throughout the body if not treated correctly, and eventually affect the chemical and mental sides of the triad. Treating the sprained ankle correctly entails follow-up evaluation for structural balance and normal nerve function in the foot after the obvious tissue damage from the sprain has been repaired.

Structural Affecting Chemical

What follows is the hypothetical background of a typical chronic health problem, which illustrates the effect that structural influences can have on chemical ones: one year previously the patient sprained an ankle, which apparently healed successfully. Unknown to the patient or his physician, there were *subluxations* of the foot and ankle which improperly stimulated the *proprioceptors* when standing, walking, or running. This improper proprioception caused structural stress in the *suboccipital* area as a result of improper facilitation and inhibition of the *upper trapezious, sternocleidomastoid*, and other muscles active during walking and running. The patient began noticing mild *suboccipital headaches*, but they would go away after a good night's rest. The continued imbalanced pull of the muscles into the cranium eventually caused *cranial faults*, which interfered with normal *vagus nerve* activity. This, in turn, reduced the secretion of *hydrochloric acid.* The reduction of hydrochloric acid depressed production of *pancreatic enzymes*, and *poor digestion* developed, with resulting *toxicity*. This weakening of the *stomach meridian* caused an imbalance in the related teeth (upper 1st and 2nd molars, bottom bicuspids) and started degeneration there as well. As the patient grew more toxic, the headaches became more generalized and severe in intensity, to the point that now they're constant.

This snowballing effect is a relatively common occurrence in many types of health problems. Already the relatively simple structural problem has affected the chemical side of the triad of health. If this patient is allowed to become chronic with severe headaches, s/he will probably do poorly at work and possibly have family problems, which ultimately would affect the mental side of the triad. Doctors specializing in one side of the triad can fail to find the primary cause because treatment directed to one side of the triad may obtain only partial results. A chiropractor may examine this patient, find the suboccipital stress, and give partial results with upper cervical adjustments, which relieve that portion of the patient's headache. A nutritionist might find the gut problem, administer hydrochloric acid and enzymes, and start a detoxification program. This would also give results but not of a permanent nature. There are many doors for entering the patient's health care arena. The best choice is to have a system that evaluates all three sides of the triad of health, to determine when corrections are obtained and if the body is capable of maintaining the corrections. The chiropractor who reduced the headache with cervical manipulation whould find that as soon as the patient walked, the corrections obtained would be lost. The nutritionist used nutrition as an allopathic approach and did nothing to eliminate the cause of the reduced hydrochloric acid secretion, which, in turn, caused the lack of enzymes and toxic gut. The dynamic evaluation that finds the problems and then evaluates the patient to determine if corrections are maintained is the answer to ultimately finding the primary cause, which is in the foot and ankle. The procedures in AK evaluation can easily track down the foot involvement, which is the underlying cause of the problem.

Chemical Affecting Structure

Chief complaint: low back pain. In this case there is no significant history to be obtained from the patient. He denies injuring himself and states the backache "just seemed to start." He used to get relief periodically, but now it is there all the time. As with all these examples, the patient has a digestive disturbance that he chooses not to discuss with the examiner, or fails to recognize as a problem. This patient has a very poor diet, high in refined carbohydrates and low in roughage. Over a period of time, he has developed a malabsorption syndrome from mucous congestion between the villi (thread-like structures that absorb nutrients) of the small intestine. The small intestine is associated with the *abdominal muscles*, as well as the *quadriceps* group (The 3rd molars are on the small intestine meridian). The abdominal muscles are very important to anterior pelvic stabilization. When weak, they allow the pelvis to rotate anteriorly, increasing the *lordotic* curve of the lumbar spine and jamming the *facet* articulations. The *oblique abdominal muscles* also give pelvic stabilization to prevent twist, important in preventing sacroiliac dysfunction.

A chiropractor can manipulate the lower spine and pelvis with some success. An orthopedist may brace the pelvis with some success. But the key is to find out why there is structural imbalance of the pelvis and lumbar spine in the first place. The only satisfactory approach to this condition is to find the bowel (lower 1st & 2nd molars–upper bicuspids) involvement and return the diet to normal. It will probably be necessary to directly treat the digestive system as well. Subjects with musculoskeletal/dental symptoms and signs are more apt to be consuming more refined carbohydrate foodstuffs than those free of such clinical findings. Returning nutrition to normal leads to a decreased incidence of musculoskeletal/ dental problems.

Chemical Affecting Mental

Chief complaint: depression. A similar example to that above is an individual on the same poor diet, high in carbohydrates and low in roughage. With the *malabsorption syndrome* he develops relative *hypoglycemia*, which is a common condition causing *depression*. Counseling or medication may give temporary relief, but again, until the digestive disturbance is corrected, the primary cause has not been treated. There are many other ways that the chemical side can affect the mental. Doctors who work with *orthomolecular psychiatry* have found that any food allergy can have this effect! Often when chemical affects mental, there is also a structural component involved. Most people who are extremely susceptible to food additives have frank allergies, in turn causing increased susceptibility to chemicals, and finally causing mental health problems. Another common condition is toxic metals from dental materials and appliances causing mental disturbances.

Mental Affecting Chemical

Chief complaint: menopausal symptoms of *hot flashes* and *severe fatigue*. The patient has severe *emotional stress* due to coping with an **alcoholic husband**, and the same *digestive disturbance* used in the other illustrations is also present. The patient feels the digestive disturbance is secondary to the emotional stress, which she does not choose to discuss with the examiner. From another physician, she is receiving hormones for her menopausal symptoms, which is treating the condition on a secondary basis. Normally, at menopause the adrenal glands increase their production of estrogen for a maintenance function. In this woman's case, they are incapable of doing so because of *relative hypoadrenia, secondary to the mental stress*. The relative **hypoadrenia is also the cause of the fatigue**, which is listed as part of the chief complaint. Recognition of the various forms of stress and their effects on the adrenal gland, gives the doctor knowledgeable about the interplay of the triad of health the ability to find the primary cause of the menopausal symptoms and fatigue, regardless of the patient's willingness to discuss them. Unless the primary emotional disturbance is removed, results will not be complete. Interestingly, as the adrenal glands begin to function in an improved manner, the patient will probably have an increased ability to control her emotional stress. Frequently, when there is a relative hypoadrenia, the blood sugar level drops to an unacceptable low. When this happens, **mental processes are reduced,** and the subject has difficulty coping with problems which may be present.

Mental Affecting Structural

Chief complaint: lower back and leg pain. The history of this patient is similar to the one above–an **alcoholic husband**, and she has *colitis*. The patient recognizes that the colitis correlates with the emotional disturbance. It is being treated by another physician, who prescribed a bland diet. She does not mention the colitis or emotional disturbance because she is seeking help for her lower back and leg pain from a structurally oriented doctor. Chronic colitis will often cause a weakness of the *tensor fascia lata* muscle by activation of the *neurolymphatic reflex* affecting both the colon and the muscle. A reflex subluxation around the second or third lumbar may also develop. The structural imbalance of the pelvis and leg as a result of the tensor fascia lata muscle weakness, as well as the subluxation, will cause *back pain*. The structurally oriented doctor may obtain temporary relief by manipulation or mechanical support to these areas. He will not obtain permanent results unless the emotional cause of the conditon is brought under control.

Structural Affecting Mental

Chief complaint: schizophrenia. The patient was in an automobile accident several years ago. This seemed to be the beginning of several general health problems, including mental aberrations eventually diagnosed as schizophrenia.

The injury from the auto accident created a structural imbalance of the pelvis. As a result of this imbalance, proprioceptive communication to the rest of the body became disorganized, developing into what is known in AK as a *homolateral crawl pattern*, (lack of cross crawl) which is present in schizophrenics. The pelvic distortion in the patient also created constant stress to the *sartorius* and *gracilis* muscles, ultimately affecting their glandular association, the *adrenals*. Hypoadrenia is quite important in blood sugar regulation. Approximately 60% of schizophrenics have hypoglycemia. Schizophrenia is like all other conditions: There is always a causative factor; which remains to be found for correction of the condition. In this case, the chemical and structural sides of the triad must be corrected to eliminate the mental factor. Another example: The toxic metals used in dentistry to structurally treat a tooth can directly enter the body's cells. Many of these (especially mercury) have an affinity for neurons and, along with the *galvanic electrical current* they generate, can cause psychological imbalances, such as hyperactivity, depression, anxiety, and even suicidal behavior. There is a definite lack of knowledge in the general health care field regarding how significantly structure, especially dentistry, affects mental health–the role dentistry plays in teh process.

The Stomatognathic System

The term *stomatognathic* usually refers to the mouth and jaw. Here we are looking at a more comprehensive unit and refer to the *stomatognathic system*, which includes components of the bones of the skull, the mandible, the hyoid, the clavicle and the sternum; the muscles and the ligaments; the dentoalveolar and the temporomandibular joints; the vascular, the lymphatic and the nerve supply systems; the soft tissues of the head; the teeth; the spinal column and the pelvis. The stomatognathic area can potentially influence the *cranial primary respiratory mechanism* in either a positive or a negative way, and the converse is true; the cranial primary respiratory mechanism is capable of influencing the stomatognathic area in either a positive or a negative way. The two are inseparable entities. The stomatognathic system interacts with total body function.

There is much disagreement and lack of general knowledge among physicians about the stomatognathic system. One of the major reasons for the controversy is that there are usually no organic findings in most stomatognathic disturbance. Most physicians are trained primarily to differentiate and treat pathological problems. Those who think in terms of functional disturbances are more likely to look for and ultimately treat the functional type of disturbances found in the stomatognathic system. The structures within the stomatognathic system interact, and a disturbance in one area can, by a domino effect, create a great many additonal disturbances. Often the *secondary* factors are treated rather than the *primary* condition. Unfortunately, many who specialize in the treatment of these disturbances have a concept that there is one primary cause of the condition and fit most patients into that slot.

Because of the great amount of interaction within the system, the kind of condition the physician usually treats may be found, but it may not be the *primary* condition. It is important that a thorough examination protocol be developed, taking into consideration the wide range of etiologic factors in stomatognathic conditions. The patient, recognizing a symptomatic pattern, often chooses his own diagnosis and treatment with his selection of a physician. Treatment may include *occlusal therapy, cervical* or *cranial manipulation, medication, psychological counseling, biofeedback, surgery*, etc. One of these therapies may actually be appropriate for the patient, but it should be the job of the physician consulted as the primary care provider to diagnose the condition and determine the approach needed for its correction. Since no profession is capable of providing all the potential therapies that might be needed, consultation and referral are often the duty of the primary care physician. It is important to emphasize again that very often the symptomatic pattern presented by the patient is an *effect* rather than the primary *cause*; in fact, sometimes the patient's symptoms are *iatrogenic,* stemming from the treatment for some other condition. The stomatognathic system can be evaluated effectively with applied kinesiology.

Muscular imbalance, which develops from occlusal disturbances, can ultimately involve the whole body. First it is important to understand that the jaw-closing muscles of mastication are part of a *closed kinematic chain*, and contribute to the chain from the mandible to the skull. The mandible, in turn, is anchored to the shoulder girdle by the *supra-* and *infrahyoid* muscles. The *neck* and head *extensor muscles* contribute to the posterior portion of the chain. Muscle hypo- or hyper-tonicity in any link of this chain disturbs its balance, and a vicious circle may develop. It may start as a result of TMJ disturbance, which causes muscle contraction, and pain of muscular contraction produces further muscle contraction over the short reflex arc, and this contraction, in turn, increases pain and furthers more contraction. This inappropriate muscle contraction causes reactions in remote areas of the body by way of stimulating the muscle's neuromuscular *spindle cell* and, depending on the location of the muscle, possibly *equilbrium proprioceptors*; the vicious circle begins.

Information about the inappropriate muscle contraction is sent by the *afferent system*, which causes reaction in another muscle. The reaction becomes an action that sends information to cause an additional reaction. The far-ranging effects of the disturbance in the closed kinematic chain can go on and on. Not only are the equilibrium proprioceptors of the cervical spine and head-balancing muscles involved, the *hyoid muscles* are very important in the equilibrium and centering of the body. The hyoid and its associated muscles work like a gyroscope in the body. Disturbance in the stomatognathic system can influence structure throughout the body. The question should arise as to whether malocclusion is the primary cause of disturbance in the stomatognathic system, or if it is secondary. The orthopedic influence points out that the TMJ syndrome can be caused by postural imbalance.

A short leg or a pelvic disturbance can create secondary imbalances in the stomatognathic system. The influence may be to the neck and head extensors–one area of the closed kinematic chain–ultimately causing imbalance in the temporomandibular joint. Strachan and Robinson, at the Chicago College of Osteopathy, were the first to observe a short leg's influence on malocclusion. Evaluationg the pattern of masticatory muscles by electromyography, they removed a three-eights inch heel lift from a standing subject's shoe and found an altered firing sequence of the muscles of mastication during chewing. When the lift was worn, the muscles showed the firing pattern of normal occlusion; with it removed, the firing pattern was one of a severe malocclusion.

The healing powers of nature rest upon balance and the restoration of balance, and whenever and wherever man has interfered with that balance, he has paid the penalty. Total structural balancing is a priority in the applied kinesiology approach to the stomatognathic system. The interrelationship of the stomatognathic system with the rest of the body does not have to correlate with jaw function and occlusion. In some cases, the only evidence of trouble is pain. Cranial nerves V, VII. IX, and X are all involved in some way. The tongue can become the seat of referred pain from a distant source of irritation in any organ innervated by the *trigeminal, facial, vagus*, or *glossopharyngeal* nerve. The primary cause may be remote from the site of the symptom. This is true whether the direction of involvement is from the stomatognathic system to remote areas, or from remote areas to the stomatognathic system.

By using plethysmography on the digits of the feet and hands and by Doppler ultrasonic evaluation of arterial flow, improved circulation has been demonstrated after occlusal adjustment with a *wax bite* or with cotton roll supports. By thus changing the mandible's position, improved circulation was demonstrated on both the arterial flow and the capillary flow, indicated by the Doppler and the plethysmograph respectively. Influence of the stomatognathic system on general body function can be seen by its influence on muscle function as observed by manual muscle testing. This was originally demonstrated clinically by Goodheart.

Many in the dental profession have used applied kinesiology procedures to evaluate the stomatognathic system. Some have done a very credible job of applying this system in the dental field. It is necessary to have a good working knowledge of manual muscle testing; a great number of errors can potentially develop as a result of its improper use.

History of Kinesiology and Biomechanics

Kinesiology monitors and tests the energetics of the body and balances its structural, biochemical and electromagnetic aspects, It also can aid in distinguishing the truth from the false.

From original muscle response research called Applied Kinesiology, developed by Dr. George Goodheart, D.C., in 1964, simple body movements were used to evaluate physical functioning. All forms of kinesiology use manual muscle testing as a fundamental tool. The basic principle of Applied Kinesiology is that testing the tension in specific muscles reveals all stresses, imbalances and blockages in the nervous system. All muscles in the body are connected to different internal organs, endocrine glands, spinal vertebrae and nerve roots, teeth, specific nutrients, thoughts and feelings, acupuncture meridians, and other parts of the body's electrical system.

Dr. Robert Lovett and the American physiotherapists Henry and Florence Kendall originally developed manual muscle testing. In 1949, Kendall & Kendall published a classic reference work on the subject that has become the foundation of all muscle testing. The Kendalls used around 100 manual muscle tests in their work. Now Kinesiologists are further developing manual muscle testing applications. Especially in Clinical Kinesiology where Dr. Alan Beardall developed another 250 - 300 new manual muscle tests. In 1968, Dr. Alan Beardall became one of Dr. Goodheart's most brilliant protégés. Dr. Goodheart developed all of the groundwork on Applied Kinesiology muscle testing based on the Chinese acupuncture philosophy. In 1975, Beardall began innovating and testing the Clinical Kinesiology method, discovering over 250 specific muscle tests, while concentrating primarily on related muscle reflexes.

Dr. Beardall integrated all major chiropractic techniques, numerous adjunctive therapies such as acupuncture, nutrition, and homeopathy, including flower remedies and Chinese five element diagnostics into his Clinical Kinesiology system. Clinical Kinesiology includes the testing component for each individual, which translates what is going on energetically in the body. Goodheart's and Beardall's original research on kinesiology was given wider application by Dr. John Diamond, whose books brought the subject of *Behavioral Kinesiology* to the public. Diamond determined that **a positive or negative response occurs with stimuli both physical and mental**.

In 1975, the well-known psychiatrist and physician, Dr. David Hawkins began research on the kinesiological response to truth and falsehood. Through 20+ years of research, Hawkins was able to analyze the full spectrum of the levels of human consciousness developing a fascinating map of the geography of man's experience. This "anatomy of consciousness" produces a profile of the entire human condition, allowing a comprehensive analysis of the emotional and spiritual development of individuals, societies, and the race in general. This allowed kinesiology to become a guide for all of us as to our place on the ladder of spiritual enlightenment and on our own personal journeys to reach our potential.

A great degree of accuracy and reproducibility is achieved in manual muscle testing when done by individuals knowledgeable in the science and proficient in its art. Although manual muscle testing is a reliable indicator of function when done properly, this diagnostic tool is no better than the person performing the test. It could be compared with a time-honored diagnostic tool, the stethoscope, which functions no better than what is between the earpieces. A stethoscope in the hands of a poorly trained practitioner, deficient in both the science and art of its use, will consistently give erroneous information, jeopardizing the patient's health and damaging the examiner's reputation.

Physiology of Muscle Testing

Dietrich Klinghardt, M.D., and Louisa Williams, M.S., D.C., N.D. have discovered that the skin's normal *electrodermal* activity is always measured as a negative polarity. In fact, the skin of the palms of the hand and the soles of the feet is actually 10-25 millivolts more negative than the rest of the body. However, the skin over a diseased organ or an injured area has a positive charge. The theory of an *injury current* was first described by Luigi Galvani in 1794 and then confirmed by Robert Becker M.D. in the early 1960s. Thus, when the examiner holds the negatively charged palm of his hand over a positively-charged skin surface–at the location of a patient's functional disturbance–a *capacitor* is formed. Physics describes the ability of two parallel plates to store an electrical charge and thus serve as a capacitor. As soon as the two plates (hand & skin) come in contact, an electric current flows for a short time.

This increased electron flow stimulates the *unmyelinated* autonomic and sensory nerve fibers in the corresponding region. As a result of recent research, it is now believed that **up to 80% of all autonomic nerve fibers are *sensory* not *motor***. This flood of sensory action potentials excites *core* regions of the *posterior horn* of the spinal cord. There exist, from this point, nerve fiber connections with the sympathetic *motor* region of the *lateral horn* and the *alpha* and *gamma motor neurons* of the *anterior horn*. The sympathetic motor fibers innervate the *intrafusal* muscle *spindle fibers*. The *alpha motor neurons* innervate the *extrafusal fibers*, which are directly connected with the *Golgi tendon organs*.

These structures are responsible for the muscle tone of the corresponding muscles. Changes in the "electrical state" of these receptors determine whether a test muscle will be strong or weak. The latest investigations have shown that **only the sympathetic** innervations of the muscle spindles–independently of the activity of the alpha and gamma motor neurons–**can be responsible for an increase or decrease in muscle tone**. The Golgi tendon organs have a remote inhibiting effect: spinal interneurons send *collaterals* to motor neurons that communicate, via *internuncial fibers*, over a number of spinal cord segments, and trigger muscle weakness there.

The impulses, which reach the spinal cord, communicate within milliseconds with higher centers, in particular with the *reticular activating system* and the cerebral cortex. From here, impulses can again reach the test muscle via descending inhibitory nerve pathways to the motor anterior and lateral horn cells, which leads to a weakening of the previously strong muscle. Chronic diseases usually have a significant common component, namely latent chronic ischemia (diminished blood flow). This is caused by the sympathetic innervations of the arterioles in the disease region. The cause of this is a disease-induced dysregulation of the autonomic ganglia.

Therapy Localization of Disturbances

The examining hand should generate an increased tissue pressure in the disease region, in order to increase the ischemia briefly. If the *superordinate ganglia* are fully functional, this triggers a swift local counter reaction (loss of sympathetic tone) without the participation of the higher reflex pathways. If local regulation has rigidified due to ganglial illness, then the ischemia signal will be transmitted to higher centers via the above-mentioned reflex pathways, which will then trigger a *counter-regulation* via the intact *collateral pathways*. **This leads to a loss of muscle tone in a number of segments or even in the entire body.** In order to generate sufficient afferent ischemia signals, moderate to strong pressure during therapy localization is recommended. A diseased region or diseased ganglion will reveal itself by the weakening of the previously strong test muscle.

American physiologist Irvin Korr has measured the *sympathetic sweat gland reaction* (damp regions of the skin), which shows itself through a reduction in skin resistance. This is an indication for a high *vasomotor tone*, which leads to chronic *vasoconstriction*. In every case, Korr found a correlation between *sympathetic hyperactivity*, low skin resistance and *visceral* pathology. This is also the basis for the EAV (electro-acupuncture according to Voll) measurements. This form of kinesiological therapy localization is a test of the functional competence of the sympathetic system. Positive therapy localization signifies: overburdened or diseased ganglion and associated autonomic nerve pathways, ischemia and chaotic *afferent* autonomic and sensory nerve signals. *Blocked regulation* is a rigidification of the *mesenchyme* due to medications, surgical intervention, chemotherapy and radiation therapy, chronic emotional stress, food and environmental allergies, toxic ganglia and, most widespread, **silver/amalgam fillings**. These stresses primarily affect the autonomic nervous system, whose fibers begin or end in the extracellular space.

Actually, it is these fibers and their associated ganglia whose regulation becomes "rigid." Your brain filters the unconscious information into your unconscious mind, storing the data in your *reticular activating system*–the part of your subconscious mind that regulates the special software in your body.

The reticular activating system functions as a filtering system, working to filter data into either your conscious or unconscious mind as needed. This needed information lies just below the surface for recall for the purpose of monitoring the body. If the system records an imbalance, you're notified immediately–**the body-mind works together to create a symptom**. The reticular activating system continually evaluates, sorts, and prioritizes possible dangers: It signals the feedback or "body language" interpreted through the muscle testing. You need not depend on chemical drugs or risky surgery to obtain answers. **Your body can talk, if you simply communicate with it.** Kinesiology provides a fascinating way of communicating and healing through the inseparable energy linking mind, body and spirit.

Information from your body's computer software system relays hidden, energetic messages to the surface for consideration and indication of healing through muscle testing. The energy/organ system so intertwines that it's not unusual to experience knee pain, for example, when the kidney becomes unbalanced. The reason? The knee is located along the course of the kidney meridian. If a pathway is blocked, off balance or "complaining" a bit, the condition is usually connected to a problem in a related organ or tooth. The knee can become painful if the *adrenals* (*sartorius, gracillus, soleus*, and *gastrocnemius* muscles) or the *gallbladder* meridian (popliteus muscle) is in trouble (canines), with the large intestine (hamstrings), through muscular reflex hypertonicity and weakness, creating instability of the knee joint, etc.

Manual Muscle Testing

Manual muscle testing has been used for structural and neurologic evaluation since the early 1900s. Recent texts on the subject offer considerable information on the art and science of manual muscle testing. Specific procedures are described thatare continually being improved as technology, such as *electromyography*, provides more evidence about the prime action of muscles. The greatest potential weakness in kinesiology is lack of quality muscle testing. A great degree of accuracy and reproducibility is achieved in manual muscle testing when done by individuals knowledgeable in the science and proficient in its art.
Although manual muscle testing is a reliable indicator of function when done properly, this diagnostic tool is no better than the person performing the test.

The correct attitude is to accurately perform a test **without concern for the outcome** of the procedure. When the practitioner is trying to "prove" to a patient that s/he has a specific condition, the enthusiasm for the information being imparted to the patient may, on a subconscious level, alter the results of the test. The tester's mental attitude also enters the testing procedure when s/he believes very strongly in some specific "principle." There must be an accurate knowledge of the science of muscle testing.

This includes the anatomy and physiology of the muscle being tested, and also of joint movements and other muscles that play a role in the testing procedure. Any peculiarities of the patient being tested, such as joint pathology, should also be known.

A practitioner knowledgeable in muscle testing probably gains as much information from observation as he does from the actual forceful muscle testing. Knowledge of the subtle movements the patient makes and what they mean is a significant part of the science of muscle testing. Another aspect is the *art* of muscle testing. The only way this can be acquired is by **practice**, keeping uppermost in mind the potential of operator prejudice. Practice includes not only learning to observe the scientific information of the muscle activity, but also the mechanical aspects and the feel of the muscle testing procedure. Accurate muscle testing requires *knowledge* in the science and *practice* in the art.

To apply the science of manual muscle testing, the examiner must have knowledge of the anatomy of the muscles involved in the test, the tendon attachments, the actions of the muscles, and the physiology of muscle contraction. Applying this knowledge, s/he can observe the patient's attempts to recruit other muscles to substitute for the *prime mover* being tested. The examiner must have knowledge of the stabilization necessary for the patient to be able to use the prime mover to the best advantage. Furthermore, the examiner must know the dynamics of his/her own body and how they influence the evaluation of the muscle strength exhibited by the patient. **The patient's hands should always be placed away from the body during testing.** *Therapy localization*, which is the placing of the patient's hands on specific areas of the body to stimulate nerve endings and other factors, may change the results of a muscle test.

Testing a muscle or weakness with nothing being done to influence either its strength or weakness is called testing the muscle *in the clear*. The examiner should constantly observe the location of the patient's hands, keeping them off the body when it is intended that the patient be tested in the clear. Continued testing of an individual while looking for an abnormality can possibly fatigue the patient's muscle. Thus the examiner may conclude that an additional parameter to the test is positive when it is not. It is easy to determine whether or not fatigue is a factor in test results when a muscle weakens from some additional factor placed into the test. When the muscle weakens, simply reverse the additional factor to determine if the muscle regains its original strength. A fatigued muscle will not immediately regain its strength; it remains weak until it is rested.

It is important to isolate the specific muscle for testing as well as possible. This is accomplished when the structure is placed in a position that gives a specific muscle the best advantage to be the prime mover in the activity.

The basic fact that muscles cannot generally be isolated gives the experienced muscle tester a considerable amount of information about muscle strength from observing the patient's activity as the test is performed. Testing specific muscles gives experienced examiners the ability to obtain excellent reproducibility in muscle testing. *Generalized* tests, such as the "arm pull-down test" or the "leg test" are of groups of muscles; they are not *specific* muscle tests. They are used for tests requiring group evaluations, such as the gait mechanism.

There are four muscle categories which must be understood and evaluated in any specific manual muscle test. The **prime mover** is the muscle being tested; the starting position of the test is one that gives greatest isolation and opportunity for that muscle to be the major factor in performing the procedure. **Synergist muscles** are those anatomically situated to aid the prime mover. With slight change of testing position or of movement, they can be recruited to aid the prime mover to a greater extent. In most instances, the synergist muscles are active in the testing of the prime mover; however, the object is to place them at a disadvantage so they are not a major factor in the test. The fixator muscles are those responsible for stabilizing the part or parts being tested. **Fixator muscles** are not a factor in all muscle tests, but when present they are extremely important in evaluating the outcome. Fixator muscles are sometimes located between the point of the prime mover muscle and the point of force being applied to test the muscle. An illustration of this is the necessity of normal *deltoid* function when the arm is being used as a lever to test the ability of the *serratus anticus* to hold the scapula. In other instances, the fixator is located distal to the point of muscle activity and the point of force being applied. An example of this is the reverse of the previous example; the serratus anticus must be capable of stabilizing the scapula when the deltoid is being tested. The **antagonist muscle** is usually not a factor in a routine muscle test because of *reciprocal inhibition*. It can be a factor in situations or procedures in applied kinesiology, such as reactive muscle testing.

In order to evaluate the prime mover, synergists, fixators, and antagonists, the examiner must have a high degree of anatomical knowledge. First, the exact origin and insertion of each muscle is important. This ties in with the knowledge of the muscle's action. Additional information in muscle evaluation can be obtained by palpating for tenderness and nodules at these locations. The tendon gives considerable information, especially on those muscles having long tendons which stand out during the muscle test. For example, it is easy for the experienced muscle tester to obtain excellent isolation of the *peroneus longus* and *brevis* by observing maximum tension on those tendons and minimum tension of the tendons of the *peroneus tertius* and *tensor digitorum longus*. Knowing the location of the tendons and muscle belly also gives the examiner the ability to palpate these structures for contraction during the test.

The examiner must thoroughly understand the muscle test. Sometimes a muscle test is misinterpreted because of failure to observe what the prime mover is actu ally doing. An example of this is the serratus anticus test, which uses the arm as a lever to move the scapula while the examiner's thumb lifts on the angle of the scapula. If the serratus anticus muscle is weak, the scapula is not being stabilized, and the arm will come down easily. The test, however, is actually whether the scapula moves, not whether the arm comes down. The test requires an intact shoulder, and the arm is used only as a lever to direct force into the scapula. Another test with a similar observation is the *popliteus* test. The examiner exerts force on the foot to rotate the tibia on the femur. Whether the foot turns around is insignificant; the actual test is the movement of the tibia on the femur as observed by movement of the *tibial tubercle*. The examiner cannot evaluate this test unless he is observing the tibial movement.

Laboratory Testing

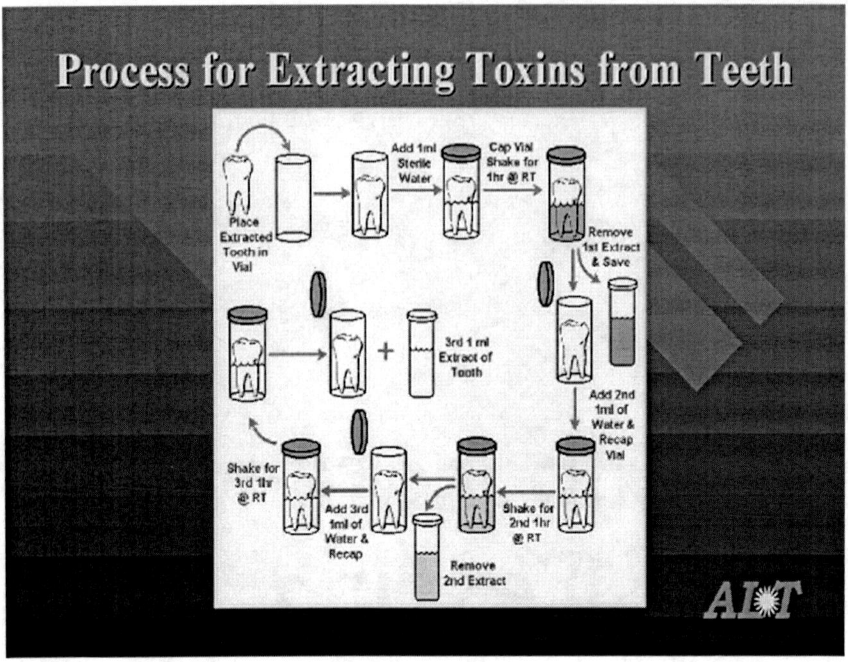

Process for Extracting Toxins from Teeth
Place Extracted Tooth in Vial
Add 1ml Sterile Water
Cap Vial Shake for 1hr @ RT
Remove 1st Extract & Save
Add 2nd 1ml of Water & Recap Vial
Shake for 2nd 1hr @ RT
Remove 2nd Extract
Add 3rd 1ml of Water & Recap
Shake for 3rd 1hr @ RT
3rd 1 ml Extract of Tooth
ALT

Laboratory Testing

Oral Toxicity Testing

ALT, Inc. (altcorp.com) was founded in 1997 by Dr. Boyd Haley, Professor and Chair of Chemistry Department, University of Kentucky, Dr. Curt Pendergrass, President and Dr. Anjan Bhattacharyya, Radiochemicals Laboratory Director. These scientists have over 50 years combined research experience in the synthesis and use of *photoaffinity nucleotide analogs* in the study of protein biochemistry, heavy metal neurotoxicology and neurodegenerative diseases. The technique of *nucleotide photoaffinity labeling* has been largely pioneered by Dr. Haley over the past 30 years and continuously supported by the National Institutes of Health.

Nucleotide Photoaffinity Labeling

Nucleotides and *nucleotide binding proteins* regulate numerous biochemical processes in the cell. Many of the nucleotide binding proteins controlling these biochemical process are the targets of *drugs* as well as *toxicants*. In addition, many of these nucleotide binding proteins are affected or altered in various disease states. The use of nucleotide photoaffinity analogs allows for the study of protein-nucleotide interactions at the molecular level. This powerful technique allows one to identify the amino acid residues actually involved in formation of the active site of nucleotide binding proteins and how mutations in that active site subsequently affect nucleotide binding. It also allows one to study how substrates, cofactors, drugs, toxicants, etc. all affect binding of nucleotides to the active site of proteins. The information gained from these studies allows researchers to determine how these nucleotide binding proteins regulate the biochemical processes in which they are involved. In addition, this technique can be used to determine which specific nucleotide binding proteins are the targets of drugs and toxicants as well as how these proteins are regulated.

Photoaffinity vs Chemical Affinity Labeling

Photoaffinity labeling differs in several ways from classical chemical affinity labeling. Chemically reactive probes normally have an *electrophillic* group which reacts with basic amino acids such as *arginine* or *lysine* or with *sulfhydryls* containing amino acids such as *cysteine*. Although this method results in higher *stoichiometry* of labeling, a large proportion of it can be nonspecific (outside the active site). This is due to the ability of chemically reactive probes to potentially react with all these available amino residues which are accessible not only those just within the active site. In contrast, photoaffinity probes have a chemically inert photactive azido group. This distinctive feature allows the study of enzymatic processes without the destruction of the azido group. The optimal bound analog in the enzyme active site can then be photoactivated by brief exposure to UV light. The reactive intermediate has a short half life and reacts indiscriminately to form a covalent bond with amino acid residues within the active site.

The Photolabeling Procedure

The photolabeling procedure involves initial incubation of the radiolabeled photoprobe with the protein or a crude mixture of proteins. (i.e. cell lysate or tissue homogenate). Brief (1-2 min.) *photolysis* with a low intensity (2000-6000 μW), hand held 254 nm UV light produces a covalent linkage within the active site. Immediately after photolysis, the photolabeling reaction is quenched with a thiol reagent such as *dithiothreitol* or *beta mercaptoethanol* (10 mM or greater). The photolabeled protein is then separated from the unbound photolyzed probe by several methods such as *precipitation with acid*, *ammonium sulfate, polyethylene glycol*, etc. or by *gel filtration* or *ultrafiltration*. The photolabeled proteins can then be analyzed by virtually any biochemical method. Quantification of the degree of *photoincorporation* of radioactivity can then be simply determined by any of a number of commonly used techniques such as *autoradiography, imaging analysis* or *scintillation counting*.

Materials Reactivity Testing

Because each of us possesses a unique biochemistry, substances we come in contact with daily effect each of us differently and in varying degrees. For some, the effects of certain substances (and their corrosion byproducts) can be toxic and hazardous, and may result in serious health problems. A substance which causes little or no reaction in one individual can prove harmful to another. Since these effects may vary in each of us, it is vital that these factors be considered when choosing dental and other materials for use in the body, especially in patients with special or unique health concerns. The *Clifford materials reactivity testing* (www.ccrlab.com) provides dentists and other professional health care providers with extensive information about their patient's individual sensitivities so that least offensive materials can be chosen and used in their treatments.

When we come in contact with harmful substances, the body's natural defense system produces antibodies to counter these agents. Among other things, these IgG, IgM and IgA antibodies provide an immunological record of chemical families which have proven offensive. The Clifford materials reactivity test, developed by Walter J. Clifford, screens patient blood samples for these antibodies. Antibodies which have been specifically formed against harmful agents are detected and analyzed. The agents against which these antibodies were formed are then cross referenced against a list of over 2600 dental and medical trade-named products and narrows it down to a list of "suited: materials for personal suitability.

The Clifford materials reactivity test results allow a dentist or physician to quickly determine from an extensive list of materials that can be used with the least degree of risk in meeting needs. The report also lists trade-named products with simple *suited/not suited* indicators for rapid spot checks of products in question. It does not address issues of mechanical performance nor electro-activity between materials.

TMJ
Dysfunction

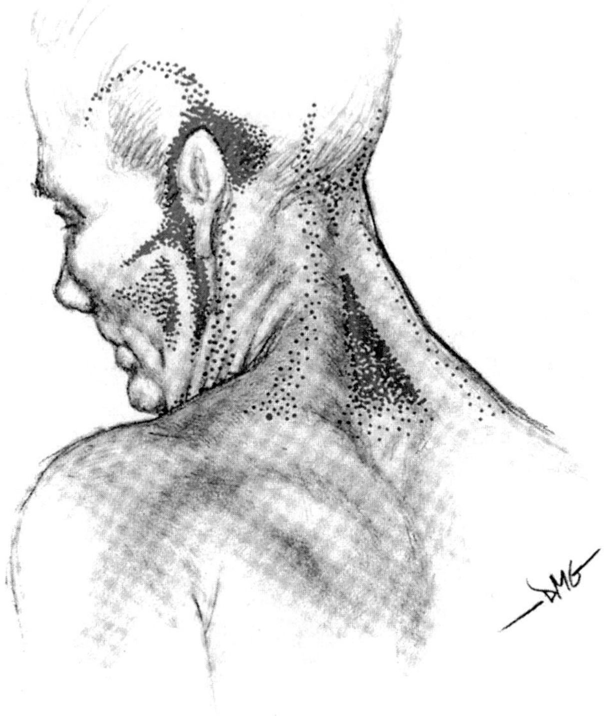

TMJ Pain Patterns

TMJ Dysfunction

TMJ dysfunction is a disorder of the jaw joint and related structures where the ball (condyle), socket (fossa), and cushioning disk (*meniscus*) of the joint are damaged or misaligned. Over time, the meniscus becomes increasingly compressed and torn, allowing the bony structures of the ball and socket to deteriorate at an accelerating rate due to the grinding wear on the joint and the loss of cushioning effect of the meniscus. This grinding (*crepitus*) and concurrent pressure on the capsular ligament surrounding the joint can cause head pain, and may create difficulty in opening or closing of the mouth. The body attempts to realign the joint using the musculature in the face, jaw and neck. As these muscles become fatigued, additional muscles in the shoulders and back attempt to help this condition, then become stressed themselves. This can cause symptoms of generalized muscle pain and weakness that are diagnosed as *Myofascial Pain Dysfunction Syndrome* (Fibromyalgia) and/or Chronic Fatigue Syndrome.

"TMJ" is a popular term commonly used to describe the same group of symptoms. TMJ stands for *Temporomandibular Joints*. These are the two joints (TMJ) that connect your jaw to your skull. When these joints are out of place, they can cause many problems, such as: Clicking or popping of the jaw joints. Pain in or around the jaw joints. Locking or limited opening of your mouth. The misalignment of the joint can also affect the nearby ear structures, due to pressure on the petrotympanic fissure and tympanic bone. The tympanic bone separates the jaw joint from the ear canal. The mandibular malleolar ligament (disco-malleolar ligament) connects the malleous as this ligament traverses through the fissure to attach to the meniscus and the capsular ligament of the TMJ. The capsular ligament is the sac surrounding the joint

The anterior tympanic artery, which is responsible for supplying oxygenated blood to the tissue around the tympanic membrane (ear drum) travels through this fissure. The chorda tympani nerve traverses through this fissure. This nerve gives pain sensation to the tongue. Pressure on these structures can cause dysfunction and symptoms such as *ear pain, tinnitus* (ringing in the ears), *vertigo* (dizziness), *subjective hearing loss, hyperacusis* (increased sensitivity to sound), *Chronic Fatigue Syndrome, tongue pain, muscle pain, sinus headaches, migraines, neck and shoulder stiffness,* and other symptoms.

In 1934 Costen, a medical doctor, reported that headache and ear symptoms often result from disturbed function of the temporomandibular joint. His report received enough attention for the pattern of involvement ot become known as *Costen's Syndrome*. The mechanisms which Costen related as causing the symptoms have been discredited. Although his mechanisms may have been incorrect, it seems apparent today that many of the conditions which Costen related to the temporomandibular joint are, in fact, caused by dysfunction in that mechanism and in surrounding tissues. Various theories have replaced Costen's. Dechaume described a major cause of the symptoms of TMJ dysfunction to be a result of intervention of the sympathetic system. This relates to the high concentration of *terminal vascular nerves* in the articulation being irritated. In addition to Costen's *overclosure* theory and Dechaume's *neurologic irritation* theory, there have been several who have proposed other theories, all of which are currently being practiced in varying degrees.

The tooth theory primarily deals with malocclusion causing displacement of the mandible. The tooth-muscle theory also relates with malocclusion but brings into the picture the neuromuscular system disturbed by stimulaiton to the periodontal ligament proprioceptors. The psychophysiologic theory primarily relates the myofascial pain syndrome to psychological causes that increase muscle tension. The *cavitational osteonecrosis* theory addresses the bone marrow lesions that silently destroy nerve and blood vessels and can cause TMJ and other facial pain.

Various terms are used to describe this disorder. Distress patterns have been referred to as the *temporomandibular joint syndrome* (TMJS), *dental distress syndrome, masticatory myalgia syndrome, psychophysiologic theory,* as well as many other names. Treatment approaches have been called *cervico-oro-facial orthopedia* and/or *dental orthopedics*, and *cranio-sacral therapy,* among other names. Such symptoms may relate to your bite and how they can successfully be treated by a health care professional that has special education in managing these disorders. *Craniomandibular Dysfunction* is a term, which describes a collection of symptoms, which result when the chewing muscles and jaw joints do not work together correctly. Muscle spasm goes hand-in-hand with displaced jaw joints. Because the nerves and muscles are so complex in this area, when these muscles are in spasm the problems can be far-reaching.

People suffer from TMJ symptoms they would never think to associate with their bite, such as: *headaches, pain behind the eyes, dizziness, ear-aches or ringing of the ears, clenching or grinding of the teeth, neck, shoulder, or back pain, numbness*, or *tingling of the fingers*.

TMJ Diagnosis

It is necessary to have a knowledgeable clinician perform a complete diagnosis before a successful treatment program can begin. This diagnosis should include the following:

* A complete medical and dental history.

* A complete clinical examination including:

* *Cavitat* sonic immaging.

* *Transcranial Lateral Oblique* X-Rays (8-view), Tomograms (3 cuts) and MRI procedures are necessary to evaluate the condition and shape of the joint bones and meniscus of the TMJ.

* *Electromyographic* evaluation of the tension (hyperactivity) in the jaw and facial muscles surrounding the joint.

* Range-of-motion studies and jaw tracking tests to determine the condition of the joint during function and at rest. (Myotronics, Seattle, Washington).

* Examination of posture and body symmetry.
In some cases, the clinician may request a MMPI (Minnesota Multiphsic Personality Inventory) to evaluate possible psychogenic factors.

* Ear, nose and throat examination to rule out other conditions when necessary (acoustic neuroma).

* Neurological examination when necessary.

* Orthodonic examination when necessary.

* General internal medical examination when necessary.

TMJ Treatment Procedures

Non-surgical treatment

The diagnostic procedures enable the clinician to assess the severity and the cause(s) of the condition. In many cases, the symptoms are related to muscle hyperactivity and/or dental and skeletal mal-relationships with minimal joint damage. Successful non-surgical treatment may include:

* Application of moist heat and cold spray.

* Injections of a local anesthetic into muscle trigger points.

* Physical therapy (passive and active jaw exercises).

* Medication, in extreme cases (muscle relaxants, anti-anxiety medication, anti-depressants, anti-inflamatories, and pain relieving medication).

* Nutritional supplementation and wholesome diet.

* Neuro-muscular orthotics to restore the proper vertical, lateral, anterior-posterior muscle resting length and the most comfortable position of the condyle to the eminence-fossa-meniscal complex.

* Biofeedback and acupuncture.

* TENS (transcutaneous electrical neural simulation) Myomonitor.

* Coronoplasty (reshaping anatomy of tooth structures)

* Orthodontics to restore proper relationship between the upper and lower jaw and teeth; after this relationship has been established by use of a neuro-muscular orthotic.

* General dentistry to restore missing teeth and maintain proper relationship of the maxilla and mandible by use of partial and complete dentures, crowns, bridgework, and dental implants after this relationship has been established with a neuro-muscular orthotic.

* Local anesthetic and cortisone injections into the joint to relieve pain and swelling.

Surgical treatment

In other, more severe cases, surgery is necessary to correct bone and tissue damage caused by disease, trauma, chronic dysfunction, and iatrogenic causes, i.e., Proplast. These may include:

* Arthroscopic examination (*lysis* and *lavage*) and arthroscopic surgery to treat early and less severe damage to the joint.

* Surgery to repair *cavitational ischemic osteonecrosis* when present.

* Surgery to repair damaged bony joint and meniscal surfaces due to osteoarthritis. This is a wear and tear arthritis. This is done by use of a *Vitallium articular eminence* device. The device has been used over 30 years. There have been multiple long-term studies of its bio-compatibility and efficacy.

* Total jaw joint implants are needed to restore extensively damaged joint surfaces. These devices are a *Vitallium ramus* and *acrylic condylar head functioning* against a Vitallium articular eminence device. This system has been in use for 30 years.

Books

TMJ: Its Many Faces, also explains why the patient may need to consult with other health care professionals such as a neurologist, chiropractor, physical therapist, massotherapist (medical massage therapist), an oral surgeon, and ENT doctor, or psychologist. Dr. Shankland's description of disorders that mimic TMJ emphasizes the importance of obtaining an accurate diagnosis from a knowledgeable and experienced practitioner. Chapter 9, "The Concept of Pain," presents an in-depth discussion of emotional elements of chronic pain and helps remove the stigma of getting the psychological care that is often so necessary in restoring a chronic pain sufferer to health.

Face The Pain

Dr. shankland wrote theis book as a follow-up to *TMJ: Its Many Faces*. Even with the outstanding reception the first book received, he felt more information needed to be written for the general public. Billions of dollars are spent each year for healthcare, much for the diagnosis of the cause of pain.

Pain sufferers will do and pay anything for some hope of relief. Unfortunately, insurance companies don't share such enthusiasm for pain relief, and it's going to get worst, at least in the United States. Because most doctors both don't understand, nor pursue, the numerous causes of pain, the medical profession won't demand reasonable payment from insurance companies for adequate pain treatment. It's funny how doctors and insurance executives alike change their attitudes when a loved one is in pain!

The Dental Restorative Diet

The Dental Restorative Diet

In this section we will explore a diet to restore, rebuild and educate not only the dentally challenged, but prople recovering from all degenerative disease as well as principles that need to be understood by all to ensure a healthy vital functioning of the human vehicle. The first section contains principles on how to eat, understanding the importance of proteins, the proper time to consume foods, stress factors of foods, and how to go about creating a diet to support health rather than detract from it. Contrary to popular belief our body's do not work like a garbage disposal, nor do we have a set of teeth in our stomachs. Knowing this and some of the rules of eating, according to our body's physiology not manufacturing conglomerates and clever and entising advertising we can make smart choices when it comes to consuming foods. Most of the recipes are based on creating food for someone that cannot chew very well, but can be utilized by anyone interested in improving their health and well being as principles of attaining and maintaining great health are explained.

Protein Foods

Algae–spirulina, blue green algae, chlorella

Animal products– conch, eggs, fish, fowl, shrimp, dairy products; cottage cheese, cultured cheese, kefir, feta cheese from goat or sheep milk, kefir, milk, ricotta, sour cream, yogurt

Barley grass

Beans–sprouted and cooked under a boil. When beans are boiled their protein nature is destroyed and they become a carbohydrate food.

Beet leaves

Dairy Products (not including butter as it is a fat)

Gelatin

Miso - a fermented paste made from the breakdown od soybeans, other beans and sometimes some grains

Nuts–almonds, cashews, pine nuts, walnuts, pecans

Nut butters–peanut butter, tahini (sesame butter)

Nut milks–almond, cashew soaked and blended

Raw red potatoes

Rice Protein powder - the separated protein part of rice made into a powder

Seaweed–agar, arame, dulse, hijike, kelp, nori, wakame. Nori (or laver) is the highest in protein

Seeds–sunflower, pumpkin, squash, flax, chia, radish

Soy proteins–tofu, miso, tempeh
Sprouts–alfalfa, mung, sunflower, pumpkin, radish, flax.-excellent sources of assimilable proteins, and are one of the highest energy foods known.
Tempeh- a cultured protein made from soybeans acted on by a culture similiar to what creates cheese
Tofu- the protein part of the soymilk separated from the fiber and coagulated into a block form
Wheat Grass
Wheatmeat (*seitan*) is made from the glutinous portion of wheat, which is a protein. The bran, germ and starch is washed away, leaving the gluey mass, which is chewy and used to imitate many meats.
Whey- the watery portion of milk after the separation of from the curds
Wild rice (a seed, not a grain) like beans, the protein remains if it is sprouted and or cooked below a boil.
Young green **coconut milk**.

Protein Guidelines

1) These foods are best eaten for breakfast and lunch **without the addition of any starch foods**. If proteins are eaten with carbohydrates (breads, crackers, pasta, rice, etc or with fruit, **digestion is severely compromised**. **Proteins are digested in an acid medium**, where the digestive system sends out gastric juices with a pH of 3, to be able to break down the complex molecules of a protein. Where **carbohydrates are digested in a more alkaline medium**.

When proteins and carbohydrates are eaten together, the body opts to digest the carbohydrate, to ensure the basic survival needs of the body by supplying immediate energy, at the expense of giving the body raw and vital components to create new cells and to repair old cells. Then to make matters worse, the protein food that isn't digested goes into the system and **rots and putrefies**. It is undigested and deposits in the colon, where it becomes the "spare tire" that is so commonly seen in people. **Undigested proteins clog the lymphatic system** of the body setting the stage for disease. All of this contributes to high cholesterol, allergies, high blood pressure, foul breath, teeth with cavities, and a host of degenerative diseases. Since proteins and carbohydrate foods do not mix, **neither one is digested** well.
Day after day, year after year of eating poorly combined meals takes its toll on our health and a myriad of symptoms develop. The human body

cannot efficiently digest both types of food groups together, especially when the live component is left out the veggies! Poorly digested and malabsorbed refined sugar laden food is what accounts for the massive degeneration and premature aging taking place so rampantly in the diets of our western cultures. Therefore, if 18% or less of a protein meal is carbohydrate, the body recognizes that it needs to supply an acid medium and can function properly to digest the protein.

2) Eat protein with both cooked and **raw vegetables**. The raw vegetables will help to digest the protein and the lightly- cooked vegetables supply the inner cell (*chromatin*) factors, rich in RNA and DNA, which are the vital factors of body revitalization. Lightly means lightly, not overcooked. Quick steaming, gentle stir frying, briefly sautéing, break down the indigestible cellulose covering that surrounds the cell nucleus in the vegetables, thus the body can absorb the vegetables DNA/RNA material

3) It is important to eat 6 out of 7 days per week this way. On the 7th day, rest from eating protein foods. It is important to give the body a rest from all protein one day per week. You can have a traditional breakfast of cereal, toast, bagel, oatmeal or pancakes, fruit, fruit juice or better yet , fresh vegetable juice.

4) If you don't eat protein for breakfast, don't eat it for lunch either. If you consume a carbohydrate breakfast then a protein lunch, you will alter your pH balance in such a way that will make you feel tired and lethargic after the protein meal and throughout the afternoon. This creates cravings for sugar and refined carbohydrate foods as well as stimulants like coffee, soda and other caffeine containing items, and does not contribute toward building strong structural proteins.

5) Proteins build tissues, which are the matrix of the body. Teeth, bones, muscle, blood, organs, skin, etc are all made up of proteins. By having 4-5 sources of proteins in the meal, the body has a wide range of available parts to build and repair itself, as well as providing strength and stamina. It is optimal to have 0-1 cooked protein and 3 -5 raw proteins.

6) Have a large amount of RAW vegetables with the meal. Since protein is a heavy food it needs enough enzymes from raw foods to be fully digested.

7) Proteins and essential oils are a great pair. When we eat protein foods with healthy oils (known as *essential fatty acids* or *E.F.A.'s*) we get double the benefit of both.

a) We need to avoid the harmful sources of fats and oils from animal food, lard, margarine and all *hydrogenated* and *partially hydrogenated* oils.

b) These can be replaced with healthy oils such as: cold pressed flax, pumpkin, sunflower, borage, wheat germ, oat germ, rice germ, hemp, black current, and evening primrose oils. The group of essential healthy oils are important in forming the cell's membrane or the "house" that each cell lives in, if you will.

The proper building blocks in the cell will keep out the *extra cellular elements*, as the proper building materials keep our houses free from rain leaking in from the roof or wind blowing in the windows excessively, or lack of insulation letting it get too hot or too cold. The E.F.A.'s also allow optimum functioning of the heart by supplying it with components to let it beat efficiently every second, every minute and every year, year after year without any vacations or breaks, hopefully.

They also help keep the circulatory system running smoothly, where the arteries aren't subject to plaque and clogging from over-consumption of saturated and hydrogenated fats. The E.F.A.'s are also important for the endocrine glands, as they regulate proper hormone function; to the eyes, by supplying the specific fatty acid chains that the eye uses to see; to the sex organs through maintaining a healthy prostate and its functioning in a man and proper ovarian-uterine and breast functioning in a female.This is a sample of what the E.F.A.'s do in the body.

8) Eat protein meals for breakfast and perhaps lunch and carbohydrate based foods for lunch or dinner. Lunch is a pivotal meal, and can be protein if you're increasing your protein pool or rebuilding your body. Lunch can be a carbohydrate meal also if you are maintaining your weight or need simple meals to digest if the digestion is weak or challenged.
9) Digestion is a tremendous process requiring 80% of our energy to break down a meal. So it makes sense to let this process be as efficient as possible. Also it would make more sense to give the body the vital com

ponents that supply it with nutrition, while not creating additional work to wear it out prematurely, i.e. aging.

10) When proteins are eaten for breakfast, they have all day to be digested and absorbed, so that late in the afternoon when most people need a "pick-me-up," you don't, because the proteins eaten for breakfast are entering the blood stream, giving you fuel and energy.

11) Sometimes the body's digestion is weak and would benefit from "digestive enzymes" to help the stomach create the correct medium for digestion and also trigger the pancreas to produce its enzymes as the partially digested food is readied for the next phase of digestion.

Good digestive enzymes include betaine HCl, *bromelain*, a protein digestive enzyme extracted from pineapple, *pancreatin*, *ox bile*, *protease*, which continue protein digestion and includes *trypsin* and *chymotrypsin* which actually break bonds between specific amino acids, *papain*, from papaya and may also include *amylase*, an enzyme continuing starch digestion and *lipase*, an enzyme that breaks fat molecules into smaller components, and *cellulase* which breaks down plant fibers.
The best available form of digestive enzymes will improve function of:

(1) The stomach, by providing the optimum digestive medium.
(2) The pancreas, to supply more enzymes of digestion.
(3) The small intestines ability to absorb.
(4) The gall bladder to concentrate bile for fat emulsification.
(5) The colon, to eliminate waste and toxicity.

Recommended to be taken with all meals until digestion is much improved. Available at health food stores.

More On Proteins

There are three types of proteins; high stress, medium stress, and low stress proteins. The high stress types are very hard on the digestive system thus requiring more energy to break down and be processed through the system than the medium and low stress types, which give energy to the system because of their ease in digestibility.
Plant proteins are almost all of the low stress type, where animal foods are mostly high stress and some medium stress. The flesh of the animal is higher stress than products made from milk, ie yogurt and cheeses.

These are also cultured/ fermented, which aid in their digestibility. In the following lists of stresses, they are listed from the highest stress to the lowest, or from the hardest to digest, in each group, to the easiest.

High Stress Proteins

These are the hardest to digest, takes more energy from the body, than it gives and is basically an inefficient form of protein.

Pork
Beef, Veal
Lobster
Crab
Lamb
Venison
Isolated soy protein and non-fermented soy products including: soy flour, soy protein powders
Peanuts, dry roasted
Raw nuts if eaten in large quantities

Medium Stress Proteins

These are proteins that are somewhat more digestible, especially to people with a strong digestion and are borderline in energy that they give to the body. The vegetarian nut and nut butters are more digestible especially if soaked, or sprouted first and combined well.

Poultry: turkey and chicken

Game birds like Cornish hen, pheasant, quail, dove. (If the animal is *organically raised* and not mass-produced it is a lower, medium stress protein). Hard cheeses: Asiago, Parmesan, Romano are lower, medium stress than: cheddar, Swiss, jack, munster and others like these. The former are often made with sheep or goat milk and cultured better and aged longer where the latter are made with hormone-laden, toxin-rich commercial cow's milk. Nuts and nut butters: peanut, cashew, and almond. These are much more digestible if they are soaked in water first then blended into butters.

Low Stress Proteins

These are the best sources of protein to humans.

Beans, sprouted, cooked without boiling -boiled beans are a carbohydrate
Beet Leaf
Chicken, organically grown (low to medium stress)
Chlorella & other algaes if mercury free
Ocean fish; Steinberg's (1990) list of 'green light' seafood includes; Cod from Denmark, Canada, Iceland, New Zealand; Dover Sole from California, Washington, France; English Sole; Flounder (not from Boston Harbor!); Grouper; Haddock; Halibut from Alaska or Iceland; Mahi Mahi; Marlin; Orange Roughie; Red Snapper; Pacific Salmon
Octopus and Squid
Conch, mussels
Scallops
Shrimp, cooked in garlic, ginger or beer to remove puricines
Yard, or free range eggs where the yolk is intact; soft boiled, poached, sunny side up, or over easy
Quality Dairy (preferably raw) cultured dairy including: yogurt, kefir, cottage, ricotta, feta...
Fermented Soy products: tofu, miso, tempeh (best for Type A blood)
Sesame tahini
Soaked nuts
Nutritional Yeast
Wild rice (cooked under a boil)
Soaked peas and beans cooked under 200° F.
Raw red potato juice
Seaweeds
Soaked seeds (sunflower and pumpkin are the easiest)
Sprouts (alfalfa, lentils, mung bean, sunflower, broccoli, radish clover)
Spirulina and other blue green algae

Essential Oils

*A good quality oil like flax seed oil or better yet a blend of oils called *Udo's Choice*, by Flora Inc. Box 950 Lynden WA. 98264. This blend contains oils of flax, sunflower, sesame, wheat germ, rice germ, oat germ, lecithin and d-alpha tocopherols. Another excellent oil blend is *Essential Balance* by Arrowhead Mills and it contains; flax, sunflower, pumpkin, sesame, and borage. Arrowhead Mills Inc. Box 2059 Hereford, TX 79045 (806)-749-0730 or The Totao EFA by Health From the Sun, PO Box179 Newport NH 03773 www.healthfromthesun.com 800-447-2249

These oil combinations contains the right ratio of omega-3 and omega-6 fatty acids for human beings (3:1 omega 6's to omega 3's), as currently available. They are mechanically pressed under low heat and in the absence of light and oxygen, thus supplying the best form of oil currently available. Flaxseed is high in the omega 3's also peanut and sesame contain some omega 3's; where borage and evening primrose is high in the Gla-rich omega 6's. Also sunflower, safflower, pumpkinseed, soy, grapeseed, and sesame are rich in the omega 6's. Olive oil is high in the omega 9 monounsaturated fatty acids.

The perfect oil for long term use is said to be hempseed oil, as it contains the best balance of 6's to 3's, and is rapidly being market out of Canadian companies and shipped to Health food stores in the U.S. These oils are then packaged in brown glass or inert plastic to further protect them from light, and can be found in the refrigerated section at most health food stores. It is best to **minimize cooking of oils** for whenever heat is applies to oils they start to degrade.The oils that withstand heat the best are: butter, peanut, sesame, and olive oils as well as refined oils. But refined oils are not the best for health. Most oils that are sold in clear bottles on the shelves of grocery stores are refined. Olive oil is the only oil at present that is not refined and is available for consumer use.

Olive oils come in several grades. Extra Virgin is the first pressing of the olives. Virgin the second and pure, the third. Light olive oil is a joke as it is the lowest grade available. It is best to only buy the extra virgin olive oil

Non-cooking Oils

For salad dressings, mayonnaise or marinades;
Sunflower, Safflower, Walnut, Olive, and all of the delicate oils listed in the essential oil blends; like flax, borage, pumpkin, hemp, pumpkinseed etc Since oils are delicate in nature, it is best to olny cook with butter, olive, sesame and peanut oils. And it is a good idea to add a little liquid to the oils when sauteeing to keep the temperatures down below 212 F, so reduce the destruction of the oils and formation of trans fatty acids, rancid factors and carcinagens. Frying should be very, very minimal and sauteeing as mentioned. Liquids added to oils can be water, wine, vegetables, stock, and rice or other milks.

Cod Liver Oil

This oils is best taken with proteins, in the morning. The emulsified kind is best absorbed and taken cold. They are flavored and quite palatable. They are best taken down-the-hatch followed by a beverage. 1-2 tablespoons daily as a source of Vitamins A and D. These are only found in the animal kingdom. Something important to know is that the body converts beta carotene into vitamin A, but not very well. If the liver is compromised with toxins, heavy metals and other pollutants it is very hard to get enough conversion from beta carotene rich foods, bad news for vegans and vegetarians. The liver itself is dependant on vitamin A for normal function. Vitamin A is only found in animal sources and these people are often very deficient in true vitamin A and D, so necessary for respiratory and epithelial tissues (those lining the entire digestive tract and respiratory tract.) Also the eyes need the retinol provided by real vitamin A. Children and babies cannot convert beta carotene into vitamin A and an adult's ability is compromised with the toxins from amalgam fillings, root canals, cavitations, etc., and other toxins we accumulate from our ever-increasingly toxic environment. So liver flushing is very important to restore this ability to the liver, especially for vegans and vegetarians.

Superfood Drinks

In this section nutritious drinks will be covered to add much nutrition to the diet without having to chew. This is especially important when the molars are missing or compromised, after dental work (drilling, cutting, pulling, suturing of tissue, etc), gum and cavitation surgery, when the teeth are soft, or when more cavities are present, reduce infections or to build up the nutrition, and greatly add vital nutrition to the body.

Vegetable Juices

The live extracted juice from vegetables can be used as a concentrated source of nutrition whenever the body is conpromised in health. By extracting off the juice portion from the pulp, many pounds of vital nutrients can be consumed by the person recovering from dental proceedures (or from other illnesses) Fiber is still consumed with the blended soups and salads, but the volume of food that would have to be consumed to get the vital componants is provided by the use of a juice extractor. The masticating types versus the spinner types are better, but use what is available and cost effective. Also for extra nutritive benefit a juice press can be utilized to squeeze out the remaining juice from the pulp. See the Appendix for equipment and further information.

Carrot Juice Blends

These are usually sweet and very palatable to most people. Use organic carrots or California carrots when possible as they are very sweet and tasty. Organic produce is also 10-15 times more nutritious. Another concideration is when people are full of mercury they usually have candida, which is sometimes aggrivated by sweet things. In this case see the next section on mixed vegetable juices.

Carrot--1 pound of carrots usually produces about 1 8 oz glass of juice
Carrot-Celery-Add several ribs to the lb of carrots 1 to 5 or 6. Celery is high in good or organic sodium, needed by the stomach to make digestive juices and to take to strain off a sluggish liver, by helping the formation of bile
Carrot-Ginger- Add 1 thumbsize of fresh gingeroot to the juice for zest and to increase circulation. Ginger is helpful for combating nausea, and increasing digestion also.
Carrot-Celery-Beet-5-7 carrots, 3-4 ribs celery and 1/2 medium sized beet. The beet is high in iron and will build the blood as well as support the functions of the liver. Beets are also sweet in taste and delicious.
Carrot-Spinach 5-7 carrots and 1/2 lb spinach. Spinach is rich in iron , and like most greens high in magnesium rich chlorophyll.
Carrot with other Greens- Kale, collards, dark green lettuces, parsley, cilantro, turnip greens and beet greens (beet greens are higher in iron that the beet root!) Parsley is rich in Vitamin C, necessary for gum healing. Cilantro helps to move mercury out of the brain, and kale is similiar to spinach. Collards and turnip greens are rich in potassium as well.

Mixed Vegetable Juices

Use **Tomatoes, Cucumbers** and/or **Celery** as a base. Say 1-3 tomatoes or 1-2 cucumbers or 5-8 ribs of celery, and add: **spinach**, **kale**, any other greens (greens are high in calcium for bone formation as well as magnesium or muscle and soft tissue repair), also **sprouts** (rich in protein and enzymes) like mung (the ones in Chinese food), alfalfa or any of the kinds available, by the handfuls (1 or 2), also add **radishes-**3 or 4 or a big piece of daikon radish 2-6 inches (good for all mucus membranes and the respiratory tract), 1-2 **sweet red pepper or green peppers** (high in silica-for the skin, hair, nails and and bones). Also put in 1-3 cloves of **garlic** for infections, vitamin C and the sulfur compounds to chelate out heavy metals and for homocysteine metabolism. Use leaf lettuces, parsnips for kidney support.

Grass Juices- Wheat grass or other grass juices (barley, rye, kamut)are highly beneficial and if you have a juicer that will juice grasses please include these as they are so nutritionally dense that they can stand alone. They are an abundant source of alkaline minerals (calcium, magnesium, potassium and the trace minerals as well. They are excellent sources of protein, B vitamins and vitamin C. They are worth the effort and investment in a juicer that can juice grasses as well as vegetables. (the Sampson or Green life or a stand alone wheat grass jyuicer either electric or manual)

Superfood Morning Drink

6-8+ oz fresh juice
2-4 oz rice or almond , goat or regular milk
2 T Essential Oil (the Total EFA or others)
1 raw free-range Egg -optional or 2 T soaked seeds
optional-1/2 oz Colloidal Silver or germanium extract to counter any salmonilla the egg may have
1 T+ Spirulina powder
1 T+ Green Phyto Power (see appendix companies) or Green Magma or Barley Green or Powdered Wheat grass (Sweet Wheat), etc...
1 T Intestimax (an l-glutamine powder to support the intestinal lining 5,000mg see appendix for more information)
1 T+ ground Flax meal (lignans, soluble fiber, proteins and omega 3"s)
Optional-1-3 tsp kelp and/or dulse powders (I find these more palatable in foods than this drink)

Blend well and enjoy! It is nutrition dense, tasty and alive! This concoction can be consumed more than once per day. It is so rich in vital nutrition that once you begin to drink these superfoof drinks, you will rapidly build up your nutritional bank account and become way ahead of the factors responsible for degenerating health!

Seeds and Nuts

These usually include hulled (without the shell) sunflower and pumpkin seeds. Some other seeds can be used such as flax, sesame and chia, but the first two are consistently better, and easier to find. Also almonds benefit greatly from soaking. These are quality proteins and since their are enzymes inhibiting the seed, the human digestive tract cannot get the nutrition from nuts and seeds without them being first soaked and germinated. Seeds will germinate and most nuts will not, but they will become much more digestable when soaked.

This is why most people do not digest them very well. They are like miniture coconuts, with the hard hull still on! They go through the digestive tract and wreak alot of havok, unless soaked first. They become more crunchy and enjoyable. Nuts can be soaked for a few hours and seeds can be soaked from 4-8 hours. It is best to use sunflower and pumpkin seeds with almonds. Soak about 1/2 to 1 cup of seeds in water in a bowl overnight or at least 6 hours. Then they are rinsed of the carbonic acids given off during the soak. For the dental patient blending them into the salad dressings or into the blended salads is the best way to use them.

The desired amount (1-4 T per meal) is eaten and the remaining are covered with fresh water and placed in the refrigerator until the next day. Repeat when low. They will last about a week this way and will only continue to sprout ever so slowly, which increases its available food energy, so the longer they sprout the better! They are rich in available proteins (amino acids), and vitamins E and F, as well as certain minerals. Pumpkin seeds are high in Zinc, so necessary for healing, especially the tissues of the mouth. Walnuts are high in manganese, especially black walnuts and those that come from Missouri. Manganese is needed for energy production of the body and to support healthy joints.

Seed Salsa

1/2 C soaked seeds
1-2 cloves Garlic (good for healing and infections)
4 chopped mushrooms or 1 plum tomato or 1/2 Zucchini or combo all
2 T Onion
2 T Essential Oil
2 T Olive Oil
2-3 T Vinegar, lemon or lime juice-depending on you liking for sour
Seasalt- pinches to season

Place all in blender and puree/ blend. Serve as a main dish or with soup.

Pumpkin Seed Pate'

1/2 -3/4 C soaked Pumpkin seeds
1 plum tomato
1/2 tsp+ seasalt
1-2 T essential oil
1 tsp Honey or 1 date
Black pepper to tasts
2-3 T Mayonnaise

Blend all until smooth. Will keep several days in refrigerator.

Sprouted Almond Hummas

1 C soaked Almonds
2-3 T Essential Oil
1-3 T Olive Oil
1/4 C fresh Lemon juice
1/4-1/2 C Water
1/2-1 tsp Seasalt
1-3 cloves Garlic
Optional- 1 T Tahini (sesame butter), and cayenne powder/or hot pepper

Place all ingredients in a blender, using the lesser amount of water and adding more if necessary, or put through a homogenizing juicer like a Champion, Sampson or Greenlife with the blank in place. Process or blend until smooth

Lively Sunflower Seed Pate

1 C soaked sunflower seeds (or pumpkin or almond or a mix)
1/2 C Olive and Essential Oils
1/2 + tsp Celtic Seasalt or 1 T Tamari Soysauce
1 tsp Dulse Flahes (a seaweed rich in minerals)
2-3 T Lemon or lime juice or 1 T Balsamic Vinegar
1/2 C fresh Parsley or Cilantro or a bit of both
2-4 T or more of Water or stock
Optional- 1/2 tsp curry powder or cumin or chili powder: pinch of cayenne pepper or a clove of garlic, a piece of onion or garlic powder.

Place all in blender and pulse blend, stopping to stir down and adding a bit more water if necessary.

Seed Dip

1/2-3/4 C Sunflower or pumpkin seeds or almonds or combination
1 T Tamari Soysauce
2-4 T Mayonnaise
1 egg yolk
1-2 T Nutritional Yeast
1 T Lemon Juice

Blend all until smooth.

Seaweeds

There are several kinds that are very good, with little to no taste, that are a gold mine of mineral rich nutrition. Seaweeds are high in potassium, iron, iodine, calcium, magnesium, as well as the trace minerals: manganese, chromium, copper and zinc. They also contain vitamins B1 (thiamine) B_2 (riboflavin), B3 (Niacin), B_6 (Pyroxidine) and B_{12} (cyanocobalamin), and contain vitamins C and E and protein. *Arame* and *hijiki* can be soaked in room temperature water for about 10 minutes or until soft. Save the water for broth, soup stock or miso soup.Then blend into soups, salads, and seed pate's. *Kombu*, a type of kelp, need to be softened longer or warmed first. Wakame and Dulse can be softened in water then blended into soups and dressings and pates. *Nori*, comes in sheets and is usually toasted. This is the type used to make *sushi*, because it is rolled up with different foods inside. It is also eaten as a snack in the toasted sheet form. *Dulse* and *kelp* can also be bought in flakes, granules and powder and sprinkled onto foods. There are many of these on the market at health food stores in shakers, usually combined with ginger, garlic and salt. Thesecan be used in dressings, sprinkled over foods, mixed ½ and ½ with seasalt in a shaker or put in soups or other prepared foods.

Healing Broths

Potassium-Stock Broth
8 C WATER
7-8 POTATOES use peeling only
1-2 cut BEETS
5-8 CARROTS
3 handfuls GREENS (collards, kale, chard, parsley...)
2-4 cut ONIONS
1- 2 blended bulbs GARLIC

This recipe is a potent mineral rich broth that people consume when they are "sick", or rather cleansing. During times of illness or imbalance the body benefits from vitamin and mineral rich foods.

Smack bulbs of garlic to break apart. Disguard the hard part and place all cloves in a blender with papers still on. Pour 2 cups water in and whiz. Pour remaining water in a large stockpot with all veggies, and garlic water. Simmer about 1 hour. Strain, squeeze and use stock for soup, or a healing drink.

Healing Onion Soup

8 C POTASSIUM STOCK
6-8 T TAMARI
3-4 medium ONIONS
1 tsp SEASALT
3-5 cloves GARLIC sliced
Combine all, cutting onions into rounds. Simmer 10-15 minutes. Serve with croutons or toast on top! *For added nutrition reduce tamari by ½ and add 1-2 T miso before serving or spoon directly into bowls of soup at the table according to personal taste.

Soups

The ability to carry nourishing healing broths when appetite is poor and you want to give a nutritive rich source of food. Potassium broth is also a basic stock that is highly nutritious also vegetable stock or miso mixed in water is used as a carrier and to this, a number of powdered superfoods can be added. The following are a partial list of these foods: Nutritional yeast, celtic seasalt, goat whey, garlic, onions, cayenne, essential oils, seaweeds, an array of vegetables, legumes and grains, blended nuts/seeds, tomatoes, chlorophyll, sardines, coddled egg etc...

Better Broth

This is basically your own homemade stock, the essence and source of an abundance of nutrition for your food. 2 methods are given.

*Never ending toss-in-bag Method—In this method you save all edible skins, peels, tops, bottoms, etc of veggies, toss into a ziplock bag and accumulate in the freezer and eventually cook in water ½-1+ hours to extract the nutrition & flavor.

**Potassium Broth Method- This method is specific and concentrates nutrition. Use a large stock pot and fill with ¼ potato peelings, ¼ chopped carrots and beets, ¼ onions and garlic, and ¼ Greens like celery, kale, turnip or collards (no spinach as the cooking creates oxalic acid) Simmer 1-2 hours and strain.

Stone-Soup

This soup is like that old children's book "Stone Soup" where a one poor village member adds a large stone is added to a pot of water, and other village members add whatever they can to make a pot of soup so all can share. This soup starts with one can of soup and other ingredients are added to it to enhance in into a stew, a one-dish casserole or a thick soup to pour over steamed broccoli, a baked potato or a tortilla-style roll up.

Try *lentil or split pea over a baked potato served w/ a greens salad or **non-dairy cream of mushroom over steamed broccoli on top of a piece of sprouted grain bread or toast w/ a greens salad or coleslaw, or ***quick steamed or sautéed veggies and raw grated veggies (onion, zucchini, carrot, mushroom…), a can of chili or refried beans or bean dip or mashed potato, mashed yam or avocado w/ lemon, or leftover or fresh rice or quinoa, rolled into a burrito-style wrap. Serve w/ salsa or a variety of dressings. This 1-can idea is the stone to base the meal around!

Puree of Fresh and Steamed Bisque

Previously baked veggies like potatoes, onions, garlic, carrots, parsnips, beets can be used as the base for blending in some liquid. Liquids can range: water, broth, almond or rice milk. Add fresh vegetables for enzymes, water-soluble vitamins and life quality: carrot, zucchini, mushrooms, red sweet pepper, and celery… Next, season with sea salt, tamari soy sauce, miso, fresh or dried herbs and spices: basil, garlic, gingerroot, chili, curry, garlic, or onion powder, leftover rice, noodles…

Miso

Miso, is a tasty, full flavored, fermented paste of broken down soybeans, barley or rice, seasalt and the enzyme culture that breaks down, chemically, these nutritious foods. It tastes of a very strong bouillon and is used to flavor foods and enrich them with usable amino acids (broken down proteins), minerals, trace minerals, vitamins, and enzymes! Quality miso should be made with seasalt only. Many of the commercial types are made from inferior salt. This kind of salt is mined from the Earth and super heated to dry it. It is not the same as seasalt, for it is a cooked substance without the completeness of natural occurring seasalt. Miso has a range of flavors and colors, from deep chocolate brown, reddish browns, amber, cinnamon red, creamy beige, and light yellow. The darker types have heartier, saltier, almost meaty flavors and the lighter kinds are sweeter, more delicate tasting.

Miso is one of East Asia's most important soy foods. In Japan alone over 70% of the population start each day with this wonderful healthy, nutritious and warming food as a beverage. The quality protein that miso contains combines with essential oils, vegetables, some sea vegetables and tofu chunks making this the cereal of the future! It supplies a steady high-quality source of energy. Miso also contains the much sought after vitamin B_{12}, lactic acid-forming bacteria, that is much like yogurt, and other microorganisms, and digestive enzymes

It is a live culture and needs to be refrigerated. Miso is valued by cooks for its unlimited versatility. It can be used as a bouillon or a rich meat-like stock in soups, gravies and stews. It can be an essential ingredient in sauces and used to thicken. It can be used as a cheese substitute in casseroles, and spreads. It is spread on bread, made into chutneys and relishes for veggies, toppings for grains and even used for pickling.

A Cup Of Miso Soup

The basic miso soup is simply miso, stirred into hot water. From this broth, you can add many other foods. Makes 1 serving.

8-10 oz WATER, POTASSIUM BROTH or SOUP STOCK
2-3 tsp MISO

Heat water or stock. Add miso and stir well. Drink as a beverage, stirring the bottom because the miso settles. Or make into one of an infinite variety of soups.

Optionals

1 oz TOFU diced
sprinkles of dulse or kelp flakes or a small handful of arame
1T ESSENTIAL OIL (Flax w/ Borage, Hempseed, etc)
GREEN ONIONS sliced into little pieces
1-2 T NUTRITIONAL YEAST
1-2 Shiitake or other MUSHROOMS
Sauteed onions, celery, carrot...

Brothy Miso Soup

In the traditional Japanese method of miso soup making, the liquid portion would be a combination of a seaweed like kombu or wakame, simmered in water with the addition of dashi flakes: tiny fish, dried and shaved.
Sometimes shiitake mushrooms were added to the simmering broth. This ancient way of eating follows the principles of eating low stress proteins with vegetables early in the day!

16 oz WATER *2 servings*
1 large piece of KOMBU seaweed, cut into pieces
2 sliced SHIITAKE MUSHROOMS or other mushrooms
1 -2 tsp dried BONITO or DASHI flakes, or a small sardine or 2 tsp TAMARI Soysauce, or a pinch of Celtic Seasalt
1 T MISO

Add all except miso, to a 1-2 qt. saucepan and gently simmer 15-20 minutes. Cool slightly, add miso and drink. From this basic traditional broth add other vegetables and health giving components. Serves 2.

Essential Oils And Miso Soup

16 oz WATER or BROTH
1 sliced or grated MUSHROOM and/or 1 clove GARLIC
2-4 tsp MISO
1-3 tsp ESSENTIAL OIL BLEND
½ to 1tsp DULSE flakes or a handful of dulse seaweed (whole form)

Heat water to hot but not boiling, remove from heat. Add the clove of garlic, mushroom, dulse, miso and stir well, then add the oil, stir and serve. Shiitake mushrooms are good in this soup.

***Shiitake mushrooms** are available fresh and dried and are a rich source of immune enhancing componants.

***Garlic**-Rich in sulfur compounds to create a condition hostile to unwanted forms of bacteria. Garlic is anti-bacterial, anti-fungal, anti-viral and anti-cancer. It also speeds up healing time by enhancing immune function.

Ginger Miso Soup

Add 1 tsp grated GINGER to the previous soup. Grate ginger and squeeze in juice.

***Ginger** is good to help quell nausea, it also supports the heart warms the body.

Chicken, Fish or Tofu Miso Soup

16 oz. WATER
2 tsp TAMARI
1 T ESSENTIAL OIL
1 small piece of WAKAME or DULSE
1-2 oz piece of cooked chicken, or raw fish as fish cooks very fast, or a slice of TOFU
1-2 sliced white MUSHROOMS
several slices off the end of a bunch of GREEN ONIONS
1-2 tsp MISO

In a bowl, add tamari to tofu chunks or meat to marinate and to coat. Bring water to boil. Add fish if using and cook through; or add meat or remove from heat, and add tofu. Then add the green onions, wakame or dulse, mushroom, miso and oil. Serve. (Add 1 to 4 tsp nutritional yeast for a more savory taste, also 1-3 teaspoons of butter or ghee)

Creamy Vegetable Soup

3 T BUTTER, GHEE or OLIVE OIL
1 ONION diced
3 cloves GARLIC chopped
1-2 C chopped VEGGIES: Any variety: celery, carrots, zucchini, or yellow squash, mushrooms, tomato, broccoli, cauliflower, red pepper...
about 4 C WATER, POTASSIUM BROTH or STOCK

Sauté onion and garlic in oil, add vegetables and cook about 5 minutes covered. Cook enough to warm but not cook excessively. Blend vegetables, salt or tamari with 2 cups of water or stock in blender until smooth; add remaining water or stock to blended soup, season to taste. Serve.

Sprouted Lentil Soup

When a bean or legume is soaked in water and allowed to sprout, then cooked under a boil, it retains its protein qualities. When the bean is heated and boiled all, of the protein qualities are destroyed and the bean now is a carbohydrate. Sprout lentils by soaking them in water overnight. Then rinse well. This usually will start the lentil sprouting. It may need to sit for 6-8 additional hours in the jar to sprout if the water or air temperature is cold. Use about 2 Cups of sprouted lentils or beans. If you use other beans, they will require 2-3 days to sprout, usually, and the taste is very beany!

2 C SPROUTED LENTILS
6 to 8 C WATER
3-4 T TAMARI
½ to 1 tsp Celtic SEASALT
½ to 1 tsp OREGANO
sprinkles of SAGE, BASIL or THYME
4 cloves crushed GARLIC
1 diced ONION
2-3 ribs chopped CELERY
½ chopped CARROT
MISO at end to further flavor if necessary

Combine all in a large soup pot and cook over medium heat about 1 hour. It is important to not let this boil. If soup begins to boil, remove from heat and turn down. Also everything except the lentils can be cooked first. Then add the lentils and turn off. Just let them warm through without excess cooking. Note-- The onion, celery, garlic, salt and spices can be sauteed first for a few minutes to create a different more savory taste before the other vegetables, lentils and stock are added. This can then be blended for easier assimilation.

Note-- If you want a harty, carbohydrate, traditional lentil soup, continue to cook the lentils until they are tender and fall apart, anywhere from 45 minutes to 2 hours depending on cooking temperature.

Non-dairy Cream Of Broccoli Soup

Sauté 1 ONION in 2 T BUTTER, GHEE or OLIVE OIL
Then blend the following in a blender and add to onion:
2 C BROCCOLI (use cut stems and flowerettes)
2 C WATER
6 oz. soft or silken TOFU or 1 C cooked RICE or MILLET
1 tsp SEASALT or a little more to taste
1 tsp. DULSE Seaweed or flakes (optional)
5-8 MUSHROOMS or 1/2 C ZUCCHINI blend before serving
1-2 T NUTRITIONAL YEAST (optional)
2 T OLIVE OIL or ESSENTIAL OIL

Add the blended mixture to the onion. Cook 5 minutes, then add the sliced mushrooms or zucchini, tofu or rice, seasalt, dulse, and nutritional yeast. Warm through without "cooking" too long as to preserve the live enzyme quality of the vegetables, a few minutes and serve. Add 2 T olive oil or essential balance oil just before serving for added richness. Note-- the dulse is a tasty seaweed rich in protein, trace minerals, especially potassium, chromoium, iron, manganese, zinc and vitamins B 6 and 12.

Sea Vegetable Soup

4 C WATER
4-6 T MISO at end of cooking
Several large pieces of KOMBU
handful dry or soaked ARAME or HIJIKI
1 large piece of WAKAME or DULSE or both
2-6 T OLIVE OIL
3-4 cloves GARLIC, 1 ONION, 1 piece CELERY 1 CARROT, SHIITAKE or other MUSHROOMS
1-4 T ESSENTIAL BALANCE Essential Oil (Arrowhead Mills)
1/-1 tsp CELTIC SEASALT
optional-1 to 2 T NUTRITIONAL YEAST per cup

Saute onions and garlic in olive oil until transparent. Next add celery, carrots, saute a minute or two and add the salt, kombu and water. Simmer 12-15 minutes. Add the arame, hijiki, wakame or dulse and let absorb a few minutes then serve. If you add the seaweeds dry, they will take a few minutes to hydrate and absorb the broth. Then blend the soup and serve. Blending can help when the digestion is weak.

Optional- ingredients can be added such as: noodles, cooked rice or millet, a piece of garlic toast or crackers, as they will absorb the broth and give a soft item to "chew" on!s

Warm Gazpacho Soup

This soup contains the fresh taste of tomatoes, sweet peppers, onions & carrots into a raw but warm soup. It is very nutritious as it is raw , live vital and full of enzymes so necessary for healing and recovering form trauma.

Sauté the following briefly to extract and concentrate the flavors:
1 ONION
4 cloves GARLIC
2 T OLIVE OIL or GHEE
1 tsp SEASALT

Blend:
2 1/2 C WATER
1-3 tsp DULSE flakes or kelp or whole dulse
1 sweet RED PEPPER (green peppers are unripe red peppers)
1 small CARROT
1 large TOMATO or 1 med-sized ZUCCHINI or 1 C CAULIFLOWER
1-3 tsp TAMARI SOYSAUCE or more seasalt
1-2 T OLIVE OIL or ESSENTIAL OILS
Optional–1/2 to 1 C SOAKED SEEDS or ALMONDS or cooked rice or millet

While the onions and garlic are briefly sautéing (about 5 minutes) cut the vegetables into chunks, and put in blender with water, additional seasonings and blend (also add the seeds or almonds or grain if desired.) Add to onions and garlic. Then just warm through. Do not heat excessively, for this will destroy the live enzyme quality.

Optional–Add 1 large handful of arame and hijiki to the soup and turn off. Allow this to absorb the soup and soften before serving. Or presoak in water and blend with the rest of the vegetables.

Breakfast Foods

Understanding Proteins Recap

Breakfast is the best time of the day to consume your proteins and oils. Contrary to the breakfast scene so popular in creating degenerative disease, the real old fashioned meals of proteins without starches are the best to support good health. There are several reasons for this.

#1. Eating fruit or carbohydrates (croissants, bagels, cereal, pancakes, potatoes, grits...) for breakfast disrupts the bod's natural pH cycles and interferes with its proper use of proteins.Building strong cellular proteins is a function of the pH cycle of the body. The body is naturally more acid in the early part of the day and then swings more alkaline as the day goes on. This means that since the body is naturally more acidic early, it can better digest acid and heavier foods-namely proteins! In the course of 24 hours, three 8-hour cycles ensue: they are:

7 a.m.-3 p.m. Process nutrients (eat and digest)
3 p.m.-11p.m. Use nutrients (build and exercise)
11 p.m.-7 a.m. cleanse cellular waste (rest)

#2 The body digests and processes proteins best from 7am to 2 pm, with proteins eaten the earlier the better. Breakfast at 7-9 am is better than eaten at 11-1pm.

#3. The largest protein meal should be eaten earliest, followed by a small er protein meal for lunch if desired.

#4. Enzymes which digest food can only function within a certain range. Example being pepsin in our stomach is not active in an environment higher than a pH of 5. This means that to digest meat or other proteins, if milk (pH of 7.2) is taken along or a piece of bread (pH 7.5) or other carbohydrates, the pH raises, pepsin will not work and the food leaves the stomach undigested only to putrify and toxify the body, setting the stage for degenerative disease, bad teeth, gums, bones, and other body tissues.

Rules of Eating

1) Eat all proteins early in the day, between 7 am and 2 pm. The earlier the better.

2) Eat several proteins together for complete protein combinations (maximizing all daily requirements for the needed amino acids) Not all proteins are created equal. Example: most vegetarian sources of protein are

very low in methionine and lysine, with the former so necessary in liver detoxification, especialy ridding heavy metals.
3) Eat protein away from carbohydrates.
4) Have non-starchy vegetables with proteins.
5) Consume high-quality oils with proteins.
6) Avoid proteins as snacks. Eat then as meals.
7) Avoid excess liquids with protein meals.
8) Eat more low and medium stress proteins than high-stress proteins.

The more these rules are observed, the more the digestive powers will build as well as tissue integrity, health and vitality. This is the premise of the meals in this section.

Non-Starchy Vegetables

Bok choy
Cauliflower
Celery
Chinese cabbage
Cucumber
Green beans
Greens: beet and carrot tops, chard, cilantro, collards, dandelion, kale, mustard, parsley, spinach, turnip
Lettuces: arugula, bibb, Boston, butter crunch, cress, endive, escarole, frizzie, radicchio, red and green leaf, romaine
Radishes
Red and green cabbage
Summer squash and zucchini
Sprouts (double as a vegetable and a protein source)
Sweet red pepper
Tomato
Technically anything with a seed is considered a fruit, i.e. tomato, cucumber, pumpkin. Due to the low natural sugar content of these "quasi fruits," they act more as a vegetable.

Medium Starchy Vegetables

Artichoke
Beets
Carrots
Corn
Daikon radish

Egg plant
Jicama
Okra
Parsnips
Squash (large yellow squash, small spaghetti; the larger types become a starchy vegetable; acorn, butternut, Hubbard, spaghetti...)
Turnips
Water chestnuts
Zucchini (large, not the smaller ones)

Egg Meals

*Eggs are a great food full of vital nutrition including protein, lecithin, vitamin A, D, and E. All eggs are not created equal. Commercial eggs are very void of this vital nutrition as the hen is in very bad living conditions. She is placed in a small cage, just slightly larger than her body, for the duration of her life. The cages are stacked one on top of the other and often the beaks are cut as to keep the hens from pecking at each other in these stacked cages. The hens are never allowed to go outside and be a normal chicken. Chickens peck and scratch for bugs and greens. They are then fed an abnormal diet low in the vital greens and nutritive rich sources of foods, so they therefore lay inferior, weak, pale tasteless eggs. Chickens that are free- range or roaming fed an organic diet rich in vital greens and allowed to be outside are quite a different product. Spend the extra time and dollar to find and purchase these type of eggs, as the others simply are not worth the energy spent consuming them.

*Eggs are best is poached, soft-boiled or served over easy, as this preserves the most vital part of the organic egg - the yolk. Less often, they can be served scrambled or made into an omelette.

Raw Egg (or Rice Protein) Shake

4-6 oz. ALMOND MILK
1 EGG (free range/ organically fed) and/or 1-2 T RICE PROTEIN
pinch NUTMEG, CINNAMON, CARDAMOM
OPTIONAL- 1 T ESSENTIAL OIL, 1T FLAX SEED MEAL, 1 T SPIRULINA POWDER, 1 tsp WHEAT GERM, 1 T LECITHIN GRANULES...
Place all in a blender and whizz up.

Poached Eggs

1 SKILLET
1 inch WATER in skillet
desired amount of EGGS

Cook eggs in water slowly, ideally between 170°-200°F, until the white is firm and the yolk is still soft. This way of preparing eggs makes it more alkalizing to the metabolism, whereas fried, scrambled or overheated eggs are acid forming. Poaching and soft boiling is the ideal way to prepare eggs because they are heated gradually and ready to eat when firm. Most of the value is in the yolk, which is rich in minerals, lipids, lecithin, and sulfur proteins.

Soft Boiled Eggs

These eggs are cooked slowly as the water temperature gradually increases. Put eggs into a pot of water and bring up to a boil. When it starts to boil remove from heat and drain. Crack in half and remove egg with a spoon.

Egg white should be cooked firm and yolk soft. You may adjust the cooking time slightly for your own preference of snottiness to the egg.

Eggs Over Easy

Butter, Olive, Peanut, or Sesame Oil
Water
Eggs

Heat pan over medium heat and add oil and a tablespoon or two of water. The water cools the oil and steams the egg. Crack the egg carefully into the pan. Cook about 3 minutes and turn carefully. Turn off or remove from heat and serve.

Egg Delight Omelette

4 Eggs
Butter or Oil
Water
Veggies (onions, mushrooms, peppers, zucchini...)

Saute veggies in the butter or oil a few minutes. Meanwhile whip eggs by hand or in blender. (For fluffy omelette–separate eggs and whip whites until foamy then add back in the yolks). Pour over the vegetablesand cook over medium heat, lifting up so the runny eggs on top can seep underneath the cooked part. Do this until their is little runny part on top. Then flip the whole thing over in one piece or cut in half and flip both halves separately. Or place the whole thing under the broiler and finish the top ths way rather than flipping.

NOTE- Soft Boiled, poached or over easy eggs are best served with a blended salad and only 1/2 to 1 piece or no toast as to not have a bad food combination. Proteins and starch foods are best eaten separately. Some people can digest a small amount of whole grain toast dipped into the egg yolks and taken with digestive enzymes that contain protease (to digest proteins) and amylase (digests starches) and lipase (digests fats).

Blended Salads and other Salads

Basic Blending of a Salad

Put romaine or mixed green lettuces (a big handful) into a blender and add favorite salad dressing or yogurt- about 2 to 3 tablespoons or 1 Tablespoon of Sesame Tahini, 1 teaspoon Honey and 1-2 Tablespoons of Lemon juice along with a little water for blending- about 1/8-1/4 cup, and blend until smooth. Season with sea salt and or pepper if desired. Optional- add other vegetables that you may enjoy and that are in season, like: spinach, other lettuces, tomato, cucumber, red pepper, carrot and celery.

Avocado Cream

1/2 Avocado
1-2 T healthy Mayonnaise
1 T Lemon Juice
Pinches of Seasalt to taste
Optional-1 clove crushed Garlic

Mash ripe Avocado with the salt, lemon juice and mayonnaise. If adding the garlic use a garlic press or smash up and add to avocado. The small ugly fleshed and other small ones are usually from California and are an oilier kind.The large ones are usually from Florida and are less oily, both are delicious. Adjust the lemon juice and mayonnaise for the size of the avocado and your personal tastes. It should be delicious and not to tart or salty. It also does not even need the mayo! This makes it more of a cream than a guacamole
Optional- add chopped tomato or diced onion

Yummy Salad Dressing

¼ C Olive Oil and ¼ C Essential Oil
¼ C soaked Almonds (or sunflower or pumpkin seeds)
¼ C Lemon or Lime Juice or Balsamic Vinegar
¼ C Water
2 T Maple Syrup or Honey
1-2 T Tamari soy sauce or ½-1 tsp Celtic Seasalt
optional- 1 small Slice of Beet, 1 T Dulse/Kelp, a clove of Garlic
+Other Optional-Adjunctive ingredients- Yogurt, mayonnaise, rice parmesan or other dry cheeses, dry deaweeds like:Kelp, Dulse, & Nori, aloe gel, lecithin granules, rehydrated seaweeds like Arame and Hijiki, miso paste, wet mustard, prepared horseradish, spirulina powder or powdered green juice (wheat grass, barley grass…), garlic or garlic powder, chili or curry powder.

Blend all together and serve with salad. Use a variety of red and green lettuces, raddichio, red cabbage, etc

Vegan Caesar Salad

1-2 Cloves Garlic
½ tsp Umeboshi (plum or paste)
Pinch course Celtic Seasalt
3 T Essential Oil Blend
5 T Extra-virgin Olive Oil
¼ Lemon wedge-squeezed
4 T Rice Parmesan cheese
Black Pepper to taste
5-6 Sliced Romaine lettuce leaves

Mash the garlic with the umeboshi and salt, in a wooden bowl preferably. Add oils, stir well and add lettuce and coat well. Add the lemon juice and stir lightly. Finish by adding the parmesan and black pepper. Arrange additional vegetables if desired. Red peppers, carrot shreds, radishes, and cucumbers are all delicious. Place some in the Blender and blend. Save the remaining for the next day.

Vegan Ranch Dressing

3/4 C Vegenaise Mayonnaise or other favorite mayo or yogurt
2 T Essential Oils (flaxseed oil, essential balance, the total efa, udo's choice…)

¼ C Rice Vinegar or Lemon Juice
2-4 T Water or Aloe Gel
1 T Honey
½ tsp Celtic seasalt or more to taste & big pinches of kelp granules, black or white pepper or dry mustard

Blend or stir all together. Delicious as a dip for vegetables and bread or rserve over rice, pasta or mashed steamed vegetables. **Also omit the vinegar and substitute 1/3 C rice parmesan cheese and ½ C artichoke hearts for a great artichoke dip!

999 Island

1/3 C Vegenaise or yogurt
2-4 T Essential Oil (see above list)
1/3 C natural Catsup or Salsa
2 T chopped Dill Pickles
1-2 T Honey
1-2 T Aloe Gel or water
big pinch Kelp or Dulse flakes and seasalt to taste

Stir and store in a jar. Delicious as a dressing or a dip for vegetables, pita pieces, rice cakes or crackers.

Apple-Apple Sauce

1 C Apple sauce
2 T Apple Cider Vinegar and 2 T Balsamic Vinegar
2 T hydrated Arame seaweed
optional-1 T Honey and 1 T Aloe gel
Stir all together and use as a dressing or a sauce.

Savory Breakfast Scrambled Tofu

1 lb. Tofu
1 Onion
1 to 2 C diced or chunked Vegetables: Celery Zucchini, Cabbage, Carrot, red pepper, mushrooms, Others–Mung Bean Sprouts, Tomato, Kale, Spinach
Seasalt- about 1/2 tsp. or 1 T Tamari Soysauce
Turmeric- a heavy sprinkling (1/4 to 1/2 tsp)
1-3 T Nutritional Yeast
Optional Mustard 1 tsp wet type– Garlic powder to taste

Sauté the onion in about 1 T oil or butter and 1-2 T water or soup stock, while a few other veggies are cut and lightly sautéed. Add seasalt to veggies, stir, and then add the tamari, turmeric, nutritional yeast, and mustard. Add optional garlic powder or fresh garlic if desired. Squish the tofu over the pan and stir into mixture. Sauté 5 minutes and serve.

Fish

Fish that are from clean waters, not near chemical factories or intercoastal waters or the major rivers near manufacturing plants, that are not bottom feeders, or that are farm raised and fresh provide a better source of protein and essential fatty acids. Fish is best poached or broiled. To poach fish pour a few tablespoons of olive oil in a skillet and cover with sliced onions and/or other vegetables. Place fish on top salt or season with herbs like basil, tarragon, thyme or parsley fresh or dried. Add a splash of water, wine or soup stock to help create steam and cook the fish.

Cover pan and cook over medium heat. Turn fish once or twice until desired firmness is reached. The rule with fish is less cooking as it tends to get rubbery or dry if overcooked. Slice into flesh to check for doneness. Favorites include: salmon, steelhead trout, rainbow trout, grouper, haddock, cod, tilapia, monkfish, or other soft fleshed fish. Serve with a blended salad for fiber and enzymes.

Broiled fish can be prepared the same way and placed under the broiler and turned once and seasoned on the other side and then served. Most fish is usually soft enough for the person to eat.

Poached Fish over Braised Onions

(2 servings)
1 medium Onion
4 Tablespoons Butter or Olive Oil
Seasalt and pepper to season
1 tsp Herbs like Tarragon, thyme, basil or garlic powder, also nutmeg
two 4 oz Fish Fillets (Salmon or rainbow trout)

Melt butter in saute pan add 1-2 T water and onions.Cover. Begin to saute while you rinse and salt the fish. Sprinkle salt on both sides also add any herb seasonings to fish and place on top of onions. Keep covered to steam. You may also want to add 1/3 cup of stock, wine or water to steam better. Cook 5-7 minutes and shake pans to keep onions loose.

Flip fish, cook several minutes more (about 5) depending on thickness of fish. Test for doneness by cutting into center and then serve immediatly. Most fish is very soft and can be easily over cooked- it gets rubbery.

Oven-Steamed Fish

(2 servings)
1 C Vegetables-Onions, Zucchini, Mushrooms, Tomato...
two 4 oz. Fish Fillets (Salmon, or Grouper)
2-4 T Butter or Olive Oil
Herbs and Spices
Salt and Pepper

Place butter or olive oil in bottom of a cassarole dish. Add vegetables, then fish. Season with salt and herbs. Cover and bake 12-20 minutes at 325 F, or until you see the white fat begin to emerge on top of the fillet.

Teriyake Marinated Broiled Fish

(2 servings)
6 T Tamari Soysauce
3 T Water
4 T Balsamic, Rice, or Wine Vinegar
3T Honey or Maple Syrup for a different taste
two 4 oz Fillets of Fish (Steelhead Trout, Salmon or Haddock)
2 T Olive Oil

Marinate fish in the teriyaki sauce for 20-40 minutes, turinig once. Remove and brush or coat with olive oil on both side. Place on a pan undr broiler and cook about 5 minutes per side. Fish should have the white fat globules appear on top and begin to sizzle. Turn over and broil the other side 5-7 minutes or until desired crispness. Check for doneness. Fish should be flaky when tested a fork. Serve with any remaining teriyaki sauce brushed on top before serving, or you can brush the fish with the sauce after you have turned it over.s

Vegetables

Mushroom -Pepper Pate

½ lb Mushrooms or 2 Portobello's
¼ C diced Onion
1-2 Cloves Garlic
2-3 T Butter or Olive Oil

2-4 T Olive oil or Essential Oils
¼-1/2 tsp Seasalt
Fresh ground Black Pepper

Sauté ½ of the mushrooms in the butter or olive oil;, add garlic and salt. Combine in a blender with remaining mushrooms, oil, and pepper. Blend to smooth. Serve over pasta, rice or millet, or as a side dish for lunch.

Scallion-Brown Gravy w/ Pine Nuts

4-6 T Olive oil, ghee or butter
¼ C Scallions diced
black pepper
½-2/3 C Spelt or Rice Flour (or ½ & ½)
1 C + Stock or Water w/ 1-2 T Tamari added or Rice milk and tamari, miso or salt
Handful of Pine nuts

Sautee the scallions until soft, then add the black pepper and flour. Stir a couple of minutes then add the liquid, a little at a time, stirring into a paste and thinning as you add more liquid. Adjust to desired thickness and saltiness. Add pine nuts before serving.

Emerald Greens & Yukon Gold Potato Swirl

4-6 Yukon Gold Potatoes
3-4 T Butter, Olive oil or ghee
½ C Rice milk
Sea salt to taste
4 large leaves Kale

Cook potatoes and mash with oil and salt. Blanch the green in hot water 30-45 seconds. Place in blender with the ricemilk to blend. Add to the potatoes. Using a butter knife cut in the greens in a swirling manner.

Acorn Squash Salad

Baked squash, olive oil or organic butter or ghee and veggies (sautéed onion and finely chopped cauliflower/corn, or raisins, cinnamon/nutmeg, & grated carrots.

Sweet Yam Salad

Baked or steamed yam or sweet potato, yogurt or mayo and veggies (fennel/celery, pineapple/pear pieces, toasted sesame seeds/caraway/fennel or cumin seeds also-slightly toast & crush to release flavor)

Baked Root Vegetable 1-dish

In a casserole dish w/ a cover, cut the following in layers: Olive oil or butter, Yukon gold or red skinned potatoes, onion chunks, carrot chunks, —note make 1 version w/ seasalt sprinkled on top, garlic powder and nutritional yeast, and another version baked w/ no flavorings until serving. Amazingly they taste very different. The 1st makes a roasted taste, w/ a natural gravy, and the 2nd makes a more pure or clean, watery tasting vegetable dish.

Maple Sweet Potatoes

4 Sweet Potatoes or Yams
½ C Maple Syrup
¼ C Butter or Grape seed Oil

Bake or boil the yams. Mash them with some of the peels. Add the butter and maple syrup, continue to mash and stir together. Serve

Cranberry-Apple-Raisin Bake

4-6 Apples or apples and pears
1 C raisins
Pinches of: Cinnamon, nutmeg, ginger-all or any
1 jar of Cranberry preserves, jam, jelly or the like

Slice fruit in half. If using apples, peel and scoop out the core: if pears, no need to peel, just scoop out the core. Arrange in a casserole dish with a tight fitting cover. Place fruit in dish, sprinkle with desired spices. Then place raisins in the centers of the fruit, followed by a dollop of cranberry. Place remaining raisins around bottom of dish, and a few scoops of cranberry here and there. Cover and bake 15 minutes 350 F.

Grains

Best if cooked with more water until very soft or blended in a blender. Can be served with butter or olive oil, herbs salt and pepper, in soups or as a gruel or cereal. As a hot cereal, serve with raw honey as a sweetener and with whole milk or rice or almond milk.

Rice

Brown rice is better than white rice as it has many nutrients in the bran layer (fiber, B-vitamins, minerals, that are lost in the milling process) Basmati brown is very tasty and fragrant, also or long, medium and short grain can be used. The longer the grain the less starch. Longer grains are better in hot climates and weather and shorter grains are better in colder climates and weather because of the warming qualities of the higher starch content. The Italian *aborio* rice is from northern Italy and is short fat grains that cooks up very creamy and stickt, it is usually served with butter or olive oil salt and other flavorings like olives, cheese, tomatoes, etc. Basmati rice is from India and is very fragrant, and cooks up where the grains do not stick together, it is the rice that is best as a stir fry or what most people are used to. Rice is usually cooked with twice the amount of water to grain, but for softer, mushier rice fior the dental patient use 3-4 times more water. Cook rice from 30-40 minutes at medium heat. The seasonings on top will greatly add to the creamy texture.

Basic Rice

makes 2-3 servings

1 C Rice of choice
3 C Water
1-2 T Olive Oil
1/2 tsp Seasalt
1 tsp: garlic powder, or onion powder, or nutritional yeast or heabs like oregano, basil or curry powder or several combined.

Put olive oil in a large sauce pan, turn on meadium heat and add salt and any seasonings or spices. Sautee a few minutes then add rice. Stir around and saute about 3-5 minutes to coat and flavor rice. Add water and cover. Bring to a boil then turn down to medium and cook about 35 minutes until most of the water is absorbed and rice is tender. Turn off heat, keep covered and allow rice to absorb the water.

Sweet Rice

For a sweet, pudding like rice use cinnamon, ginger or nutmeg spices and 1/2 water and 1/2 ricemilk (or regular milk or almond milk). Also add about 1/2 C raisins to the mixture. Cook over medium heat. Also this can be blended into a rice cereal. Prunes can be add or any other dried fruit. This will also help in producing bowel movements!

Millet

Millet can be made like rice and serve in similiar ways. It is a more alkaline forming grain and is very tasty. It can be pureed or used in soups as well.

Basic Millet

1 C Millet
3 C Water
1/2 tsp Seasalt
1-2 T Olive Oil
Spices- See rice

Cook as you would rice, only a little longer about 40 minutes or until the grains are very soft

Barley

This is a great grain to add to soups, as it is very mucilaginous and thickens the soup. Pearl barley has had some of the outet hull removed and is generally the easiest to use. Add about 1/2 C to soups or stock containing at least 4 cups of liquid. Cook at least 30 minutes.

Oats

Oatmeal is a very good grain since it is very easy and quick to cook. Oats are best when allowed to soak in water to which a little (capful) of apple cider vinegar has been added to alleviate the ill effects of the phytates and to make it more digestable. Soak from 1/2 hour to overnight then cook as usual. The longer it is soaked the less cooking time is needed to absorb the water. Sweeten with honey and ricemilk or whole milk on top.

Oats can be the quick cooking or regular type. The quick cooking type is a small thinner flattened oat flake. If the regular oatmeal is soaked, the quick cooking type is not needed.

Oatmeal

(2 servings)
1 C regular flake Oatmeal
3 C Water
1 tsp apple cider vinegar
pinch seasalt

Soak oats in water and vinegar 1-2 hours or over night. Add salt and cook about 10-15 minutes over medium heat until smooth, creamy and water is absorbed. Serve with butter on top, some rice milk or regular milk and honey to sweeten if needed. Also good with salt and pepper.

Grits

Corn grits are very tasty and a great grain meal for the afternoon. Cook according to package directions and serve with butter, salt and pepper. Also steamed vegetables are good with grits, like cauliflower or broccoli. Mash then up in the grits.

Quinoa Pudding

1 C Quinoa-ground in blender
2 C Rice milk
½ C Water
1 T Ghee or Grape seed Oil
Spices ½ tsp total-pinches of ginger, nutmeg, allspice and or cinnamon
3-5 T Honey, rice syrup or dehydrated sugar
½ tsp Vanilla extract (or Almond extract)

Grind Quinoa in blender until powder consistency. Heat ghee or oil and a bit then add the spices. Stir a minute or two to release the flavors then add the quinoa flour. Combine with the spices, then add the rice milk, sweetener and water. Cook over medium low heat. Stir as the liquid is absorbed, about 5-10 minutes. Turn heat off, add vanilla. Stir. Serve with sweetener drizzled over the top, or chopped nuts, carob chips or dried fruit.

Cooking Quinoa

1 T Ghee or Olive Oil
2 cloves Garlic chopped
½ -1 tsp each: garlic granules, basil, seasalt
1 1/4 C Quinoa
2 C Water

Place spices in hot oil and simmer a minute or two, then add the quinoa and stir to coat. Sautee several minutes, stirring. Then add the water, cover and bring to boil over med-high heat. Stir once or twice so the bottom doesn't stick. Cook 12-15 minutes, until water is absorbed.

Arrowroot Brown Gravy

2 C Cool Water
3-4 T Arrowroot Flour
3-4 T Tamari Soy sauce

Stir the arrowroot into the cool water, and then add the soy sauce. Stir over medium heat until clear and thickened. Sautéed onions, garlic or mushrooms can be added.

Additional Resources

Additional Resources

Books

"It's All In Your Head"
by Hal A. Huggins DDS, MS

"Uninformed Consent"
by Hal A. Huggins DDS, MS
Thomas E. Levy, MD, JD

"Root Canal Cover-up"
by George E. Meinig DDS, FACD

"Tooth Truth"
by Frank J. Jerome, DDS

"Whole Body Dentistry"
by Mark A. Breiner, DDS

"Beyond Amalgam"
NeuroCranial Restructuring"
by Susan Stockton

"Dentistry Without Mercury"
by Sam Ziff
Michael Ziff, DDS

"Dental Mercury Detox"
by Sam Ziff
Michael F. Ziff, DDS
Mats Hanson, Ph.D.

"Infertility And Birth Defects"
by Sam Ziff
Michael F. Ziff, DDS
"How To Save Your Teeth"
by David Kennedy, DDS

"Healthy Teeth For Kids"
by Jerome Mittelman DDS, FAPM/
Beverly Mittelman BS, CNC/Jean Barilla, BA, BS, MS

"The Missing Link"
by Michael F. Ziff, DDS

"Amalgam Illness Diagnosis and Treatment"
Andrew Hall Cutler, PhD, PE

"Mercury Free"
Dr. James E. Hardy

"Where There Is No Dentist"
by Murray Dickson

"The Smile Method"
by Vasilios Gardiakos

"The Complete Bood of Dental Remedies"
by Flora Parsa Stay, DDS

Fluoride The Aging Factor"
by Dr. John Yiamouyiannis

"The Mercury In Your Mouth"
by Quicksilver Associates

Available from:
Dental Amalgam Mercury Syndrome (D.A.M.S.)
PO Box 7249
Minneapolis, MN 55407-0249
800-311-6265 or 612-721-1144

"Elements Of Danger"
by Morton walker, DPM

"Nutrition And Physical Degeneration"
by Weston A. Price, DDS

"Death And Dentistry"
by Martin H. Fischer

"Hypothyroidism: The Unsuspected Illness"
by Broda O. Barnes, MD/Lawrence Galton

"The Plague Makers"
by Jeffrey A. Fisher MD

"Applied Kinesiology" Vols. I & II
by David S. Walther

"Traditional Chinese Acupuncture"
by J.R. Worsley

"Medical Physiology" 10th Edition
by Arthur C. Guyton

"Anatomy As A Basic For Clinical Medicine"
by E.C.B. Hall-Craggs

"Human Anatomy & Physiology"
by John W. Hole, Jr.

"Biochemistry"
by Donald Voet/Judith G. Voet

"Textbook of Endocrinology" 5th Edition
by Robert H. Williams

Videotapes

"A Physician's Holistic Overview of Toxic Dentistry"
by Roy Kupsinel MD VHS 1:56:00

"Osteo Cavitation"
by Susan Stockton VHS 1:58:00

"The Holistic Dental Practice"
by Michael Margolis VHS 1:50:00

"Diagnosis & Treatment of Cavitational Osteonecrosis"
Wes Shankland, DDS, MS, PhD VHS 1:50:00

"Systemic Detoxification" (2-tapes)
Brenda Watson, CT, and Leonard Smith MD VHS 2:50:00

"Kinesiologic Testing of the Dental Patient"
by Robert Broe VHS 0:50:00

"The Detection & Treatment of Cavitational Ischemic Osteonecrosis"
(3-tape set)
by Jerry Bouquot, DDS, MSD, Wes Shankland, DDS, MS, PhD and Michael Margolis, DDS VHS 5:00:00

"Cavitational Osteonecrosis"
Diagnosis, Treatment & Recovery Program
by Ray G. Behm DDS & Robert Broe VHS 1:33:00

Available from:
Tuberose Video Productions
PO Box 603
Aripeka, Fl 34679
(352) 688-1356
www.health-equip.com

Websites

Consumers for Dental Choice
www.swankin-turner.com/projects.html

International Association of Oral Medicine & Toxicology
www.iaomt.com

Cavitat Medical Technologies
www.dentalhelp.org

Affinity Labeling Technologies
www.altcorp.com/

Susan Stockton
www.healthcarealternatives.net

Dentist Directory
www.dentalfind.com/Holistic_Dentistry

Holistic Dental Association
www.holisticdental.org

Mercury Free and Biological Dentists International
www.talkinternational.com/mfdsindex1.htm

Temporomandibular Dysfunction
www.TMJ-treatment.com

Health Equipment and Educational Resources
www.tuberose.com

International College of Applied Kinesiology
www.icak.com

Chiro Plus Kinesiology Association USA
http://www.cpkusa.org